MEDICAL MASTERCLASS

Neurology, Ophthalmology and Psychiatry

Disclaimer

Although every effort has been made to ensure that drug doses and other information are presented accurately in this publication, the ultimate responsibility rests with the prescribing physician. Neither the publishers nor the authors can be held responsible for any consequences arising from the use of information contained herein. Any product mentioned in this publication should be used in accordance with the prescribing information prepared by the manufacturers.

The information presented in this publication reflects the opinions of its contributors and should not be taken to represent the policy and views of the Royal College of Physicians of London, unless this is specifically stated.

Every effort has been made by the contributors to contact holders of copyright to obtain permission to reproduce copyright material. However, if any have been inadvertently overlooked, the publisher will be pleased to make the necessary arrangements at the first opportunity.

Medical Masterclass

EDITOR-IN-CHIEF

John D. Firth DM FRCP
Consultant Physician and Nephrologist
Addenbrooke's Hospital,
Cambridge

Neurology, Ophthalmology and Psychiatry

EDITORS

Nick Ward BSc MBBS MRCP
Wellcome Clinical Research Fellow and Specialist Registrar
Institute of Neurology
University College London
London

Peggy Frith MD FRCP FRCOphth
Consultant Ophthalmic Physician
The Eye Hospital
Radcliffe Infirmary
Oxford

Maurice Lipsedge MPhil FRCP FRC Psych
Consultant Psychiatrist
Guy's Hospital
London

**Blackwell
Science**

© 2001 Royal College of Physicians of London, 11 St Andrews Place, London NW1 4LE,
Registered Charity No. 210508

Published by:
Blackwell Science Ltd
Editorial Offices:
Osney Mead, Oxford OX2 0EL
25 John Street, London WC1N 2BS
23 Ainslie Place, Edinburgh EH3 6AJ
350 Main Street, Malden
  MA 02148-5018, USA
54 University Street, Carlton
  Victoria 3053, Australia
10, rue Casimir Delavigne
  75006 Paris, France

Other Editorial Offices:
Blackwell Wissenschafts-Verlag GmbH
Kurfürstendamm 57
10707 Berlin, Germany

Blackwell Science KK
MG Kodenmacho Building
7–10 Kodenmacho Nihombashi
Chuo-ku, Tokyo 104, Japan

Iowa State University Press
A Blackwell Science Company
2121 S. State Avenue
Ames, Iowa 50014-8300, USA

First published 2001

Set by Graphicraft Limited, Hong Kong
Printed and bound in Italy by
Rotolito Lombarda SpA, Milan

Catalogue records for this title are available from the British Library and the Library of Congress

ISBN 0-632-05868-4 (this book)
      0-632-05567-7 (set)

Commissioning Editors: Mike Stein and
  Rachel Robson
Project Manager (RCP): Filipa Maia
Editorial Assistant (RCP): Katherine Bowker
Production: Charlie Hamlyn and Jonathan
  Rowley
Layout and Cover Design: Chris Stone

DISTRIBUTORS

Marston Book Services Ltd
PO Box 269
Abingdon, Oxon OX14 4YN
(*Orders*: Tel: 01235 465500
          Fax: 01235 465555)

USA
Blackwell Science, Inc.
Commerce Place
350 Main Street
Malden, MA 02148-5018
(*Orders*: Tel: 800 759 6102
          781 388 8250
          Fax: 781 388 8255)

Canada
Login Brothers Book Company
324 Saulteaux Crescent
Winnipeg, Manitoba R3J 3T2
(*Orders*: Tel: 204 837 2987)

Australia
Blackwell Science Pty Ltd
54 University Street
Carlton, Victoria 3053
(*Orders*: Tel: 3 9347 0300
          Fax: 3 9347 5001)

For further information on
Blackwell Science, visit our website:
www.blackwell-science.com

Contents

Psychiatry

List of contributors

Peggy Frith MD FRCP FRCOphth
Consultant Ophthalmic Physician
The Eye Hospital
Radcliffe Infirmary
Oxford

Gillian L. Hall BSc BMBCh MRCP PhD
Specialist Registrar
Addenbrooke's Hospital
Cambridge

Aroon D. Hingorani MA MRCP PhD
Senior Lecturer and BHF Intermediate Fellow
Centre for Clinical Pharmacology
University College London
London

John P. Patten BSc FRCP (Illustrator)
Latterly Consultant Neurologist
King Edward VII Hospital
Midhurst
West Sussex

Vincent Kirchner MBChB FCPsych
Locum Consultant
St Pancras Hospital
London

Sivakumar Sathasivam MB BCh MRCP
Clinical Research Fellow
University of Sheffield and
The Royal Hallamshire Hospital
Sheffield

Hamish M.A. Towler FRCPEd FRCSEd FRCOphth
Consultant
Department of Ophthalmology
Whipps Cross Hospital
London

Nick Ward BSc MBBS MRCP
Wellcome Clinical Research Fellow & Specialist Registrar
Institute of Neurology
University College London
London

Foreword

Medical Masterclass is the most innovative and important educational development from the Royal College of Physicians in the last 100 years. Throughout our 480-year history we have pioneered and supported high-quality medicine, and while *Medical Masterclass* continues that tradition, it also represents a quantum leap for the College as it moves into the 21st century.

The effort that the College has put in to improve the Membership Examination, which started 150 years ago and is now run by all three UK Royal Colleges of Physicians, will now be matched by its attention to basic learning in general medicine—the grounding and preparation for the exam.

Teaching and learning for the exam have changed little over the past 50 years, relying on local courses, word-based teaching and commercial courses. *Medical Masterclass* is a completely new approach for those wishing to practise high-quality medicine. It is an imaginative multimedia programme with paper and CD modules covering the major areas of medicine, supported by a website which will provide summaries and links to the latest articles and guidelines, and self-assessment questionnaires with feedback. Its focus is on self-learning, self-assessment and dealing with realistic clinical problems—not just force-feeding facts. The series of interactive case studies on which the modules are based entail making diagnostic and treatment decisions, closely mimicking the situations found in the admission suite or outpatient clinic.

Medical Masterclass has been produced by the RCP's Education Department together with Blackwell Science. It represents a formidable amount of work by Dr John Firth and his team of authors and editors and is set to be the jewel in our crown. It also signals very clearly our intention to lead in the field of learning and to be supportive to our future members. I anticipate the package will also be invaluable for continued learning by our specialist registrars and consultants as part of continuing professional development.

I congratulate our colleagues for this superb product and commend it to you without reservation.

Professor Sir George Alberti
President of the Royal College of Physicians, London

Preface

Medical Masterclass comprises twelve paper-based modules, two CD-ROMs and a companion website. Its aim is to help doctors in their first few years of training to improve their medical skills and knowledge.

The twelve paper-based modules are divided as follows: two cover the scientific background to medicine, one is devoted to general clinical issues, one to emergency medicine and practical procedures, and eight cover the range of medical specialities. Medicine is often fairly straightforward when the diagnosis is clear, but patients rarely come to their doctor and say 'I've got Hodgkin's disease': they have lumps. The core material of each of the clinical specialities is defined by case presentations in the first part of each module: how do you approach the man who has lumps? Structured concise notes on specific diseases follow later. All practising doctors know that medicine is much more than knowing lots of facts about diseases: how do you tell someone they've got cancer? How do you decide when to stop treatment? Most medical texts say little about these issues: *Medical Masterclass* does not avoid them, nor does it talk in vague and abstract terms.

The two CD-ROMs each contain 30 interactive cases requiring diagnosis and treatment. The format is remarkably close to real life: you see the patient and are told the story; you have to decide how to investigate and treat; but you can't see all the results before you start to make decisions!

The companion website, which will be regularly updated, includes literature and guideline updates and review, and self-assessment questions. How much do you know, and are you improving? You will see how your score compares with your previous attempts, and also how your performance compares with others who have logged on to the site.

The *Medical Masterclass* is produced by the Education Department of the Royal College of Physicians of London and published by Blackwell Science. It is not a crammer for the MRCP exam and not written by those who set the exam. However, I have no doubt that someone putting effort into learning through the *Medical Masterclass* would be in a strong position to impress the examiners, although I am afraid that success—like much else in medicine and in life—cannot be guaranteed.

John Firth
Editor-in-Chief

Acknowledgements

Medical Masterclass has been produced by a team. The names of those who have written and edited material are clearly indicated elsewhere, but without the efforts of many other people *Medical Masterclass* would not exist at all. These include Professor Lesley Rees and Mrs Winnie Wade from the Education Department of the Royal College of Physicians of London, who initiated the project; Dr Mike Stein and Dr Andy Robinson from Medschool.com and Blackwell Science respectively, who have enthusiastically supported it from the beginning; and Ms Filipa Maia and Ms Katherine Bowker, who have run the office with splendid efficiency and induced authors and editors to perform to a schedule rarely achieved. I and the whole of the team of editors and authors are immensely grateful to all of these people for the energy that they have poured into *Medical Masterclass* in various ways.

John Firth
Editor-in-Chief

Key features

We have created a range of icon boxes to help you identify key information and to make learning easier and more enjoyable. Here is a brief explanation:

 Clinical pointer

This icon highlights important information to be noted.

 Further information

This icon indicates the source of further information and reference.

 Hints

This icon highlights useful hints, tips and mnemonics.

 Key points

This icon is used to highlight points of particular importance.

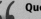 **Quote**

This icon indicates useful or interesting citations from notable individuals, including well-known physicians.

 Think about

This icon indicates what the reader should reflect on after having read a passage from the text.

Warning/Hazard

This icon is used to indicate common or important drug interactions, pitfalls of practical procedures, or when to take symptoms or signs particularly seriously.

Neurology

AUTHORS:
**G. Hall, A. Hingorani, J. Patten,
S. Sathasivam, N. Ward**

EDITOR:
N. Ward

EDITOR-IN-CHIEF:
J.D. Firth

1 Clinical presentations

1.1 Numb toes

Case history

A middle-aged man has developed numbness and tingling in his toes and feet, and more recently his fingertips. He also complains that he trips up more frequently.

Clinical approach

This man has distal sensory symptoms and motor symptoms. You have to decide whether this is due to a peripheral (polyneuropathy or mononeuritis multiplex) or central (myelopathy) cause, or to a combination of the two (e.g. subacute combined degeneration of the cord), and must take particular care to look for a treatable problem.

History of the presenting problem

Is this an urgent case?

Does this case require urgent attention or not? Could it, for instance, be due to cervical cord compression or to Guillain–Barré syndrome? Key points in the history are to establish:
• duration of symptoms
• rate of progression
• presence of any worrying associated symptoms, e.g. sphincter disturbance of recent onset, difficulty in breathing.

Symptoms of short duration that are progressing rapidly clearly need more rapid assessment than those that are long-standing and gradually worsening.

Is the problem due to peripheral or central nervous system dysfunction?

Although the examination will be the most useful aid in answering this question, some features of the history will also be helpful. Peripheral nervous system dysfunction would be suggested by description of:
• tingling, numbness and burning in the feet (see Fig. 1), together with a description of feeling as if walking on cotton wool (peripheral neuropathy)
• numb fingertips (peripheral neuropathy)

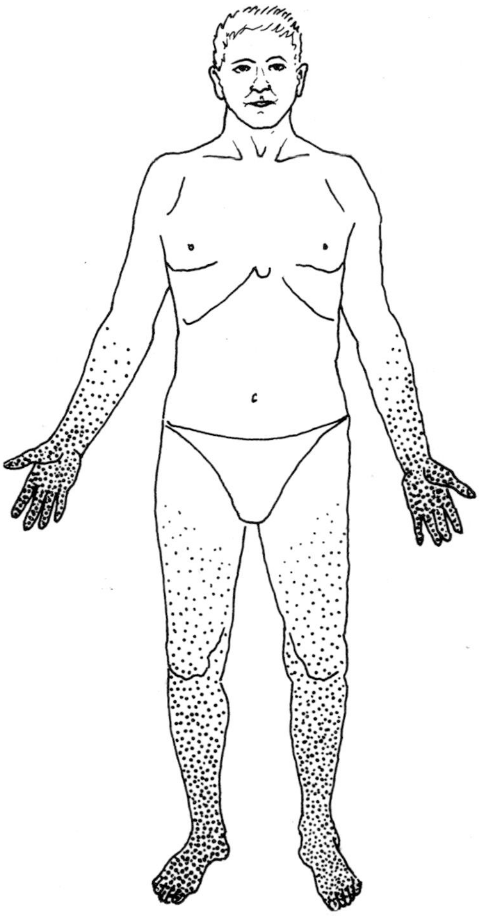

Fig. 1 Sensory loss in peripheral neuropathy. All modalities should be equally affected, but the transition phase to light touch, pain and temperature sensation is not a sharp cut-off—it gradually fades.

• catching his feet on uneven ground (foot drop/distal weakness), or difficulty in rising from a chair and going up and down stairs (proximal weakness).

By contrast, a spinal cord lesion (myelopathy) would be suggested by an account of:
• legs and feet feeling stiff and heavy
• clumsy, stiff hands
• a sensory level, often described as tightness around the chest or abdomen (cervical myelopathy)
• new-onset sphincter disturbance
• neck pain (cervical myelopathy).

If a neuropathy, then what type is it? The duration of symptoms and the rate of progress is important.
• If acute, consider Guillain–Barré syndrome.
• Subacute symptoms may also indicate a neuropathy

3

associated with vasculitis, systemic inflammatory disorders or malignancy [1].
- Very long-standing symptoms may be hereditary [2].
- Painful neuropathies may also indicate serious underlying pathology.

For further information see Section 2.1, p. 57.

Relevant past history

Ask specifically about the following, which may give clues to the cause of neuropathy or myelopathy:
- diabetes mellitus [3]
- alcohol intake
- current medication
- dietary history (vegetarian or vegan)
- pernicious anaemia
- hypothyroidism
- weight loss
- smoking
- neck trauma (cervical myelopathy)
- rheumatoid arthritis (atlanto-axial subluxation).

Examination

Peripheral or central nervous system disorder?

This distinction is easier to make from the physical signs than from the history. Examine the legs carefully, looking for the following patterns.

Peripheral nervous system

Typical findings are:
- distal weakness
- absent ankle reflexes (± knee reflexes)
- stocking distribution sensory loss
- wasting (if the problem is severe).

If there is loss of sensation to pain, but preservation of proprioception, power and reflexes, consider a small fibre neuropathy (see Section 2.1, p. 57).

Central nervous system

Typical findings are:
- spastic tone
- weakness both proximally and distally, but predominantly in leg flexors
- brisk reflexes
- extensor plantars
- possible sensory level.

The arms may also provide useful information:
- distal blunting to pinprick with absent reflexes indicates a peripheral neuropathy

- loss of dexterity and inverted supinator/biceps reflex pattern suggests cervical cord compression at C5/6 (see Section 1.12, p. 25).

Subacute combined degeneration of the cord

Vitamin B_{12} deficiency may cause a peripheral neuropathy, but may also lead to additional corticospinal tract and dorsal column degeneration, leading to combined upper and lower motor neurone features. The clinical picture can be variable, but remember that this is a treatable condition and must not be missed.

Are the signs symmetrical?

In this case, asymmetry in the context of an upper motor neurone syndrome would represent a Brown-Séquard syndrome, with loss of proprioception ipsilateral to the weak leg, and loss of pain and temperature sensation contralateral to the weak leg. Asymmetric lower motor neurone findings suggest mononeuritis multiplex or entrapment neuropathies.

Look for evidence of the peripheral nerve lesions discussed below.

Common peroneal (or fibular) nerve palsy

Leads to foot drop with loss of ankle and toe dorsiflexion, and ankle eversion. Numbness occurs over the lateral aspect of the lower leg and dorsum of the foot. It is usually due to pressure over the fibular head.

Posterior tibial nerve palsy (tarsal tunnel syndrome)

Causes burning sensation in the toes and the sole of the foot, with reduced sensation on the sole. Wasting may occur in the intrinsic muscles of the foot, leading to weakness of toe flexion. Entrapment usually occurs behind and below the medial malleolus.

Sciatic nerve lesion

The sciatic nerve splits to form the common peroneal nerve and the posterior tibial nerve, and so damage to the sciatic nerve encompasses both of the above. Weakness occurs in all muscles below the knee, as well as knee flexors. There is sensory loss over the lateral border of the lower leg and entire foot, except the medial malleolus, which is supplied by the saphenous nerve.

Are there associated cranial nerve palsies?

If so, then specific diagnoses should be considered.
- Deafness (CN VIII) is associated with some hereditary neuropathies.
- Bilateral facial weakness is seen in Guillain–Barré syndrome and sarcoidosis.
- Malignant infiltration of the basal meninges may lead to multiple cranial nerve palsies.

General examination

Is the patient systemically well? Are there indications of any of the conditions discussed in Section 2.1? Look in particular for:
• cachexia—which may suggest malignancy or alcoholism
• evidence of alcoholism/chronic liver disease (see *Gastroenterology and hepatology*, Sections 1.6 and 1.7)
• vasculitic rash—probably indicating systemic vasculitis in this context
• signs of hypothyroidism (see *Endocrinology*, Section 2.3), which can produce mild neuropathy
• postural hypotension—which is likely to indicate an autonomic component.

Approach to investigations and management

Investigations

History and examination may allow focused investigations; see Section 2.1, for the details.

Management

See Section 2.1, it may be possible to prevent any further damage but regeneration of nerve axons is slow.

See *Endocrinology*, Section 2.6.
1 Grisold W, Drlicek M. Paraneoplastic neuropathy. *Curr Opin Neurol* 1999; 12: 617–625.
2 Reilly MM. Genetically determined neuropathies. *J Neurol* 1998; 245: 6–13.
3 Said S. Diabetic neuropathy: an update. *J Neurol* 1996; 243: 431–440.

1.2 Back and leg pain

Case history

A middle-aged woman presents with back and unilateral leg pain.

Clinical approach

There are many causes of back pain. Radiation to a leg implies involvement of nerve root or lumbosacral plexus and limits the differential diagnosis (Table 1). L5 and S1 are the most commonly affected nerves in degenerative disease; L4 is involved occasionally, but L2 and 3 rarely,

Table 1 Causes of back and leg pain.

Radiculopathy	Disc disease
	Degenerative spinal disease
	Infective spinal disease (pyogenic abscess, TB)
	Malignant spinal disease (secondary tumour, myeloma)
	Intrinsic, e.g. secondary tumour, myeloma
	Extrinsic, e.g. extramedullary, nerve sheath tumour, meningeal infiltration
Plexopathy/sciatic nerve lesion	Pelvic retroperitoneal mass
	Tumour
	Haematoma
	Abscess
	Hip fracture
	Misplaced deep muscular injection

and if they are the diagnosis is not likely to be simple degeneration. Your approach should be to: (a) define the site of the lesion if possible (Figs 2 and 3); and (b) determine its cause.

History of the presenting problem

Ask about the following if the details do not emerge spontaneously.
• How did the pain come on? Was it sudden? Did it develop when bending or lifting? These would suggest a 'mechanical' cause, e.g. disc prolapse.
• Is the pain positional? Sitting and bending cause increased stretch of the nerve. Root pain is often worse when sitting, and improved on walking.
• Is the pain worse at night? Nocturnal pain with radiation should make you think about nerve or root involvement; if persistent and severe consider the possibility of malignant infiltration.
• What is the pain like? Sciatica is described as burning in the buttocks, and stabbing, shooting or lancing in the leg.
• Is there any associated numbness or weakness? This is suggestive of nerve or root involvement.
• Does the pain radiate and if so where? Radicular pain starts in the back and radiates along the course of the nerve (Table 2).

Beware bladder dysfunction as this implies interruption of S2–4, either centrally (spinal cord compression, conus lesion) or peripherally (cauda equina lesion, pelvic pathology, autonomic dysfunction).

Relevant past history

Is there a history of any of the following, which might indicate the cause of the problem?

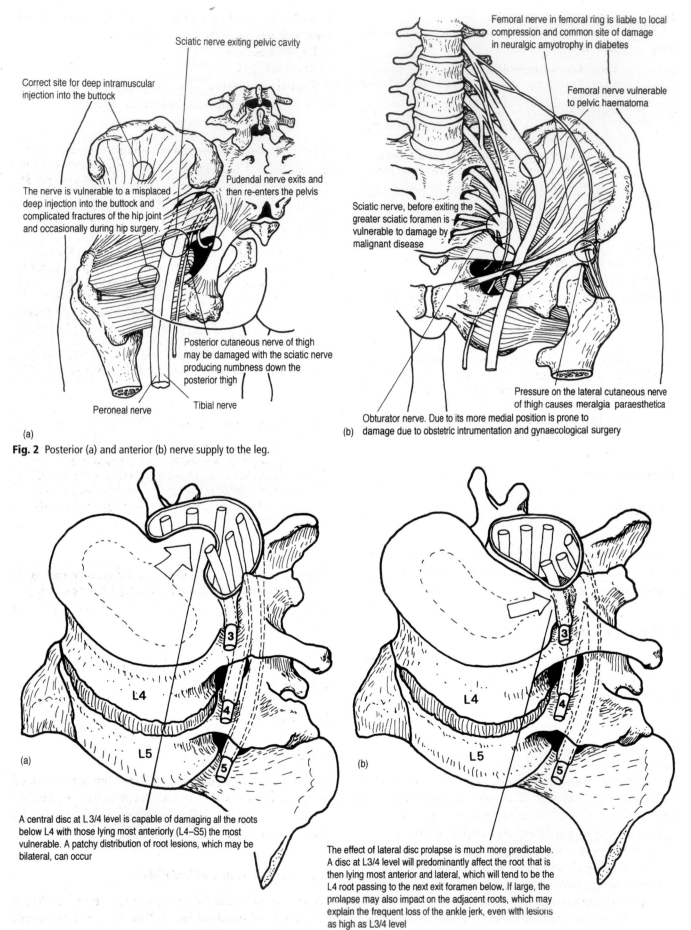

Correct site for deep intramuscular injection into the buttock

Sciatic nerve exiting pelvic cavity

The nerve is vulnerable to a misplaced deep injection into the buttock and complicated fractures of the hip joint and occasionally during hip surgery.

Pudendal nerve exits and then re-enters the pelvis

Posterior cutaneous nerve of thigh may be damaged with the sciatic nerve producing numbness down the posterior thigh

Peroneal nerve

Tibial nerve

(a)

Femoral nerve in femoral ring is liable to local compression and common site of damage in neuralgic amyotrophy in diabetes

Femoral nerve vulnerable to pelvic haematoma

Sciatic nerve, before exiting the greater sciatic foramen is vulnerable to damage by malignant disease

Pressure on the lateral cutaneous nerve of thigh causes meralgia paraesthetica

Obturator nerve. Due to its more medial position is prone to damage due to obstetric intrumentation and gynaecological surgery

(b)

Fig. 2 Posterior (a) and anterior (b) nerve supply to the leg.

3

L4

4

L5

5

(a)

A central disc at L3/4 level is capable of damaging all the roots below L4 with those lying most anteriorly (L4–S5) the most vulnerable. A patchy distribution of root lesions, which may be bilateral, can occur

3

L4

4

L5

5

(b)

The effect of lateral disc prolapse is much more predictable. A disc at L3/4 level will predominantly affect the root that is then lying most anterior and lateral, which will tend to be the L4 root passing to the next exit foramen below. If large, the prolapse may also impact on the adjacent roots, which may explain the frequent loss of the ankle jerk, even with lesions as high as L3/4 level

Fig. 3 Anatomy of a central (a) and lateral (b) disc protrusion.

Table 2 Pain radiation in radicular lesions.

Nerve	Pain radiation
L2, 3	Pain radiates to anterior thigh
L4	Pain radiates through the knee and down the medial side of the calf to the medial malleolus
L5	Pain radiates through the buttock, down the posteriolateral aspect of the thigh, lateral aspect of calf and across the dorsum of the foot to the big toe
S1	Pain radiates through the inner buttock to the posterior aspect of the thigh, posteriolateral aspect of calf to the lateral border of the foot

- trauma
- previous degenerative back disease or arthritis
- malignancy, myeloma
- clotting disorder or poorly controlled anticoagulants
- osteoporosis.

Do any concurrent or previous medical conditions make you think of the following?
- malignant infiltration of the meninges or plexus
- vertebral metastases or collapse
- pelvic or psoas muscle haematoma.

Examination

The back

Check for:
- local tenderness—consider vertebral collapse or fracture
- paraspinal muscular spasm (in response to pain)
- restricted movement.

Straight leg raising

Unilateral restriction may signify sciatic tension, but may be limited by pain in the absence of nerve or root compression.

Legs

Check carefully for the following:
- Is there wasting or fasciculation of the affected muscles?
- Is there any weakness? If so, what is the distribution?
Specifically check for lesions of the following roots:
 L2 weakness of hip flexion and thigh adduction;
 L3 weakness of thigh adduction and knee extension;
 L4 weakness of knee extension and ankle inversion;
 L5 weakness of ankle dorsiflexion, inversion and eversion and dorsiflexion of the great toe;
 S1 weakness of plantar flexion, eversion and knee flexion.

- Reflexes—are they normal? Hypo- or areflexia is only seen with lesions of the following roots:
 L3, 4—knee jerk
 S1—ankle jerk
- Sensation—sensory abnormalities in a well-defined distribution will help with localization (Fig. 4).

In assessing a weak leg, remember the following:
- Because muscle groups receive innervation from more than one root, weakness may be minimal in someone with a single root lesion.
- In the case of severe weakness, e.g. complete foot drop, a peripheral nerve lesion or multi-level radiculopathy must be implicated.
- Differentiation between a common peroneal nerve lesion and a L5 root lesion is a common clinical dilemma: a common peroneal nerve lesion will cause weakness of ankle dorsiflexion and eversion but will not affect inversion.
- A complete sciatic nerve lesion will cause weakness of knee flexion (hamstrings) and all muscle groups below the knee (through the peroneal and tibial divisions).
- Weakness that does not appear to conform to a simple pattern may be due to a lumbosacral plexus lesion.

Lumbar canal stenosis

If weakness, e.g. foot drop, is associated with pain and only comes on with exercise, then consider this diagnosis (see Section 1.6, p. 14). In the outpatient clinic, the patient with this history but no physical signs should be asked to walk until the symptoms come on, as this may reveal abnormal signs.

A common clinical mistake is to expect loss of the ankle jerk with foot drop. If this is the case it suggests involvement of both L5 and S1.

Approach to investigations and management

Investigations

Imaging

Magnetic resonance imaging (MRI) of lumbar and sacral spinal cord and exiting roots, and if indicated, lumbosacral plexus and pelvis, should be reserved for those with neurological deficit.

Nerve conduction studies/EMG

These may be indicated to help differentiate between a peripheral and proximal lesion. Sensory action potentials (SAPs) will be normal in radicular lesions proximal to the

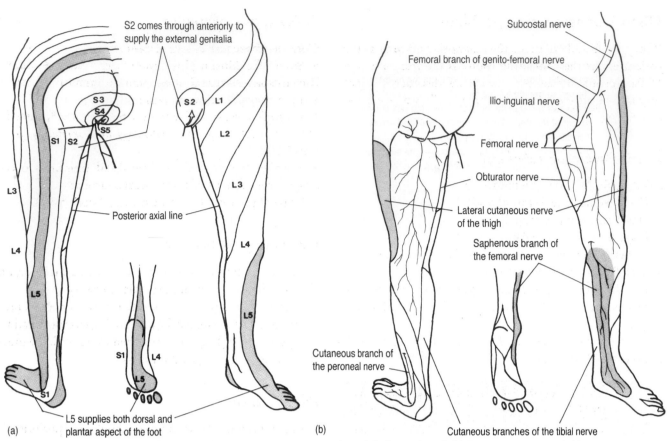

Fig. 4 (a) Cutaneous nerve root supply of the leg (note the sensory areas spiral round the leg as shown). (b) Cutaneous nerve supply (the sensory areas are vertically distributed) of the leg.

dorsal root ganglion but may be diminished in a plexopathy. Electromyography (EMG) can show the distribution of denervated muscles. Paraspinal denervation is a useful pointer to a lumbar radiculopathy rather than a peripheral lesion.

Management

Management will depend on the nature and severity of the lesion. Minor disc bulges may settle with gentle mobilization and anti-inflammatory medication, whereas lesions associated with clear neurological deficit may require surgical intervention [1]. MRI scanning should therefore be reserved for those with neurological deficit, as abnormalities in those without may be asymptomatic [2].

See *Haematology*, Section 1.15.
See *Rheumatology and clinical immunology*, Section 1.17.
1 Kerr RS, Cadoux-Hudson TA, Adams CB. The value of accurate clinical assessment in the surgical management of the lumbar disc protrusion. *J Neurol Neurosurg Psychiatry* 1988; 51(2):169–173.
2 Jensen MC, Brant-Zawadzki MN, Obuchowski N, Modic MT, Malkasian D, Ross JS. Magnetic resonance imaging of the lumbar spine in people without back pain. *N Engl J Med* 1994; 331: 69–73.

1.3 Tremor

Case history

A 60-year-old man presents with tremor.

Clinical approach

The main differential diagnosis of tremor is shown in Table 3.

Whether a tremor is maximal at rest or on action is of extreme importance diagnostically.

Table 3 Common causes of tremor.

Resting	Parkinson's disease (4–5 Hz)
Action/intention	Cerebellar (3 Hz)
Postural	Benign essential tremor (5–8 Hz, sporadic or familial)
	Enhanced physiological—exacerbated by anxiety

History of presenting problem

It may be possible to make the diagnosis before or as the patient enters the consulting room. If the tremor is part of Parkinson's disease or a cerebellar disorder, the gait may also be affected. Observation will allow focused history taking.

Is this Parkinson's disease?

Ask specifically about the following.
- Do movements feel slow and stiff?
- Has handwriting changed?
- Is the tremor most marked at rest?
- Is there asymmetry of symptoms? Parkinson's disease is almost always asymmetrical at onset.
- Has the gait changed? Is the posture more stooped? Are the steps shorter? All of these are typical of Parkinson's disease.
- Does the patient feel the he 'hurries to catch up with himself' (festinant gait)?

Idiopathic Parkinson's disease (IPD) can only be diagnosed if upper limb bradykinesia is present.

Is this benign essential tremor?

Benign essential tremor is a fine tremor that often starts in childhood or adolescence but presents only later when it becomes functionally debilitating. Ask about the following:
- Is the tremor worse on using the affected limb? Typically it affects the arms during activities such as using a knife and fork or holding a cup, i.e. an action tremor.
- Is there a family history? Benign essential tremor can be sporadic or can occur in the context of a family history which is autosomal dominant with variable penetrance.
- Does alcohol improve the symptoms?

Is this cerebellar disease?

Tremor is rarely the only symptom or sign of cerebellar disease. Gait disorder will be present if the tremor is due to cerebellar disease (see Section 1.4, p. 10).

Is this physiological tremor?

Physiological tremor is a small-amplitude, higher-frequency tremor, enhanced by fear or anxiety. It may be pathologically enhanced by:
- thyrotoxicosis
- hypoglycaemia
- alcohol withdrawal
- drugs (β-2 agonists, caffeine, amphetamine).

Other causes of tremor

Consider these rare causes of tremor.
- Some 'Parkinson-plus' syndromes such as Steel–Richardson–Olszewski syndrome or multiple system atrophy may present with tremor.
- Wilson's disease. Tremor may be an early feature in 30% of cases. (see *Gastroenterology and hepatology*, Section 2.10).
- Peripheral neuropathies. Fine distal tremor is occasionally seen as part of a peripheral neuropathy.
- Hyperthyroidism (see *Endocrinology*, Section 2.3).

Relevant past history

In the case of Parkinson's disease and essential tremor, no clues can be gained from the previous history.

If cerebellar disease is suspected, however, then past neurological and vascular history are important. In addition, is there anything to suggest that there could be metastatic disease in the posterior fossa?

Examination

A full neurological examination should be performed. Concentrate on the aspects discussed below.

Is it Parkinson's disease?

Look specifically for these features, remembering that many of them may be asymmetrical.
- Bradykinesia, i.e. slowness and fatigability of rapid movements. Ask the patient to open and close each hand as widely and as rapidly as possible, or to tap the thumb with each finger of the same hand in rapid succession with the widest amplitude possible. If not obviously slow, continue at least 10 times to demonstrate decrement in rate and amplitude. An extrapyramidal syndrome cannot be diagnosed without this feature.
- Hypomimia, i.e. paucity of facial expression with 'mask-like' facies and reduced blink rate.
- Extrapyramidal rigidity with 'cogwheeling', i.e. the combination of rigidity and tremor, best demonstrated by slow gentle rotation of the wrist.
- The tremor is classically pill-rolling and most marked at rest, although when severe will often be seen with posture and action.
- Rest tremor of hands best seen with the hands resting, palms facing inwards on the lap or over the edge of an armchair. The tremor may be intermittent and if not seen can be elicited by mental taxation, such as serial 3s, or it often comes on with walking.
- Tremor seen in the lower limbs is highly suggestive of Parkinson's disease.

• The glabellar tap (which involves tapping the glabella and observing whether the patient blinks) is a non-specific test that is not clinically useful, although it used to be said that failure of this response to fatigue (i.e. blinking to stop with repeated taps) indicated Parkinson's disease.
• Posture is stooped and when severe is referred to as 'simian'.
• Gait is typically short stepped, shuffling and festinant, with reduced or absent arm swing. In early disease, a slight reduction in arm swing on one side may be the only abnormality. Freezing of gait occurs later in the disease.
• Ask the patient to write a phrase such as 'Mary had a little lamb' several times until micrographia develops or you are sure it is absent (e.g. after two lines of writing).
• Ask the patient to draw a spiral, which may demonstrate tremor as well as micrographia.

Drug-induced parkinsonism may look identical, although it tends to be more symmetrical. Wilson's disease may present with parkinsonism, so look for a Kaiser–Fleisher ring, although this may only be visible with a slit lamp.

Is it benign essential tremor?

This can look quite similar to the tremor of Parkinson's disease, but notice the absence of other signs of parkinsonism. Examination may be normal except for tremor of outstretched arms, which may be worsened as the patient changes posture, e.g. to hold their hands palms downwards under their nose, or do the finger–nose test. If possible, ask the patient to hold a cup and saucer, or a glass of water, which often exacerbates tremor.

Is it cerebellar disease?

Look for:
• intention tremor
• past pointing on 'finger–nose' testing
• gait ataxia (wide based)
• cerebellar dysarthria (scanning speech)
• jerky smooth pursuit eye movements, nystagmus.

Approach to investigations and management

Investigations

Parkinson's disease and essential tremor are clinical diagnoses and no investigations are required in the context of a typical history and examination. If the parkinsonian picture is atypical, brain imaging can be performed to exclude other causes of basal ganglia disease.

Management

Management clearly depends on the precise diagnosis.
• Parkinson's disease (see Section 2.3.1, p. 72).
• Benign essential tremor; often reassurance that this is not something more serious is sufficient. If medication is desired β-blockers and primidone are the drugs of choice.
• Cerebellar disease. This will depend on the nature of the insult. See separate sections on demyelinating (Section 2.5, p. 77), malignant (Section 2.9, p. 101) and vascular (Section 2.8, p. 90) conditions.

See *Medicine for the elderly*, Section 1.3.

1.4 Gait disturbance

Case history

A middle-aged woman presents with unsteadiness and difficulty in walking.

Clinical approach

The common causes of gait disturbance are given in Table 4, together with their main characteristics. This is a rare situation in that the key examination is carried out before the history is taken, since the gait is observed as the patient enters the room and the diagnosis may become immediately obvious to the clinician. The history can then be obtained with this in mind and further corroboration sought with the examination.

History of presenting problem

Some of the diagnoses considered here are covered in detail in other sections.

Table 4 Commonly encountered abnormal gaits.

Diagnosis	Main characteristic
Parkinson's disease	Shuffling/stooped
Cerebellar	Wide based
Peripheral neuropathy	High stepping
Diffuse cerebrovascular disease	'Marche à petits pas'
Proximal myopathy	Waddling
Pyramidal tract involvement	
Unilateral	Circumduction
Bilateral	Scissor gait

Is this Parkinson's disease?

See Section 1.3.

Is this cerebellar disease?

Cerebellar hemisphere disease will result in ipsilateral limb symptoms. Truncal ataxia reflects involvement of the vermis. Most cerebellar disease affects the legs before the arms, speech or eye movements, and so absence of their involvement does not rule out a cerebellar gait.
- Is the unsteady gait wide based?
- Is there a tremor?

Is this a peripheral neuropathy?

See Sections 1.1, p. 3 and 2.1, p. 57.

Is this diffuse cerebrovascular disease?

Are there vascular risk factors [1]? See Section 2.8, p. 90.

Is this a spastic gait?

This may result from a single insult in the cord or brain stem or following bilateral cerebral hemisphere lesions. Ask about the following, which would indicate that the pathology is in the cord:
- is there back pain?
- are there other symptoms of cord dysfunction, e.g. sensory level or bladder or bowel dysfunction?

Is this a proximal myopathy?

- Has there been difficulty rising from a low chair or bath/hanging out the washing/washing hair?
- Has there been any muscle pain? If myopathy seems likely, is there an obvious cause? Is the patient taking steroids, etc.? See Section 2.2, p. 65.

General

Many of the causes of abnormal gait can be associated with malignant, inflammatory or vascular disease. Is there any suggestion of these from the history?

Examination

If you have not yet observed the gait, ask the patient to walk along a corridor as normally as possible. Try to decide what you think the diagnosis is, bearing in mind the conditions listed in Table 4, and then look for corroborating signs on examination.

Parkinson's disease

See Section 1.3, p. 8.

Cerebellar disease

The following are features of cerebellar disease:
- dysarthria
- nystagmus
- limb ataxia: upper limb (failure of rapid alternating movements, intention tremor, past pointing) and lower limb (heel–shin ataxia, wide-based gait, unable to perform heel–toe walking).

Peripheral neuropathy

See Sections 1.1 and 2.1. Is the gait high stepping, reflecting bilateral foot drop?

The main findings are:
- reduced tone
- distal weakness (foot drop)
- hypo- or areflexia
- glove and stocking sensory loss.

Diffuse cerebrovascular disease

'Marche à petit pas' of diffuse cerebral ischaemic white matter disease is commonly mistaken for the gait of Parkinson's disease. In 'marche à petits pas', sometimes called gait apraxia, the steps are small, turning requires several steps and there may be excessive arm swing. Crucially, the stance is upright with the centre of gravity being normal, as opposed to shifted forwards as in a parkinsonian gait. In the patient with diffuse cerebrovascular disease there are no extrapyramidal signs in the arms or face, as there would be in a patient with idiopathic Parkinson's disease. 'Marche à petits pas' is therefore sometimes incorrectly termed 'lower-body parkinsonism'.

Spastic gait

Is the gait stiff with circumduction and toe dragging of the stiff leg (unilateral disease)? When bilateral, it is described as a scissor gait. Look in particular for:
- tone, reflexes, plantars, power will reflect an upper motor neurone pattern of deficit
- is there a sensory level?

Myopathic

Look for the following features.
- Waddling gait. Failure to stabilize the pelvis caused by predominant involvement of pelvic girdle and proximal leg muscles

11

- Wasting of affected muscle groups
- May be prominent proximal weakness
- Reflexes may be normal or reduced
- No sensory signs.

General

If the history is compatible with metastatic disease—which might apply to some cases of cerebellar, neuropathic, spastic or myopathic gait disturbance—then a full systemic examination should be performed. Does the patient look as though they have lost weight? Is there lymphadenopathy? Are there masses in the breast, or on abdominal and rectal examination? Is the chest normal? Likewise, if vascular disease is suspected, full cardiovascular assessment is required (see Section 2.8, p. 90).

Approach to investigations and management

This will depend on the presumed diagnosis.

Parkinson's disease

See Section 2.3.1, p. 72.

Cerebellar disease

You are really looking to rule out a space-occupying lesion, but as other considerations include structural causes such as Arnold–Chiari malformations and inflammatory causes such as multiple sclerosis, imaging is best carried out with MRI, which best demonstrates structures of the posterior fossa. Don't forget the possibility of paraneoplastic cerebellar degeneration (see Section 2.11, p. 104).

Peripheral neuropathy

See Sections 1.1, p. 3 and 2.1, p. 57.

Diffuse cerebrovascular disease

See Section 2.8. Note that diffuse vascular disease is a different entity to a single vascular event affecting the cerebellum, affecting predominantly the white matter of the cerebral hemispheres in association with small-vessel ischaemic damage.

Spastic

Consider the following:
- MRI of spinal cord (brain if cord is normal)
- CSF to include oligoclonal bands, if intrinsic cord lesion is seen
- visual evoked responses (VER) if demyelination is suspected.

1 Richards CL, Malouin F, Dean C. Gait in stroke: assessment and rehabilitation. *Clin Geriatr Med* 1999; 15(4): 833–855.

1.5 Dementia and involuntary movements

Case history

A young man brings his father, who has behavioural changes, cognitive difficulties and fidgety hands into the clinic.

Clinical approach

This could be a difficult case, even for an experienced neurologist, with many rare degenerative and metabolic diseases coming into consideration. However, even without knowing the family history, the most likely diagnosis is Huntington's disease. Diagnosis of Huntington's is now simple, and if positive obviates the need for further extensive investigations, but there are many issues to consider before going ahead with testing for this condition.

History of presenting problem

Is this Huntington's disease?

Huntington's disease may present with a movement disorder (twitching or just clumsiness of the hands) or behavioural and/or psychiatric changes. Later on true chorea supervenes, associated with dementia.

Huntington's disease is an autosomal dominant disorder, therefore ask about family history, not only of previous generations but also younger relatives. These obviously include the son, for whom there may be profound implications. As a triplet repeat disorder, Huntington's disease can show 'anticipation', meaning that previous generations may have a milder picture such that the diagnosis could have been missed. Reports that the grandmother was remembered as 'having become a bit odd', 'having developed a bit of a twitch', or 'having demented a bit before she died', could all be very significant in this case.

Is there another cause of chorea?

The fidgety hands are likely to indicate chorea, hence consider the following.

Drug-induced chorea

Has the patient been on neuroleptics or anti-parkinsonian medication?

Metabolic causes

Some metabolic disorders (e.g. hyperthyroidism, hypo-parathyroidism, hyponatraemia, hypomagnesaemia and even hypo- and hyperglycaemia) can present acutely with movement disorder and confusion. Does he have any newly diagnosed medical disorders or new medications?

Cerebrovascular disease

Stroke will more often cause hemichorea. Look for a stepwise progression of cognitive deficit, with more acute onset of involuntary movements. A history of trauma should make one consider a subdural haematoma.

Central nervous system inflammatory diseases

Consider systemic lupus erythematosus, sarcoidosis, Behçet's disease and multiple sclerosis, although all these are rare causes of chorea.

Neurometabolic disorders

Wilson's disease can produce involuntary movements and dementia, although it is unlikely to start at this age.

Neurodegenerative diseases

Theses are all rare, and before considering their investigation, Huntington's disease will almost certainly need to be excluded.

Are there features of depression?

If dementia is suspected, make sure to rule out pseudodementia of depression, which is treatable (see Section 1.9, p. 19).

Examination

Both physical and cognitive examinations are required.

Neurological

Look particularly for the following.

Chorea

Rapid, random, semi-purposeful, 'dance-like' movements, usually of the extremities but also of the trunk and face. The patient may have 'flycatcher's tongue', i.e. an inability to sustain tongue protrusion, and may be unable to maintain a constant handgrip.

Eye movements

Slow saccades (fast eye movements), gaze impersistence, and an inability to initiate saccades without head thrusts are all features of advanced Huntington's disease.

Other neurological features

Pyramidal and cerebellar signs are seen in many neurodegenerative diseases as they advance, including prion diseases.

General

Look specifically at thyroid status, for evidence of alcohol abuse and for evidence of systemic disease.

Cognitive

A brief cognitive examination should be performed in the clinic: this can be very informative (see Section 3.1, p. 111).

Approach to investigations and management

Investigation

Investigations will clearly be guided by any clues found on history and examination, but in the absence of firm leads consider the following:
• Check full blood count, electrolytes, renal and liver function, serum calcium and glucose, thyroid function tests and inflammatory markers (ESR and CRP) to rule out metabolic or systemic disease. Further specific tests will be indicated if any of these show clear abnormality.
• Brain imaging, e.g. CT, especially if there is a history of trauma, but otherwise unlikely to be diagnostically helpful.

If these tests are unremarkable and another diagnosis is not apparent, as is probable, then consideration must be given to the question of genetic testing for Huntington's disease.

Genetic testing

This is likely to be the most difficult management issue [1]. If the diagnosis was previously considered, the patient and his son may have come to clinic with a good knowledge of the issues surrounding genetic testing for Huntington's disease. You need to explore their understanding of the issues. Counselling of this kind is not easy, and referral to a specialist clinical genetics service is often preferable. At this first consultation it would be reasonable to:

• explore their knowledge of the disease and the diagnostic testing that is available

• raise the fact that any test results will have widespread implications for other family members

• explain that testing may or may not clarify matters, but if the results are negative, the problem is not cured, and further investigations may be needed

• confirm that there is no treatment for Huntington's disease.

It would be most unlikely that more information than this could be handled at a first meeting, such that it will be necessary to arrange for the patient and his son to return to discuss issues further. Many questions may arise; many of the answers are difficult and not at all clear-cut.

• Why test when the disease is incurable?

• What exactly are the implications for other family members? The psychological effects of 'knowing' (either way) should not be underestimated [2].

Whilst it is difficult to produce 'black and white' rules in an area where much is grey, most physicians with experience of Huntington's disease feel that it is inadvisable to test in the following circumstances:

• children under 18

• for insurance purposes

• if the patient is reluctant

• if the result automatically reveals someone else (i.e. a parent) to have the disease without their consent.

After any test, follow-up will be required whatever the result:

• depression may follow a positive or negative result ('survivor guilt')

• suicide after a positive result has occurred, but this is no more common than for any other disease or chronic disability

• further investigations may be required.

Genetic testing in Huntington's disease

• Why test for an illness that cannot be treated?

• Remember that the test can have implications for other family members.

• If you could have Huntington's disease, would you like to know?

• Would you like to find out that you had Huntington's disease because someone else had a test?

• If in doubt, consult with a clinical geneticist before testing.

Management

For Huntington's disease and other neurodegenerative conditions there is no specific treatment and management is supportive. Both the patient and the carers need consideration. The chorea of Huntington's disease may respond to tetrabenazine.

See *Genetics and molecular medicine*, Section 4.

1 Paulson GW, Prior TW. Issues related to DNA testing for Huntington's disease in symptomatic patients. *Semin Neurol* 1997; 17: 235–238.

2 Wiggins S, Whyte P, Huggins M *et al.* The psychological consequences of predictive testing for Huntington's disease. *N Engl J Med* 1992; 327: 401–405.

1.6 Muscle pain on exercise

Case history

A young man presents with pain in his muscles on exercise.

Clinical approach

The list of causes of muscle pain is extensive, but pain occurring on exercise limits the differential diagnosis (Table 5) [1].

History of the presenting problem

In a young, otherwise fit man, the important differential is between a disorder of lipid or carbohydrate metabolism. These conditions are described in Section 2.2 (p. 65), which will explain the significance of the questions shown below.

Is this a disorder of energy production?

Find out:

• how much exercise is possible before the onset of pain?

Table 5 Causes of muscle pain on exercise.

Metabolic	Carnitine palmitoyl transferase deficiency
	McArdle's disease and other disorders of glycogen metabolism
	Mitochondrial myopathy
Other	Hypothyroidism
Ischaemia	Lumbar canal stenosis*
	Claudication*

*Muscular pain restricted to the legs, excepting rare cases of arm claudication.

- is a 'second wind' phenomenon experienced?
- are there associated painful muscle cramps?
- have there been episodes of dark urine (indicating rhabdomyolysis)?
- is there a family history? Autosomal recessive inheritance is seen in carnitine palmitoyl transferase (CPT) deficiency and McArdle's disease; maternal inheritance in mitochondrial disorders.

Is this hypothyroidism?

Ask about weight gain, lethargy, cold intolerance and other symptoms of hypothyroidism (see *Endocrinology*, Section 2.3).

Is this mechanical (lumbar canal stenosis)?

Find out if the symptoms are:
- confined to the legs
- improved by bending over.

Lumbar canal stenosis would be unusual in a young man. It is usually caused by progressive hypertrophy of the facet joints and disk degeneration leading to narrowing of the lumbar canal. Lumbar claudication (pain and heaviness of the legs, often proximal) is experienced on standing or walking. Flexion improves the diameter of the canal and therefore the symptoms, hence patients often report no problems with cycling, in which the lumbar spine is often flexed.

Is this muscle ischaemia?

Unlikely in young man, but is the patient an arteriopath with multiple vascular risk factors?

Relevant past history

Was the patient sporty as a child/teenager? If so, this suggests an 'acquired' illness rather than a metabolic myopathy, which is a lifelong condition.

Examination

Concentrate particularly on the following.
- Muscle bulk and power—may be normal (see box on metabolic myopathy below).
- Examination after a prolonged walk—whilst exercise provocation is not recommended in metabolic disorders, in lumbar canal stenosis this can be a useful diagnostic aid. Reversible discomfort and weakness may be induced by walking and relieved by flexion of the spine.
- Signs of hypothyroidism—what is the patient's general appearance? Are the tendon reflexes slow relaxing? (see *Endocrinology*, Section 2.3).

Metabolic myopathy

Examination may be normal between attacks in cases of McArdle's disease or CPT deficiency. Some cases of McArdle's disease do develop a myopathy with age. In McArdle's disease ischaemic exercise (opening and clenching fist with inflated BP cuff *in situ*) may induce painful cramps, but the test is best avoided because it can induce muscle necrosis.

Approach to investigations and management

Metabolic muscle disease

See Section 2.2 (p. 65) and [2].

Lumbar canal stenosis

Imaging and surgical decompression.

Thyroid disease

See *Endocrinology*, Section 2.3.

See *Biochemistry and metabolism*, Sections 2 and 3.
1 The metabolic myopathies. In: Adams RD, Victor M (eds) *Principles of Neurology* (5th edn). New York: McGraw-Hill, 1995.
2 Mastaglia FL, Laing NG. Investigation of muscle disease. *J Neurol Neurosurg Psychiatry* 1996; 60: 256–274.

1.7 Increasing seizure frequency

Case history

A 30-year-old woman with previously well-controlled epilepsy has had increasing frequency of seizures over several months, leading her general practitioner to ask for outpatient review.

Clinical approach

The most important points to establish are the level of previous seizure control, whether this has been achieved easily and by what means. A full and careful drug history is required. In the case described, the first question is whether increased seizure frequency has occurred despite adequate blood concentration of antiepileptics. Causes of deterioration in seizure control can be divided into those secondary to a fall in available drug and those that occur despite adequate drug levels (Table 6).

Table 6 Causes of deterioration in seizure control*.

Reduced drug level	Poor compliance
	Poor absorption
	Drug interactions
	Pregnancy
	Outdated drug preparations
Increased seizure frequency despite stable drug levels	Poor sleep
	Excessive alcohol/illicit drugs
	Non-epileptic seizures

*Note: any cause of acute illness or metabolic disturbance can cause temporary deterioration in seizure control.

History of the presenting problem

Is this due to a fall in blood concentration of antiepileptic?

Consider the following:
• is compliance good, or does the patient forget to take her tablets from 'time to time'?
• has new medication been added that would alter the metabolism of existing antiepileptics? Many drugs act to antagonize or potentiate antiepileptic affect. If in any doubt at all, always refer to the BNF.
• has there been any diarrhoea or vomiting to cause reduced absorption?
• is the patient using an inactive, outdated preparation (highly unlikely)?
• is the patient pregnant?

> Addition of new antiepileptic drugs can worsen as well as improve seizure control.

> Increased seizure frequency is seen in approximately one-third of pregnant epileptic patients, usually in the later stages of the pregnancy and related to expansion of the blood volume and changes in plasma protein binding and metabolism. Some will require an increase in drug dosage.

Are there new factors exacerbating epilepsy?

Is the patient getting sufficient sleep? Have they started working on a night shift, are they being kept awake by their young child, etc? Is there a possibility of excessive consumption of alcohol/abuse of drugs?

Any cause of acute illness, e.g. chest or urinary tract infection, can lead to a deterioration in epileptic control, in which case the appropriate history would need to be explored. There was no suggestion that intercurrent acute illness was the cause of the increased seizure frequency in this woman.

Are the new attacks epileptic?

Non-organic, 'functional', or pseudoseizures may occur in individuals with concurrent true epilepsy (see Section 2.7, p. 85). This can be a very difficult diagnosis to make—some pointers to pseudoseizures are:
• change in nature of attack
• social or financial gain
• occur in the presence of observers, often in emotional situations
• superficial injury only (e.g. carpet burns)
• non-synchronous limb movements
• unusually rapid postictal recovery.

Could there be a new or expanding lesion?

Particularly in patients in whom a structural lesion is known to be responsible for the attacks, it is essential to exclude expansion of the lesion. Warning symptoms include:
• recent headache, nausea or vomiting
• new focal symptoms.

Examination

A rapid neurological and general examination is required: no new abnormalities would be expected.

Approach to investigations and management

Investigation

In this case, with no suggestion on history or examination of intercurrent acute illness and no change in neurological examination, then unless the reason for loss of epileptic control is apparent from the history (see Table 6):
• check full blood count, electrolytes, renal and liver function tests, serum calcium and inflammatory markers as a 'screen'. Check pregnancy test if appropriate
• check drug levels. Therapeutic ranges are known for phenytoin and carbamezepine. Sodium valproate levels are useful to check compliance only
• imaging may be required if a new or expanding lesion is considered likely, but otherwise a brain scan is not necessary
• if pseudoseizures are suspected, measurement of serum prolactin after an attack can be helpful; this is raised following genuine but not following functional seizures.

Management

This will depend on the cause of increased seizure frequency:
• improve compliance

- increase dose
- more sleep, less alcohol.

If the seizure frequency remains increased despite appropriate drug levels and life style, then revisit the possibility of non-organic seizures. Ambulatory electroencephalogram (EEG) recording during an attack may help to make this diagnosis. Remember, however, that patients can become tolerant to drugs and it may be necessary to introduce new antiepileptic medication. In the case of those with hippocampal sclerosis, there is a higher chance that seizures may remain drug resistant, in which case it may be appropriate to refer for consideration of surgical treatment.

See *Clinical pharmacology*, Sections 2 and 3.
Duncan JS, Shorvon SD, Fish DR. *Clinical Epilepsy*. London: Churchill Livingstone, 1995.

1.8 Sleep disorders

Case history

A middle-aged man complains of excessive daytime sleepiness.

Clinical approach

'This patient complains of daytime sleepiness' is not an infrequent referral, but the narcoleptic syndrome is much less common, and even if the patient tells you that they have 'narcolepsy', other causes should be considered (Tables 7–9) [1].

History of the presenting problem

A sleep history is required: what time does the patient go to bed; when do they wake up in the morning; how often do they wake during the night; and what do they do when they do so? Exactly what does their 'excessive daytime sleepiness' mean? How often do they actually fall asleep, and have they ever fallen asleep when they were trying to stay awake, e.g. when driving? The answers to these questions will help to place the problem into one of two categories:

Table 7 Differential diagnosis of excessive daytime sleepiness.

Insomnia (insufficient sleep)
Non-restorative sleep
Narcolepsy

Table 8 Causes of insomnia.

Wrong environment	Noisy
	Too light/cold/hot
	Disturbed by partner
Psychophysiological	Anxiety/depression
	Bipolar affective disorders
Endocrine	Thyrotoxicosis
Physical	Pain
	Nocturia
	Parkinson's disease
Drugs	Alcohol
	Coffee
	Prescription
	Steroids
	β-blockers
	Phenytoin
	Bronchodilators
	Diuretics
	Stimulants
Hereditary	Fatal familial insomnia

Table 9 Causes of non-restorative sleep.

Obstructive sleep apnoea	Associated with obesity
Central	Brain-stem lesions
	Degenerative brain conditions
Mixed	Seen in myotonic dystrophy

- Insomnia: Table 8 lists the most common causes for an inability to get sufficient sleep; further questioning should be designed to address these issues.
- Non-restorative sleep, where the patient appears to spend a sufficient time asleep but does not awake refreshed, the main causes for which are shown in Table 9.

Could the patient have any of the conditions listed in Tables 7, 8 or 9? Further history should be directed to looking for evidence of the following conditions in particular.

Obstructive sleep apnoea

Is there morning headache? Patients with obstructive sleep apnoea retain CO_2, resulting in headache.

The observations of a partner are essential. Ask the partner:
- does he snore loudly?
- does he sometimes appear to stop breathing?
- does he resume breathing with a large gasp?

Central sleep apnoea

There will usually be a history of a brain-stem event

17

or of other symptoms to suggest more widespread neuro-degenerative disease.

Parasomnias

These are a group of disorders that usually start in childhood and can be linked to particular stages of sleep. They can either be disorders of movement, including hypnic jerks, periodic movements of sleep, sleep paralysis and sleep walking; or disorders of autonomic function with symptoms of sympathetic overdrive; or more complex abnormalities such as sleep terrors. They are rare in an adult population and can only be diagnosed by a witness account.

Narcoleptic syndrome

This is classically defined as the triad of narcolepsy, cataplexy and hypnogogic hallucinations (and other parasomnias, especially sleep paralysis) though not all patients will have all the symptoms.
- Narcolepsy—when daytime sleep attacks are often without warning, at times of emotion and after a carbohydrate load.
- Cataplexy—these are episodes of partial (often face or jaw) or complete loss of muscle tone that result in the patient falling to the ground. They are often triggered by emotional stimuli, usually laughter.
- Hypnogogic hallucinations—presleep dreams associated with sleep-onset REM activity. In sleep paralysis, which is not restricted to the narcoleptic syndrome, the patient feels completely paralysed at sleep onset (less commonly on waking), often associated with terror, anxiety and fear. Recovery is spontaneous.

Relevant past history

This is important in the case of central sleep apnoea. Adults with parasomnias may have been sleepwalkers or tooth-grinders as children.

Family history

May be relevant in some rare diseases.

Fatal familial insomnia is an hereditary disease caused by an Asp–Asn mutation at codon 178 of the human prion protein gene in the presence of a methionine at codon 129. The same mutation at codon 178 but with a valine at codon 129 results in a familial Creutzfeldt–Jakob disease (CJD). Fatal familial insomnia is a rapidly fatal disease characterized by insomnia and dysautonaumia and more widespread neurological involvement including pyramidal, cerebellar and cognitive signs.

Examination

Neurological examination may be entirely normal, excepting in those with central sleep apnoea when brainstem signs or evidence of a neurodegenerative condition may be present. Patients with obstructive sleep apnoea are usually obese with a large neck and often look cyanosed. Look for signs of thyrotoxicosis (see *Endocrinology*, Sections 1.13 and 2.3).

Approach to investigations and management

The approach to investigations and management will be determined by findings in the history. It may be that nothing more than simple advice is required.

Insomnia

It is often sufficient to improve sleep hygiene, whether that means sleeping with ear plugs, lining the curtains or not drinking coffee after 6.00 p.m. Psychiatric and physical disorders that are felt to be contributing must be addressed.

Sleep apnoea

Patients who might have sleep apnoea should be referred to a respiratory specialist with an interest in sleep disorders for further investigation and/or treatment. (See *Respiratory medicine*, Sections 1.8, 2.1 and 2.3.)

Narcoleptic syndrome

Narcolepsy has a 99% positive association with HLA DQB1 0602, which can be used as a diagnostic test [2]. Narcolepsy and hypnogogic hallucinations have traditionally been treated with CNS stimulants (amphetamines and related substances). A new drug is now available called Modafinil [3]. Cataplexy and sleep paralysis respond to tricyclic antidepressants, in particular clomipramine.

1 Parkes JD, Clift SJ, Dahlitz MJ, Chen SY, Dunn G. The narcoleptic syndrome. *J Neurol Neurosurg Psychiatry* 1995; 59(3): 221–224.
2 Parkes JD, Lock CB. Genetic factors in sleep disorders. *J Neurol Neurosurg Psychiatry* 1989; 52(supplement): 101–108.
3 Fry JM. Treatment modalities for narcolepsy. *Neurology* 1998; 50: S43–48.

1.9 Memory difficulties

Case history

A 60-year-old school teacher presents with a 2-month history of forgetfulness.

Clinical approach

You need to establish if the patient has dementia, which is the impairment of cognitive function affecting the content, but not the level, of consciousness. It is essential to obtain an independent description, e.g. from a relative, since given the nature of the complaint, the patient's history may be unreliable. There are many causes of dementia (Table 10), but it is particularly important to rule out any that are reversible or have a treatable cause [1].

 The commonest and most important condition to distinguish from dementia is depressive pseudodementia, which is eminently treatable.

History of the presenting problem

What are the characteristics of the memory impairment?

Ask the following questions if the relevant details do not emerge spontaneously:
• Was the onset of memory difficulties associated with a precipitating cause, e.g. a head injury causing a subdural haematoma?
• Was the onset of the dementia subacute (e.g. in normal pressure hydrocephalus, CJD) or chronic (e.g. in Alzheimer's disease, vascular dementia)?
• Is the course of the dementia gradual or step-wise in progression? The latter is seen in multi-infarct-type

Table 10 Differential diagnosis of dementia.

Common	Uncommon
Alzheimer's disease (AD)	Alcohol-related
Multi-infarct dementia	Hydrocephalus
Dementia with Lewy bodies (DLB)	Parkinson's disease
	Huntington's disease
	Creutzfeldt–Jakob disease (CJD)
	Frontotemporal dementia (FTD)
	Tumours
	Drug toxicity
	Hypothyroidism
	Chronic subdural haematoma
	Vitamin B_{12} deficiency
	Neurosyphilis
	AIDS dementia complex

vascular dementia. Is there fluctuating cognitive impairment affecting both memory and higher cortical functions (e.g. language, visuospatial ability) suggesting dementia with Lewy bodies (DLB)?
• Does the patient seem slow with disturbance of attention and motivation? This is more suggestive of so-called subcortical dementia. As the name implies, there is less cortical dysfunction and more disturbance of structures such as the basal ganglia and basal forebrain. Subcortical features are less likely to be seen in Alzheimer's disease, but may be seen in a wide variety of pathological processes affecting these deeper subcortical structures [2] including vascular dementia due to small vessel disease.
• Is there prominent behaviour disinhibition, loss of social skills, emotional blunting and language dysfunction? These features, together with personality change, are seen in frontotemporal dementia.

Associated features

Consider the following:
• Are there any neuropsychiatric symptoms (e.g. depression, apathy, irritability) or motor abnormalities (e.g. extrapyramidal features)? These are more common in subcortical than cortical dementias.
• Are there delusions, visual hallucinations or disturbances of sleep pattern associated with motor features of parkinsonism, suggesting DLB?
• Is there any gait disturbance or urinary incontinence, suggesting normal pressure hydrocephalus?
• Are there any associated headache with features suggesting raised intracranial pressure, e.g. worse on awakening, stooping or coughing?

Relevant past history

Ask about the following:
• Are there atheromatous vascular risk factors (e.g. smoking, hypertension, diabetes), cerebrovascular events (e.g. strokes), heart disease (e.g. atrial fibrillation) and hypothyroidism?
• Is there is a family history of dementia, e.g. familial Alzheimer's disease, Huntington's disease (see Section 1.5, p. 12)?
• A detailed drug history is essential, but drugs tend to cause confusion rather than dementia.
• Take a detailed sexual history (neurosyphilis causes general paresis, but is now extremely rare) and assess alcohol intake (see *General clinical issues*, Sections 2 and 3).

Examination

Mental state and neurological

To formally test cognition, the Mini-Mental State

Examination [3] is recommended, as it is easy to use, and has age- and education-adjusted norms (see *Medicine for the elderly*, Section 3.2). More detailed neuropsychometry is used in difficult cases (see Section 3.1, p. 111).

Neurological examination is relatively normal in Alzheimer's disease, although primitive reflexes may be elicited. These indicate widespread cortical damage or dysfunction, typically frontal, hence the term 'frontal-release signs'. Examples include the pout, grasp, glabellar, palmomental and suck reflexes, most of which may be present in a small proportion of the normal population.

Certain signs may point to a particular aetiology, e.g. papilloedema (brain tumour), myoclonus (CJD) or unsteady gait (normal pressure hydrocephalus).

General

A full general medical examination is required: are any of the conditions listed in Table 10 likely? Look in particular for evidence of chronic liver disease (see *Gastroenterology and hepatology*, Sections 1.6, 1.7 and 2.10), widespread vascular disease (vascular bruits, absent peripheral pulses) or hypothyroidism (see *Endocrinology*, Sections 1.14 and 2.3).

Approach to investigations and management

Investigations

Any clinical clue to conditions listed in Table 10 should be followed, but controversy surrounds what constitutes a cost-effective series of investigations, based on different estimates of the incidence of reversible dementias [4]. Many physicians would consider the following.

Blood tests

Check full blood count, electrolytes, renal, liver and thyroid function tests, inflammatory markers (ESR or CRP), serum vitamin B_{12} level and syphilis serology. Genetic testing may be useful in familial Alzheimer's disease.

Genetic testing raises complex ethical issues. Consequences of genetic testing must be carefully considered as significant harm can result from inadequate counselling.

Cerebrospinal fluid

Testing of the CSF is rarely warranted unless there are concerning clinical features such as systemic symptoms, rapid progression or unusual signs. The CSF cell count, protein and glucose are normal in Alzheimer's disease.

Neuroimaging

This is used to rule out structural and sometimes treatable causes of dementia such as tumours, normal pressure hydrocephalus or chronic subdural haematoma. In Alzheimer's disease, computed tomography or MRI of the brain shows cerebral atrophy, whilst single-photon emission CT (SPECT) shows temporoparietal hypoperfusion. MRI may play a role in early diagnosis of Alzheimer's disease, which will be crucial if and when treatments that are effective in slowing disease progression become available [5].

Electroencephalogram

This is not particularly useful because of the overlap in EEG patterns in different forms of dementia. In Alzheimer's disease, there is loss of alpha activity and increase in diffuse slow waves.

Management

Management will depend on the precise diagnosis. For Alzheimer's disease, see Section 2.4, p. 75.

> ! If a depressive element is suspected to be contributing to some or all of the clinical picture then a trial of antidepressants is warranted.
> See *Psychiatry*, Section 2.11.

See *Medicine for the elderly*, Sections 1.2, 2.7 and 3.2.
1 Weytingh MD, Bossuyt PMM, van Crevel H. Reversible dementia: more than 10% or less than 1%? A quantitative review. *J Neurol* 1995; 242: 466–471.
2 Whitehouse PJ. The concept of subcortical and cortical dementia: another look. *Ann Neurol* 1986; 19: 1–6.
3 Folstein MF, Folstein SE, McHugh PR. 'Mini-mental state': a practical method for grading the cognitive state of patients for the clinician. *J Psychiatr Res* 1975; 12: 189–198.
4 Geldmacher DS, Whitehouse PJ. Evaluation of dementia. *N Engl J Med* 1996; 335: 330–336.
5 Rossor MN, Fox NC. Mere forgetfulness or Alzheimer's disease? *Ann Neurol* 2000; 47: 419–420.

1.10 Dysphagia

Case history

A 66-year-old man is referred with an 18-month history of progressive dysphagia.

Table 11 Common causes of dysphagia.

Type of disorder	Oropharyngeal	Oesophageal
Mechanical	Tumour Zenker's diverticulum Neck surgery Goitre Retropharyngeal mass	Tumour Schatzki's ring Posterior mediastinal mass Peptic stricture
Mobility	Achalasia Scleroderma	Achalasia Scleroderma
Neurological	Pseudobulbar palsy (e.g. stroke, MND) Bulbar palsy (e.g. poliomyelitis, MND) Myasthenia gravis	Idiopathic autonomic dysfunction Vagal neuropathy due to diabetes
Muscular	Polymyositis Myotonic dystrophy	Polymyositis

Clinical approach

Dysphagia (difficulty in swallowing) must be distinguished from odynophagia (painful swallowing) and the globus sensation (a feeling of a lump in the throat). It is then necessary to determine if it is due to an oropharyngeal or an oesophageal cause, and whether this is attributable to a mechanical, motility, neurological or muscular problem (Table 11) [1].

History of the presenting problem

In many cases of dysphagia there are clear indications that the problem is likely to be mechanical, e.g. the patient has a long history of acid reflux or other digestive problems, is known to have a hiatus hernia or reflux oesophagitis, and oesophageal stricture is likely. The approach to such a case is discussed in detail in *Gastroenterology and hepatology*, Section 1.2. When there is no such history, the wide differential diagnosis of dysphagia must be considered. Think about the conditions listed in Table 11 when taking the history of the dysphagia itself, and of associated features.

Dysphagia

Ask specifically about the following:
• Is there choking or coughing due to aspiration? This is more likely to occur in neurological or muscular disorders than those due to mechanical or motility problems.
• Is swallowing worse with liquids than with solids? Patients with neuromuscular disorders usually complain of difficulties with liquids first, whereas those with mechanical disorders tend to complain that solid food sticks.
• Is there nasal regurgitation? This is more common in neuromuscular disorders affecting the oropharynx.

Associated features

Find out the following.
• Is dysphagia causing weight loss? This may arise because dysphagia is preventing adequate food intake, but may indicate a malignant cause.
• Is the course of the symptoms progressive? This might indicate a worsening mechanical lesion, but if the problem is neuromuscular, the time course can also give important diagnostic clues, e.g. inexorable progression in motor neurone disease (MND) [2], fluctuating course in myasthenia gravis, or static situation following stroke.
• Are there muscle cramps, which are common in motor neurone disease, or muscle weakness?
• Does the patient complain of respiratory difficulties, which might indicate MND or myasthenia gravis?
• Is speech affected? If so, how? This is likely to indicate a neuromuscular cause. Refer to Section 1.22 (p. 49) for distinction between the different speech disorders.
• Are there any sensory, sphincter or visual disturbances? If the problem is neuromuscular and yet these systems are not involved, then MND is more likely.
• Are there clues to any of the other diagnoses listed in Table 11? For instance, a history of Raynaud's phenomenon may indicate scleroderma with associated oesophageal motility disorder.

Relevant past history

A careful 'gastrointestinal' past medical history is clearly required: 'do you get indigestion?'; 'do you take any treatments for indigestion?'; 'have you ever done so?'; 'have you ever had a barium meal or an endoscopy test?'. As regards neurological causes, is the patient at increased risk of stroke? Is there a family history of neurological problems?

Examination

General

Look for the following features:
• Nutritional status—is the patient cachectic? What is their body mass index?
• Evidence of malignant disease—can you see anything abnormal in the oropharynx? Examine very carefully for cervical lymphadenopathy. Can you feel an epigastric mass? Is the liver enlarged?
• Chest signs—is there evidence of poor respiratory effort, suggesting respiratory muscle involvement, or of right basal consolidation, the usual site of aspiration pneumonia.
• Signs of other diseases that may cause dysphagia, e.g. skin changes in scleroderma.

Neurological

A full neurological examination is required, including a careful assessment of swallowing. Look in particular for the following:
• Is there bulbar weakness, e.g. depressed gag reflex, a weak cough, a wasted and fasciculating tongue? A brisk jaw jerk, spastic tongue and emotional lability suggest psuedobulbar palsy (Fig. 5).
• In the limbs, upper motor neurone signs only (i.e. spasticity, hyperreflexia, extensor plantars) are seen in primary lateral sclerosis (see Section 2.1.3, p. 63). Lower motor neurone signs only (i.e. flaccidity, atrophy, fasciculations, hyporeflexia) are seen in poliomyelitis and adult-onset spinal muscular atrophies (see Section 2.1.3, p. 63 and 2.2.3, p. 67). Both upper and lower motor neurone signs are seen in amyotrophic lateral sclerosis (ALS).

> **!** Swallowing is best assessed by asking the patient to drink a sip of water [3].

> **? Brain-stem and cerebral causes of dysphagia**
>
> A lesion in the medulla oblongata can affect the motor nuclei of the glossopharyngeal, vagus and hypoglossal nerves that supply the muscles involved in swallowing, but there will invariably be other clinical features.
> A unilateral cerebral hemisphere stroke will not usually cause persistent swallowing problems as the bulbar cranial nuclei receive innervation from each hemisphere.

Approach to investigations and management

Investigations

A full nutritional assessment is required for any patient

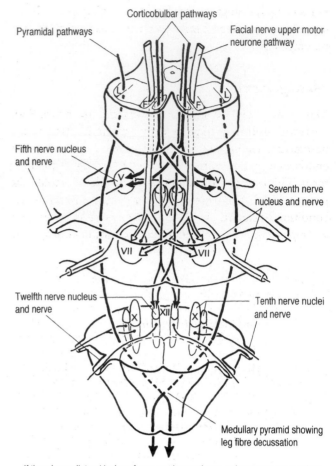

If there is a unilateral lesion of supranuclear pathway, subsequent supranuclear pathway lesion on the other side will produce sudden and complete paralysis of fifth, seventh, ninth, tenth, eleventh and twelth cranial nerves

Fig. 5 Anatomy of pseudobulbar palsy. The supranuclear pathways for the tenth nerve are not depicted, but are exactly as for the fifth and twelfth nerves as shown. (Each supranuclear pathway contributes 50% to each nucleus.) The facial nerve is different. Some 90% of fibres decussate, the right supranuclear pathways innervating the left facial nerve, hence a lesion in the right supranuclar pathway will produce significant left facial weakness, whereas corresponding lesions of the other motor cranial nerves will produce no abnormality (or at worst only transient abnormality).

whose main problem is dysphagia, and many will require investigation (barium swallow, endoscopy) to look for a mechanical cause; for details see *Gastroenterology and hepatology*, Sections 1.2, 1.10 and 2.14. Other tests may be indicated in some patients, e.g. autoimmune screen if scleroderma is suspected. The following may be useful in the differential diagnosis of neuromuscular causes of dysphagia.
• Serum immunoglobulins and electrophoresis (lymphoproliferative diseases) and thyroid function tests (thyrotoxicosis) are done to exclude diseases that may mimic MND [2].
• MRI is needed to exclude lesions in the brain stem if there is evidence of other cranial nerve dysfunction that suggests a structural cause.

• Electrophysiological studies help diagnose MND, myasthenia gravis and inflammatory muscle disease (e.g. polymyositis).

Management

Management will depend on the specific diagnosis. Poor nutrition itself may require symptomatic treatment, e.g. nasogastric feeding in the short term or percutaneous endoscopic gastrostomy (PEG) tube feeding in the long term. This can raise difficult ethical problems: should the patient with a progressive and irreversible neurological condition be started on PEG feeding? See *Gastroenterology and hepatology*, Section 1.19, for consideration of this issue.

> See *Pain relief and palliative care*, Sections 2.9 and 2.10.
> See *Medicine for the elderly*, Sections 1.4 and 2.11.
> See *Gastroenterology and hepatology*, Section 2.14.
> 1 Hughes TA, Wiles CM. Neurogenic dysphagia: the role of the neurologist. *J Neurol Neurosurg Psychiatry* 1998; 64(5): 569–572.
> 2 Hadjikoutis S, Eccles R, Wiles CM. Coughing and choking in motor neurone disease. *J Neurol Neurosurg Psychiatry* 2000; 68(5): 601–604.
> 3 Mari F, Matei M, Ceravolo MG, Pisani A, Montesi A, Provinciali L. Predictive value of clinical indices in detecting aspiration in patients with neurological disorders. *J Neurol Neurosurg Psychiatry* 1997; 63(4): 456–460.

1.11 Weak legs

Case history

A 27-year-old woman is referred urgently with a 3-day history of progressive weakness of her legs.

Clinical approach

The first requirement is to clarify what the patient means by 'weakness'. The term is often used to describe loss of energy or drive: when used properly 'weakness' means loss of muscle power. The differential diagnosis of rapidly progressive weakness of the legs, as present in this case, is shown in Table 12. The top priority is to exclude acute spinal cord compression, which is not always easy. In the acute stage it may be difficult to differentiate between upper and lower motor neurone weakness, since even in spinal cord lesions the legs may initially be flaccid. However, on the basis of the history and examination it should be possible to pick up enough clues to differentiate between a cord syndrome, acute neuropathy and muscle disease.

Table 12 Causes of acute or subacute leg weakness in a young patient.

Brain	Stroke, tumour (especially parasagittal), multiple sclerosis
Spinal cord	Spinal cord infarction, tumour, disc protrusion, transverse myelitis, abscess, multiple sclerosis, poliomyelitis
Peripheral nerve	Guillain–Barré syndrome, porphyria, diphtheria
Neuromuscular junction	Myasthenia gravis, aminoglycosides, botulism
Muscle	Polymyositis, dermatomyositis, inclusion body myositis, periodic paralysis, metabolic myopathy (e.g. hypokalaemia)

History of the presenting problem

Bear in mind the conditions listed in Table 12 as you take the history and ask about the following if the details do not emerge spontaneously.

Is this a spinal cord syndrome?

Important points to establish are:
• is there problem with the bladder? Any involvement suggests spinal cord or cauda equina pathology in this context
• is there a sensory level, or even a band of tightness (suspended sensory level) around on the torso? These features would suggest a cord lesion.

If a cord lesion is likely then sudden onset probably indicates a vascular cause (cord stroke, arteriovenous malformation): compression or transverse myelitis would typically come on over hours to a few days.

> A suspended sensory level is a band of impaired sensation below and above which sensation is normal. It may be uni- or bilateral and is indicative of an intrinsic cord lesion.

> **Weak legs**
> If it is possible that this is due to acute cord compression then an MRI scan needs to performed urgently; see *Emergency medicine*, Section 1.23.

Is this Guillain–Barré syndrome?

A history of preceding illness, particularly diarrhoea, ascending symptoms and sometimes proximal muscle aching should make you think about Guillain–Barré syndrome.

Other rare acute neuropathies may need to be considered. Are there any episodes of colicky abdominal pain or acute delirium/confusion, suggesting porphyria, which can also occasionally cause an acute neuropathy? Systemic features together with a fever should alert you to the possibility of an infective myeloradiculitis, e.g. due to tuberculosis.

> **! Back pain and weak legs**
>
> Back pain is often thought to indicate pathology in the vertebral bodies or discs, but it may equally be a feature of transverse myelitis or an epidural abscess. Most importantly, remember that back and proximal muscle pain is commonly seen in the early stages of Guillain–Barré syndrome.

Is this muscle disease?

Think about the following:
• Muscle disease or neuromuscular junction disease is likely to be generalized if it is causing this particular clinical picture, so ask carefully about symptoms in the arms and cranial nerves (particularly diplopia and dysphagia), and whether fatigability has been a recent feature (myasthenia gravis).
• Is there any shortness of breath suggesting respiratory muscle involvement? This could equally indicate progressive Guillain–Barré syndrome.
• Is there any muscle pain, e.g. in myositis?
• Is there a rash, e.g. in dermatomyositis?

Relevant past history

Ask specifically about the following:
• Take a careful drug history. Drugs may cause a motor neuropathy (e.g. dapsone) or a myopathy (e.g. zidovudine), impair neuromuscular transmission (e.g. aminoglycosides) or precipitate an acute attack of porphyria (e.g. phenytoin).
• Has she had any previous episodes of neurological symptoms, e.g. optic neuritis, to make you suspect multiple sclerosis as a cause of transverse myelitis (Fig. 6)?
• Is she known to have a connective tissue disease, which could be associated with polymyositis?

Examination

The likely diagnosis should be clear from the history: does the examination confirm this?

Is this a spinal cord syndrome?

Look for the following features:
• Brisk reflexes, extensor plantars and a clear sensory level make localization easy, but all of these may not be present. Look very carefully for any of them. If you find an extensor plantar, go back and re-examine for tone, power and reflexes, looking more carefully for upper motor neurone features.
• It is crucial to examine carefully for a sensory level, or a suspended sensory deficit, as this strongly suggests the spinal cord is the site of any lesion.

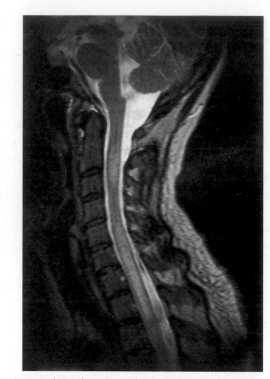

Fig. 6 Increased signal on T2-weighted sagittal MRI of cervical cord, indicative of intrinsic lesion, possibly inflammatory.

> Although demonstrating a sensory level points to the spinal cord, it is notoriously inaccurate at localizing the level of the pathology. You should therefore use all possible clinical signs to help you. For example, a patient with a sensory level at the umbilicus (T10), who also has brisk arm reflexes, is likely to have a lesion in the cervical cord above C5, rather than at T10. The significance of this is that it is the cervical cord that requires imaging, not the thoracic cord. It is generally much better to start imaging at the top (cervical) and work down, rather than the other way round.

Do not forget that:
• The presence of cranial nerve signs does not necessarily mean the lesion is in the brain stem. There may be multiple lesions, as in multiple sclerosis (acute cord syndromes are a common way for multiple sclerosis to present), and cranial nerve palsies are common in Guillain–Barré syndrome.
• Look at the back for evidence of trauma, and also for superficial vascular markings/malformations that may indicate an underlying vascular malformation as a cause of cord stroke. Auscultate over the spine for bruits: these are very rare, but if you don't, you'll never hear one!

Is this Guillain–Barré syndrome?

In the presence of a suggestive history, the finding of a symmetrical weakness of the legs (may be more proximal or more distal, as this is a demyelinating neuropathy), minimal sensory loss and areflexia is virtually diagnostic (see Sections 2.1.1, p. 57 and 2.1.2, p. 61, for discussion of the differential diagnosis).

Is this muscle disease?

If muscle disease is the cause of leg weakness:
• it is likely that examination will reveal more extensive weakness, in particular of proximal arm muscles and neck flexors
• muscle tenderness suggests myositis
• a heliotrope rash over the eyelids or extensor surfaces of joints suggests dermatomyositis
• is there fatigability of muscle power, ptosis or bulbar features, any of which would suggest myasthenia gravis?

Approach to investigations and management

Investigations

These will be dictated by the clinical diagnosis, but the following may need to be considered.

MRI spine

If an acute spinal cord lesion is suspected the patient must have an urgent MRI scan. The purpose of this is to rule out a compressive lesion that is amenable to neurosurgical decompression. A scan reported as normal should exclude a compressive lesion but does not rule out the spinal cord as the site of the lesion: cord stroke and (sometimes) inflammatory lesions may be difficult to visualize.

Further investigations

Once cord compression has been excluded, further investigations should be guided by the clinical suspicion: see 'Diseases and treatments' (pp. 57–110) on the individual conditions listed in Table 12 for further information.

Management

Treatment depends on the underlying disorder. Urgent intervention is needed in acute spinal cord compression and may include surgical decompression, high-dose steroids and radiotherapy, depending on the type of the lesion.
• Disc protrusions causing cord compression need surgical removal.
• In epidural metastasis treatment is with high-dose steroids and radiotherapy, with prognosis depending on the patient's condition at diagnosis and the radiosensitivity of the particular tumour.
• In epidural abscess, surgical decompression, drainage and intravenous antibiotics are needed in cases of spinal cord compromise.

• Neurosurgical intervention may be useful in certain spinal tumours.

For management of other conditions see the relevant sections on individual diseases.

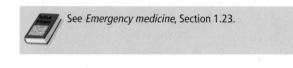 See *Emergency medicine*, Section 1.23.

1.12 Neck/shoulder pain

Case history

A 35-year-old woman presents with a several-month history of right-sided neck and shoulder pain.

Clinical approach

Presentation with neck and shoulder pain may be found in a wide range of conditions, commonly for instance in the context of generalized back pain (see *Rheumatology and clinical immunology*, Section 1.17) or in an elderly patient with general malaise (see *Medicine for the elderly*, Section 1.5). Neither of these contexts are appropriate for this woman, and when evaluating 'isolated' neck and shoulder pain it is useful to divide the causes into three major categories: radicular, deep segmental or musculoskeletal (Table 13).

History of the presenting problem

What is the pain like?

A precise description of the type of pain is essential when attempting to determine the likely cause. Pain caused by

Table 13 Causes of neck and shoulder pain.

Type of pain	Source	Common or important cause
Deep segmental	Spinal cord	Syringomyelia Tumour
Radicular	Nerve root	Disc prolapse Vertebral collapse Nerve root trauma
	Brachial plexus	Pancoast's syndrome Brachial plexopathy Cervical rib Subclavian artery aneurysm
Musculoskeletal	Shoulder	'Painful restricted shoulder syndromes', e.g. tendonitis, capsulitis, bursitis
	Neck	Spondylosis

irritation of nerve roots has a different character from that arising from the spinal cord itself or from musculoskeletal pain. When taking the history, note the following, and ask specifically if the details are not forthcoming.

• Radicular pain is caused by irritation of dorsal roots (e.g. cervical spondylosis, brachial plexopathy) and is projected to the dermatome of the nerve root, hence ask about the distribution of the pain and if there is associated paraesthesiae or numbness. The pain is sharp and stabbing in nature, and aggravated by coughing and neck flexion.

• Deep segmental pain is caused by lesions within the spinal cord (e.g. syringomyelia, intramedullary tumours). It is not as sharp or as well localized as radicular pain, and is not influenced by coughing or straining.

• Musculoskeletal pain from the neck is often associated with spasm in the trapezius, paraspinal muscles and the muscles of the scalp: dysaesthesiae may radiate to the arms in a non-radicular distribution. Pain from the shoulder is likely to be exacerbated by particular movements of the joint, in particular abduction and rotation. There is often muscle spasm of the upper fibres of the trapezius, leading to pain in the neck, and pain can also be referred to the deltoid muscle or the medial side of the elbow.

Possible causes of the pain

Also ask specifically about the following:

• is there any history of neck trauma, e.g. whiplash injury or fracture?

• is there any history of shoulder problems, e.g. previous pain, previous dislocation?

And much less likely:

• has there been abnormal posturing of the head and neck (torticollis), which may be due to spasmodic torticollis, or torticollis caused by a structural abnormality of the neck or cervical spine?

• has there been recent infection or vaccination, which are risk factors for brachial neuritis?

Relevant past history

Note the following:

• Any history of malignancy, which might lead to cervical secondaries that could present in this way. Previous breast cancer and radiotherapy might suggest a radiation plexopathy or malignant infiltration.

• Is there a family history of this problem, which might be due to familial brachial plexopathy?

Examination

Musculoskeletal

Observe how the woman moves her neck and shoulder, e.g. when removing her clothing before being examined. If movement of the neck is painful, then this will be held rigid: if the shoulder is painful then the normal scapulohumeral rhythm of movement, whereby the arm moves in the shoulder joint before the scapula moves, will be reversed. Feel for local tenderness of muscles of the back of the scalp, neck and shoulder, also for tenderness of the shoulder joint itself.

Neurological

Careful neurological examination is essential to elicit the signs of nerve root lesions (Table 14), the most common roots to be affected being C5–7. Look also for the following:

• An inverted brachioradialis jerk, which occurs when finger flexion is the only response to an attempt to elicit the normal biceps or supinator jerk. This may indicate a spinal cord lesion at C5–6, resulting in lower motor neurone signs at the level of the lesion (i.e. loss of C5–6 reflexes) and upper motor neurone signs below the lesion (i.e. brisk C7 (triceps) and C8 (finger flexion) reflexes; pyramidal signs in the legs).

• If there is dissociated sensory loss (loss of pain and temperature with intact proprioception) in a cape-like distribution (i.e. suspended sensory level, see Fig. 7) and lower motor neurone weakness, it is likely that there is an intrinsic cord lesion such as a syrinx, when other signs may include Horner's syndrome (if the lesion extends to the T1 segment) and pyramidal weakness below the level of the lesion.

Table 14 Signs in affected cervical nerve roots.

Nerve root	Weakness	Hyporeflexia	Sensory changes
C5	Deltoid, infraspinatus,	Biceps, brachioradialis	Shoulder tip, outer supraspinatus, part of upper arm
C6	Biceps, brachioradialis	Biceps, brachioradialis	Lateral aspect of wrist flexors, forearm and thumb
C7	Triceps, wrist extensors	Triceps	Middle finger
C8	Intrinsic muscles of hand	Triceps, finger	Little and ring fingers
T1	Intrinsic muscles of hand	None	Medial aspect of forearm

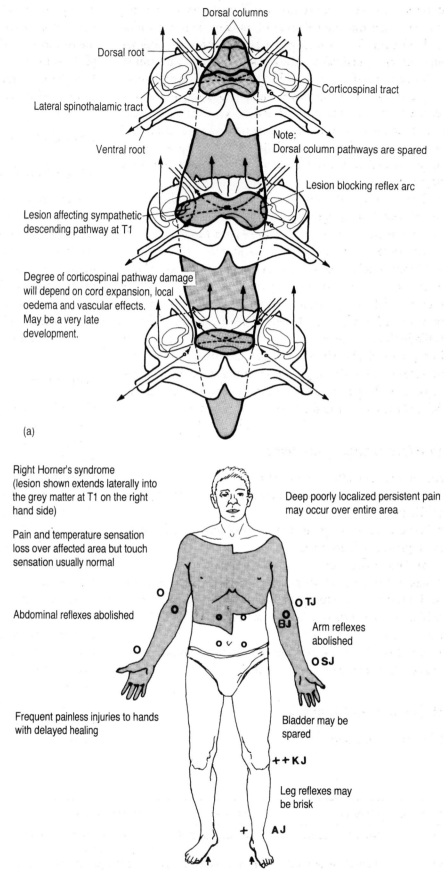

(a)

Dorsal columns

Dorsal root

Lateral spinothalamic tract

Corticospinal tract

Ventral root

Note:
Dorsal column pathways are spared

Lesion blocking reflex arc

Lesion affecting sympathetic descending pathway at T1

Degree of corticospinal pathway damage will depend on cord expansion, local oedema and vascular effects. May be a very late development.

Right Horner's syndrome (lesion shown extends laterally into the grey matter at T1 on the right hand side)

Deep poorly localized persistent pain may occur over entire area

Pain and temperature sensation loss over affected area but touch sensation usually normal

Abdominal reflexes abolished

O TJ

BJ

Arm reflexes abolished

O SJ

Frequent painless injuries to hands with delayed healing

Bladder may be spared

++ KJ

Leg reflexes may be brisk

+ AJ

Plantar responses may be extensor

(b)

Fig. 7 Lesion in central cord at C5–T6 level. (a) Anatomical diagram. Note: decussating spinothalamic pathways are blocked across the length of the central lesion. This may be slightly asymmetrical as shown, extending from C3 to T9 on the right and C4 and T8 on the left. Spinothalamic sensation below this level would be unaffected. (b) The clinical picture.

General

General examination is not likely to reveal anything untoward in this young woman, but note the following:
• Is the patient cachectic or clubbed? Is there lymphadenopathy? Any of these features would suggest malignancy.
• Check carefully for breast masses, also for any abnormal chest signs, particularly at the lung apex where a Pancoast tumour might be found (indicated by wasting of the intrinsic hand muscles and Horner's syndrome).
• Are both radial pulses equally palpable, and is the blood pressure the same in both arms? A positive Adson's test (decrease in the radial pulse when the patient turns her head to the affected side and breathes in deeply) may indicate subclavian artery compression, e.g. by a cervical rib, but the test may also be positive in normal subjects.

Approach to investigations and management

Investigations

These will be determined by the findings of the history and examination, but when no clear-cut diagnosis can be made, the following should be noted.
• Imaging of the cervical spine is essential. Cervical spine radiographs may reveal evidence of spondylosis (osteophytes, narrow disc spaces, encroachment on intervertebral foramina) or cervical ribs. MRI may reveal disc prolapse or syringomyelia.
• A chest radiograph is mandatory to exclude a Pancoast tumour (Fig. 8).
• Electromyography and nerve conduction studies can help differentiate a brachial plexus neuropathy from a root lesion due to disc prolapse or spondylosis.

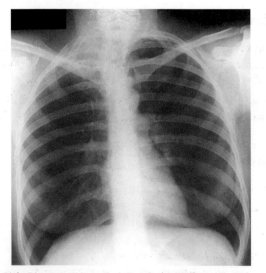

Fig. 8 Right Pancoast tumour. From Ray, Ryder, Wellings, *An Aid to Radiology for the MRCP.* Oxford: Blackwell Science 1999.

Management

Musculoskeletal pain may be helped by simple measures such as non-steroidal anti-inflammatory agents and physical methods, e.g. wearing a cervical collar may help spondylosis; infrared radiation or ice may help the painful shoulder, as can local injections of corticosteroid.

Most patients with brachial plexus neuropathy will improve spontaneously, but recovery may be incomplete in 10% of cases. Surgical intervention may be needed in cervical spondylosis, disc prolapse, cervical rib or syringomyelia, especially if the disability and signs caused are progressive.

> See *Medicine for the elderly*, Section 1.5.
> See *Rheumatology and clinical immunology*, Sections 1.17 and 1.24.
> Braakman R. Management of cervical spondylotic myelopathy and radiculopathy. *J Neurol Neurosurg Psychiatry* 1994; 57: 257–263.

1.13 Impotence and urinary difficulties

Case history

A 20-year-old man is referred with a 2-week history of sexual impotence and urinary frequency and incontinence.

Clinical approach

There are many causes of impotence (Table 15) [1], but when seen in combination with urinary symptoms you

Table 15 Causes of impotence.

Cause	Example
Neurological	Spinal cord compression (e.g. tumour)
	Conus medullaris damage
	Cauda equina damage
	Autonomic neuropathy (e.g. diabetes)
	Multiple sclerosis
	Postsurgery (e.g. interruption of pelvic nerve pathways)
Vascular	Severe atheromatous disease
Endocrine	Hyperprolactinaemia
Drugs	β-blockers
Anatomical	Deformity of the penis
Psychogenic	Depression
	Premature ejaculation
	Marital problems
	Sexual disinclination

must assume that there is a neurological cause and in particular consider lesions in the spinal cord, cauda equina or conus, and autonomic neuropathy. It is possible that the problem is psychogenic, but this should be regarded as a diagnosis of exclusion.

Before proceeding to further discussion it is appropriate to review the relevant anatomy and physiology of sexual and bladder function, as shown in Fig. 9 (overleaf).

Sexual function

In psychogenic erection (in response to thoughts) impulses from the hypothalamic centres pass down the spinal cord to the sacral centre for erection. Reflex erection (in response to tactile stimulation) is achieved by central (spinal) stimulation through segmental afferents from the genital region. Lesions of the spinal cord above the spinal centre for erection or ejaculation cause a disorder of the psychogenic phase of erection but preservation of reflex erection. Total destruction of the sacral centre for erection leads to complete impotence.

Parasympathetic efferent impulses from the sacral centre for erection pass through the roots of S2 to S4 and influence blood flow to the corpora cavernosa. Ejaculation is achieved through sympathetic activity from T11 to L2, which causes secretion of prostatic and seminal fluid and peristaltic movement, and somatic efferents that cause contractions of the striated muscles of the pelvic floor during orgasm.

Bladder function

The autonomic reflexes of micturition are mediated by the spinal cord but modulated by descending pathways from the brain (Fig. 9). Neurological disorders cause two types of bladder dysfunction—an upper motor neurone spastic bladder and a lower motor neurone flaccid bladder. Upper motor neurone lesions (e.g. stroke) interrupt the central impulses to the micturition centre at the S2, S3 and S4 levels of the spinal cord. Neuropathies or lower motor neurone lesions affect the micturition centre or the afferent and efferent parts of its reflex arc, e.g. polyneuropathy in diabetes or polyradiculitis in Guillain–Barré syndrome cause overflow incontinence. Spinal cord pathology is the most common cause of neurogenic bladder dysfunction.

History of the presenting problem

First, establish the nature of the symptoms.
• Is there failure of psychogenic erections, reflex erections or both?
• Are the urinary problems those of frequency and urgency with a small, contracted bladder (spastic bladder), or

continual dribbling incontinence with a large atonic bladder (flaccid bladder)? In practice it can be difficult to tell the difference between the two on the basis of the history, and the voluntary bladder control mechanisms may further complicate the picture.

Answers to these questions will help to determine the site of the neurological lesion: further questions should be directed to this end.

Is this a spinal cord lesion?

See Section 1.11, p. 23; note that reflex erections will be unaffected and a spastic bladder is anticipated.

Is this a cauda equina lesion?

A central lesion may present with complete impotence (psychogenic and reflex) and an atonic bladder. Leg pain and saddle anaesthesia may be seen, and bowel dysfunction may be an early feature. Weakness of the legs is often a late sign as there will be no motor deficit until S1 is involved, when the ankle reflex is lost.

Is this a conus lesion?

An intrinsic lesion of the terminal cord may produce an identical clinical picture to a cauda equina lesion except that there may also be upper motor neurone features (Fig. 10).

Is there an autonomic neuropathy?

Ask about other autonomic features, such as postural hypotension, but in practice impotence and sphincter disturbance are the earliest symptoms [2]. The commonest cause of an autonomic neuropathy is diabetes mellitus, so ask about features of this.

Relevant past history

Ask about diabetes, multiple sclerosis, vascular risk factors, trauma and previous abdominal surgery. Also enquire about any previous episodes of impotence and urinary difficulty; a psychogenic cause is likely if the patient has had similar symptoms before and recovered from them.

Examination

Is the bladder palpable?

Neurological

The most important aspects are as follows:
• Legs—the presence of upper motor neurone signs suggests a spinal cord lesion; patchy lower motor neurone

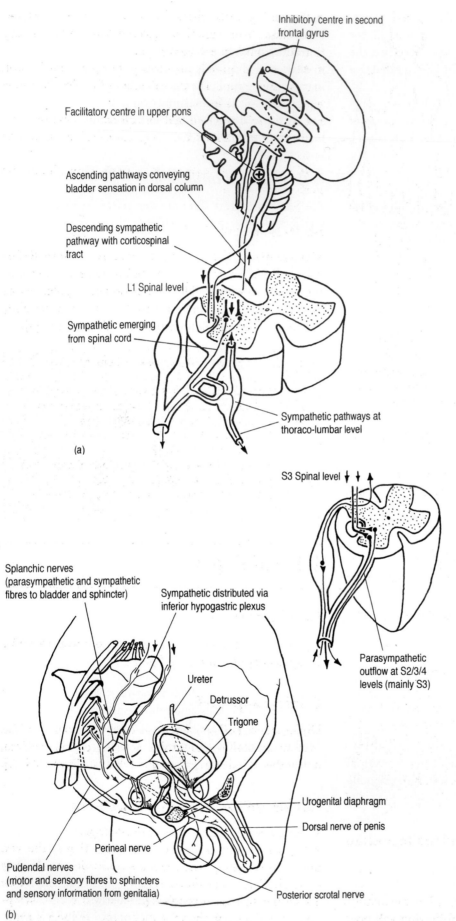

Inhibitory centre in second frontal gyrus

Facilitatory centre in upper pons

Ascending pathways conveying bladder sensation in dorsal column

Descending sympathetic pathway with corticospinal tract

L1 Spinal level

Sympathetic emerging from spinal cord

Sympathetic pathways at thoraco-lumbar level

(a)

S3 Spinal level

Splanchic nerves (parasympathetic and sympathetic fibres to bladder and sphincter)

Sympathetic distributed via inferior hypogastric plexus

Parasympathetic outflow at S2/3/4 levels (mainly S3)

Ureter

Detrussor

Trigone

Urogenital diaphragm

Dorsal nerve of penis

Perineal nerve

Pudendal nerves (motor and sensory fibres to sphincters and sensory information from genitalia)

Posterior scrotal nerve

(b)

Fig. 9 Micturition pathways. (a) Nerve supply between spinal cord and brain. (b) Nerve supply outside the spinal cord.

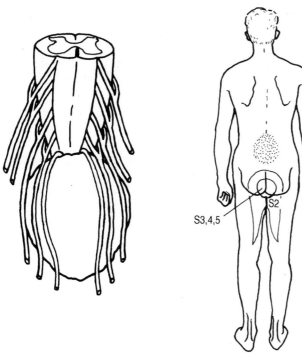

Fig. 10 Conus lesion of the spinal cord. A lesion will affect sacral roots from inside outwards, hence the peri-anal and perineal areas are involved first, with progressive numbness and often surprisingly little pain.

signs indicate a cauda equina lesion; and the presence of both points to the conus.
• Sensory abnormalities—is there a sensory level to indicate a cord lesion? Is perineal sensation intact? If not, then a cauda equina or conus lesion is possible.

In addition, look for:
• signs of autonomic dysfunction
• bitemporal hemianopia, which would probably indicate a pituitary tumour as a cause of hyperprolactinaemia in this context
• evidence of multiple sclerosis, i.e. optic atrophy, cerebellar signs, internuclear ophthalmoplegia.

> ⚡ **Examination of the patient with impotence or urinary frequency/incontinence**
>
> Never forget to examine for saddle anaesthesia (S3–5), as this may be the only feature pointing to a cauda equina lesion. Lesions in this area are often malignant, including metastatic disease (especially prostatic), primary sacral bone tumours (chordomas) and direct seeding of some CNS tumours. The usual causes of conus lesions are an ependymoma, dermoid or lipoma.

Approach to investigations and management

Investigation

The plan of investigation should be guided by the findings on history and examination, but the following will need to be considered [3].

• 'Screening' tests: check full blood count, electrolytes, renal and liver function, glucose and inflammatory markers. Check chest radiograph.
• MRI of the spine is mandatory if a spinal cord lesion is suspected, and is the investigation of choice for cauda equina and conus lesions.
• CSF should be examined for cell count, glucose, protein, oligoclonal bands and malignant cells if no structural lesion is seen on MRI.
• If metastasis is suspected, a bone scan should be performed.

Managememt

Management will depend on the underlying cause. Referral to specialists may be required if there are continuing problems with bladder dysfunction or impotence (see Section 2.5, p. 77) [4]. Sildenafil (Viagra) is certainly worth considering in chronic cases of all aetiology [5].

1 Morgentaler A. Male impotence. *Lancet* 1999; 354: 1713–1718.
2 McDougall AJ, McLeod JG. Autonomic neuropathy, I. Clinical features, investigation, pathophysiology, and treatment. *J Neurol Sci* 1996; 137(2): 79–88.
3 Jeffcoate WJ. The investigation of impotence. *Br J Urol* 1991; 68(5): 449–453.
4 Fowler CJ. Neurological disorders of micturition and their treatment. *Brain* 1999; 122: 1213–1231.
5 Sildenafil for erectile dysfunction. *Drug Ther Bull* 1998; 36(11): 81–84.

1.14 Diplopia

Case history

A general practitioner refers a 19-year-old woman with a 3-day history of worsening diplopia.

Clinical approach

Diplopia is caused by misalignment of the visual axes. You need to establish whether this is an isolated local problem, or whether it is due to neurological disease (Table 16) [1,2].

History of the presenting problem

What are the characteristics of the diplopia?
• Does covering either eye relieve it? If not, the two images are coming from the same eye, which is relatively unusual. This can be due to refractive error, in which case asking her to look through a pinhole will relieve symptoms. If it does not, then the monocular diplopia is probably psychogenic.

Table 16 Causes of diplopia.

Binocular	Physiological	At extremes of vision
	Pathological	Neuromuscular
		Any cause of third, fourth or sixth nerve palsy, e.g. multiple sclerosis
		Myasthenia gravis
		Brain-stem ischaemic event (not isolated diplopia)
		Miller–Fisher variant of Guillain–Barré syndrome
		Cavernous sinus thrombosis
		Chronic progressive external ophthalmoplegia
		Mitochondrial diseases, e.g. Kearns–Sayre syndrome
		Local anatomical
		Orbital infiltration, e.g. metastases
		Dysthyroid eye disease
Monocular	Psychogenic	—
	Pathological	Astigmatism
		Cataract
		Foreign body in aqueous or vitreous media
		Poor optical equipment, e.g. defective lenses

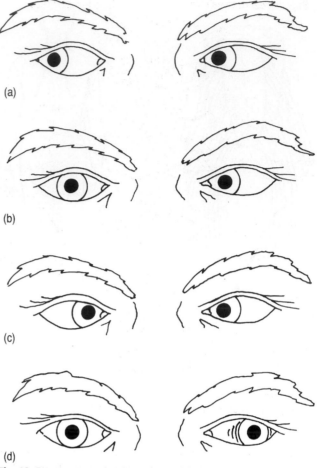

(a)

(b)

(c)

(d)

Fig. 12 Eye movements in internuclear ophthalmoplegia and sixth nerve palsy. (a) Normal. on right gaze, both eyes move normally and single vision is retained with no nystagmus. (b) Sixth nerve palsy. A lesion at position B on Fig. 13 produces a left sixth nerve palsy. At rest, the left eye will be slightly medially deviated giving a disconcerting diplopia best prevented by closing the eye or tilting the head round to the left, to line up the ocular axis with the normal right eye. (c) On attempted left lateral gaze, the right eye achieves full adduction and the left eye remains static, producing widely separated images. (d) Internuclear ophthalmoplegia. A lesion at position 'A' on Fig. 13 will prevent the activation of the right medial rectus muscle on attempted left lateral gaze. On attempted lateral gaze the left eye abducts nearly completely but shows nystagmus. The right eye makes little or no movement medially but due to minimal displacement no nystagmus occurs.

Fig. 11 The eyeball and eye movements. The left eyeball is shown from above, the optic nerve is shown cut off so that the inferior rectus muscle can be seen. Note that due to the angulation of the orbit, the superior and inferior rectus muscles have their main elevating and depressing effect when the eyeball is looking laterally, whereas the oblique muscles (superior and inferior oblique) which, respectively, depress and elevate the eyeball, are maximally effective when the eye is looking medially. The medial and lateral recti are not as complicated as they pull the eyeball inwards and outwards.

• Are the images separated horizontally or vertically? In which direction is the diplopia worse? This occurs on looking in the direction in which the weak muscle has its purest action (Fig. 11). Horizontal separation is likely to indicate sixth nerve palsy (Figs 12 and 13). The common cause of isolated vertical diplopia is superior oblique palsy, in which the patient may describe difficulty looking down, often notable when reading or walking down stairs.

• Is the diplopia worse at any particular time of the day? Worsening in the evenings suggests myasthenia gravis.

Associated symptoms

Find out about the following:

• Any other neurological symptoms that might indicate multiple sclerosis; ask specifically regarding pain in the eye, visual loss, focal weakness or paraesthesiae in a limb, unsteadiness or disturbance of bladder function.

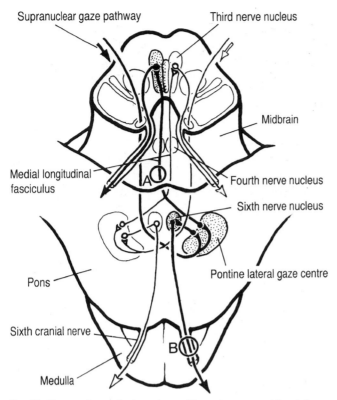

Fig. 13 Nerve pathways for lateral gaze. The pathways to achieve left lateral gaze are shown in thicker lines and stippled areas.

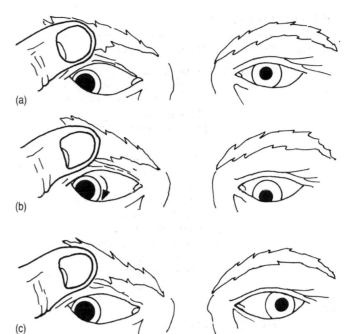

Fig. 14 Right third nerve palsy. (a) At rest when the eyelid is lifted by the examiner, the eye is looking down and out and the pupil is fixed and dilated. (b) On attempted down-gaze the affected eye ball will be seen to rotate inwards, best demonstrated by watching a conjunctival vessel during the attempt. (c) Attempted gaze to the left. The right eye remains in position while the left lateral achieves full abduction.

• Any other weakness: dysphagia, slurred speech, shortness of breath or limb weakness could indicate myasthenia gravis in this context.
• Any history of head trauma that may have caused a third, fourth or sixth nerve palsy.
• Any symptoms to suggest thyrotoxicosis, such as intolerance to heat, weight loss or agitation.
• If the diplopia is intermittent, is there a preceding headache, which might suggest ophthalmoplegic migraine (see Section 2.6.1, p. 79)?

> **Cavernous sinus syndrome**
>
> This may result in ophthalmoplegia, pain, proptosis, Horner's syndrome (resulting in a mid-sized pupil caused by the combination with a third nerve palsy, i.e. both sympathetic and parasympathetic paresis) and prominent scleral vessels. Intracavernous carotid artery aneurysm, mass lesions or thrombophlebitis may be causes. The latter may sometimes be due to mucormycosis in the case of immunocompromised or diabetic patients.

Relevant past history

Note the following:
• any history of autoimmune diseases, increasing the risk of myasthenia gravis
• drug history: certain drugs, e.g. D-penicillamine worsen myasthenia gravis
• any previous eye surgery

• any previous arterial or venous thrombotic events or risk factors for these.

Examination

On inspection, look for:
• proptosis—suggesting an orbital lesion or thyroid eye disease
• head tilt—the head tilts in the direction of action of the weak muscle
• signs of thyroid disease (see *Endocrinology*, Section 2.3)
• ptosis and a dilated pupil—indicating third nerve palsy (Fig. 14).

Neurological

The most important aspect is to check eye movements and at the point of maximum separation of an image, cover one eye.
• Loss of the lateral image indicates that the covered eye is the abnormal one; careful consideration of Figs 11, 12, 13 and 14 should then allow you to decide which muscle or nerve is causing the problem.
• Always deliberately consider the question 'is there internuclear ophthalmoplegia' (nystagmus in abducting eye and failure of adduction of the affected side), suggesting multiple sclerosis (Fig. 13)?
 A complete neurological examination is required to look

	Type of disorder	Example
Unilateral	Neuromuscular	Third nerve palsy
		Horner's syndrome
		Levator palpebrae muscle paralysis
	Local anatomical	Levator aponeurosis dehiscence/disinsertion
		Inflammation (e.g. chalazion) or infiltration (e.g. amyloidosis) of eyelids or conjunctiva
		Lost contact lens
	Congenital	—
Bilateral	Neuromuscular	Myasthenia gravis
		Myotonic dystrophy
		Chronic progressive external ophthalmoplegia
		Ocular dystrophy
		Oculopharyngeal dystrophy
		Guillain–Barré syndrome
	Congenital	—

Table 17 Causes of ptosis.

for clues to differentiate the possible causes of diplopia given in Table 16, e.g. reduced visual acuity, optic atrophy or cerebellar signs in multiple sclerosis; fatigability in myasthenia gravis.

Approach to investigations and management

Investigation

This depends on the likely cause. Local retro-orbital causes will need high-resolution imaging, e.g. coronal CT or MRI. If multiple sclerosis or myasthenia gravis is suspected, these will need to be investigated as appropriate (see Sections 2.5, p. 77 and 2.2.5, p. 70).

Management

Specific treatments will obviously depend on the cause. For multiple sclerosis or myasthenia gravis, see Sections 2.2.5 and 2.5. As regards symptomatic treatment, wearing a patch on alternate eyes may help diplopia, and prisms may be useful if the deviation is not too great. Botulinum toxin is occasionally used for strabismus. Extraocular eye surgery may be needed in some cases.

1 Brazis PW, Lee AG. Acquired binocular horizontal diplopia. *Mayo Clin Proc* 1999; 74(9): 907–916.
2 Brazis PW, Lee AG. Binocular vertical diplopia. *Mayo Clin Proc* 1998; 73(1): 55–66.

1.15 Ptosis

Case history

A 60-year-old woman is referred with an asymptomatic unilateral right-sided ptosis.

Clinical approach

Ptosis is abnormal lowering of the upper eyelid and is due to a problem with the levator palpebrae superioris muscle or its nerve supply (third cranial nerve), or involvement of the sympathetic supply of the smooth muscle fibres of the superior tarsal muscle (Table 17). In assessing this patient, remember that many of the causes of ptosis would not be asymptomatic; those that might present without symptoms include congenital ptosis, disinsertion of levator, myasthenia gravis or a Horner's syndrome.

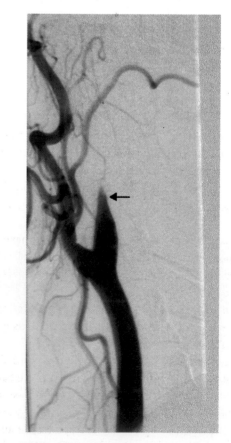

Fig. 15 Carotid artery dissection.

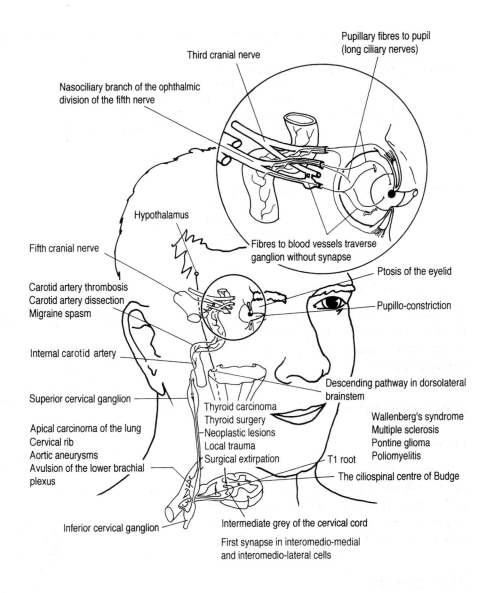

Third cranial nerve

Pupillary fibres to pupil
(long ciliary nerves)

Nasociliary branch of the ophthalmic
division of the fifth nerve

Hypothalamus

Fifth cranial nerve

Fibres to blood vessels traverse
ganglion without synapse

Ptosis of the eyelid

Carotid artery thrombosis
Carotid artery dissection
Migraine spasm

Pupillo-constriction

Internal carotid artery

Superior cervical ganglion

Descending pathway in dorsolateral
brainstem

Thyroid carcinoma
Thyroid surgery
Neoplastic lesions
Local trauma
Surgical extirpation

Wallenberg's syndrome
Multiple sclerosis
Pontine glioma
Poliomyelitis

Apical carcinoma of the lung
Cervical rib
Aortic aneurysms
Avulsion of the lower brachial
plexus

T1 root

The ciliospinal centre of Budge

Inferior cervical ganglion

Intermediate grey of the cervical cord

First synapse in interomedio-medial
and interomedio-lateral cells

Fig. 16 Horner's syndrome.

History of the presenting problem

Think about the conditions listed in Table 17 as you take the history, and ask about the following if the details do not emerge spontaneously.
• How long has the patient noticed the ptosis? Is it congenital or acquired? Does she have any old photos of herself?
• Is there any history of trauma that may have caused levator aponeurosis dehiscence or disinsertion?
• Is there any fluctuation of the severity of ptosis, which should lead you to suspect myasthenia gravis?
• Is there any associated swallowing difficulty or other muscle weakness, again pointing to myasthenia gravis in this context, or to oculopharyngeal dystrophy?
• Is there any recent history of trauma or forced extension of the neck, e.g. at the hairdressers? If there have been any other neurological symptoms such as limb weakness or speech difficulty, even if these were transient, then carotid artery dissection causing a Horner's syndrome and cerebral ischaemia should be considered (Figs 15 and 16).

• Is there a family history of neurological or visual problems?
And do not forget the banal:
• Does she wear contact lenses? A lost contact lens in the upper conjunctiva may cause ptosis.
Also:
• Are there any features to suggest a malignancy, in particular of the chest?

Examination

The eyes

The upper eyelid normally covers 1–2 mm of the cornea, and the lower lid just reaches the level of the cornea. Are the pupils normal? Are ocular movements normal (see Section 1.14, p. 31)? Look for the following patterns:
• meiosis, anhidrosis and enophthalmos with partial ptosis in Horner's syndrome (see Section 1.16, p. 36)
• complete ptosis and abnormal eye position and movement in third nerve palsy, with normal or dilated pupil

• fatigability of the ptosis on looking up persistently, which would suggest myasthenia gravis.

Other

Are there features to support any of the conditions listed in Table 17?
• Neurological—a full examination may be required depending on the context. Key features are likely to be: Is visual acuity normal? Are the fundi normal? Do the muscles look normal, is there any generalized weakness and are they easily fatigued?
• General—are there any chest signs or indications of malignancy?

> **Levator disinsertion**
>
> Disinsertion of the aponeurosis of levator palpebrae superioris from the tarsal plate is a common cause of unilateral ptosis in the elderly population, and is associated with trauma. The important clinical sign is that the crease that is normally found on the upper eyelid is lost. There are no disorders of pupil or external ocular movements. It is important to realize that these patients may complain of increasing ptosis at the end of the day, and may even report subjective (without objective) improvement after a Tensilon test, so differentiation from myasthenia gravis should be on different grounds (other neurological signs, anti-acetylcholine receptor antibodies). Surgical reinsertion can be offered for symptomatic cases [1,2].

> **!** Think of Pancoast tumour in any patient with Horner's syndrome. Look for associated wasting of the intrinsic hand muscles, consistent with a T1 root lesion.

Approach to investigations and management

Myasthenia gravis: see Section 2.2.5, p. 70.
Horner's syndrome: see Section 1.16.

>
> 1 Deady JP, Morrell AJ, Sutton GA. Recognizing aponeurotic ptosis. *J Neurol Neurosurg Psychiatry* 1989; 52(8): 996–998.
> 2 Older JJ. Levator aponeurosis disinsertion in the young adult. A cause of ptosis. *Arch Ophthalmol* 1978; 96(10):1857–1858.

1.16 Unequal pupils

Case history

You are asked to assess a 70-year-old woman with asymptomatic unequal pupils.

Table 18 Common causes of miosis and mydriasis.

Abnormality	Unilateral	Bilateral
Miosis	Horner's syndrome Iritis Pilocarpine	Argyll Robertson pupils Pontine bleed
Mydriasis	Holmes–Adie syndrome Oculomotor nerve palsy Midbrain lesion Atropine Unilateral afferent pupillary defect	Bilateral afferent pupillary defect e.g. bilateral optic atrophy

Clinical approach

The causes of unequal pupils (anisocoria) are listed in Table 18 [1]. Clinically, there is a clear distinction to be made between patients who are noticed to have anisocoria but are asymptomatic, and those in whom the unequal pupils are part of a well-defined symptomatic disorder, e.g. brainstem stroke. This patient falls into the former category. In a normal pupil, miosis is caused by stimulation of the parasympathetic efferent fibres in the oculomotor nerve, whereas mydriasis is caused by activation of the sympathetic fibres from the superior cervical ganglion [2].

> Simple or physiological anisocoria (less than 0.6 mm) is seen in about 20% of the normal population.

History of the presenting problem

This patient is declared to be asymptomatic, but make brief enquiry about any general medical problems and follow any leads that this produces. Note new chest symptoms, particularly if she is a smoker (Pancoast tumour), also vascular risk factors and take a drug history—which must include the use of eye drops!

Regarding ocular/visual symptoms, check the following, the answers to which may be 'no':
• is there any pain or redness, which might indicate iritis or acute angle closure glaucoma?
• does she have any diplopia, suggesting oculomotor palsy in this context?
• does she suffer from headache? Both migraine and cluster headache can cause episodic Horner's syndrome, which may become permanent [3]
• does she suffer from photophobia when moving from dark to light, caused by a fixed dilated pupil failing to protect the retina in bright light?
• is there a history of poor night vision in a patient with small, poorly reactive pupils?

Examination

In this clinical setting the examination may come before the history, i.e. the nature of the abnormality will be established before questioning to determine possible causes.

Which is the abnormal pupil? If the pupils respond to direct light, proceed to inspect them in bright and dim light.

• If anisocoria is greater in bright light than dim, then the iris sphincter on the side of the lesion does not work well, indicating that there is a local iris problem or a parasympathetic defect such as oculomotor palsy, i.e. the problem is on the side of the large pupil.

• If anisocoria is greater in the dim light than bright, the iris dilator muscle on the side of the smaller pupil does not work properly, indicating simple anisocoria or Horner's syndrome, i.e. the problem is on the side of the small pupil.

Having decided which is the abnormal pupil, then look for those of the following specific features that are relevant.

• Ptosis.
• Irregularity of pupil.
• Inflammation of the iris.
• Light-near dissociation, where the pupil does not react to light but does to accommodation. This is tested by asking the patient to look at something in the distance and then to focus on your finger held reasonably close to their nose (Table 19).
• An afferent pupillary defect, when the pupil will not react to light because of optic atrophy or severely diminished visual acuity from another cause. The swinging light test is used: on shining a light into the normal pupil, the normal pupil will constrict and so will the affected pupil through the consensual response to light. On quickly moving the light to shine on the affected pupil, the affected pupil will dilate because it has an impaired direct response to light.
• Ophthalmoparesis.
• Optic atrophy.

When examining this asymptomatic woman, consider the conditions listed in Table 18, but particularly the following that can present asymptomatically.

Table 19 Causes of light-near dissociation.

Small pupils	Argyll Robertson pupils
	Long-standing Holmes–Adie pupils
	Diabetic neuropathy
Large pupils	Bilateral afferent pupillary defects
	Holmes–Adie pupils/tonic pupils
	Pretectal lesions

Horner's syndrome

Consists of miosis, ipsilateral partial ptosis and sometimes anhidrosis. Enophthalmos is not a useful sign. If anhidrosis affects the entire half of the body and face, the lesion is in the CNS; if it affects only the face and neck, the lesion is in the preganglionic fibres; if sweating is unaffected, the lesion is above the carotid artery bifurcation (Fig. 16).

Argyll Robertson pupils

Almost always bilateral and consists of small, irregular pupils that show light-near dissociation (poorly reactive to light, better constriction to accommodation).

Holmes–Adie syndrome

There is usually unilateral pupillary dilatation with poor constriction to light and accommodation, occurring in association with depressed deep tendon reflexes. Commonly affects young women. The pupil may become small over time.

Approach to investigations and management

This depends on the findings on history and examination. Remember the following:

• Any patient with bilateral tonic pupils, poorly reactive or irregular pupils, or pupils with light-near dissociation should have VDRL checked.
• Chest radiograph in cases of Horner's syndrome (especially if preganglionic).
• Imaging of the carotid artery in postganglionic Horner's syndrome.
• Imaging of the head is only required if other neurological features are present.

See *Ophthalmology*, Section 3.1.
1 Selhorst JB. The pupil and its disorders. *Neurol Clin* 1983; 4: 859–881.
2 Wilhelm H. Neuro-ophthalmology of pupillary function—practical guidelines. *J Neurol* 1998; 245(9): 573–583.
3 Tomsak RL. Ophthalmologic aspects of headache. *Med Clin North Am* 1991; 75(3): 693–706.

1.17 Smell and taste disorders

Case history

A 75-year-old man is referred because he is unable to smell or taste his food normally.

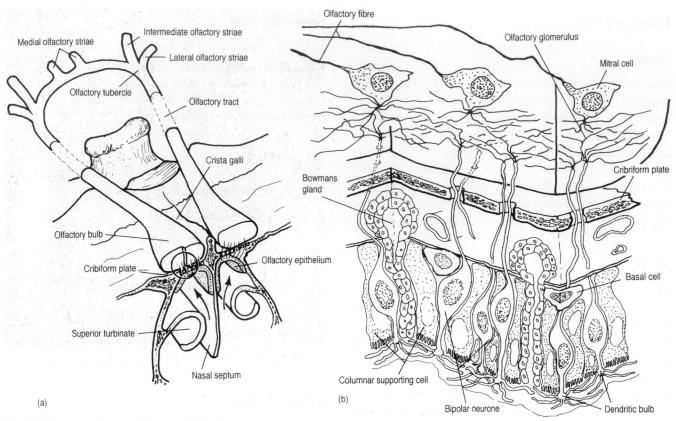

(a)

(b)

Fig. 17 Olfactory mechanisms. (a) Axons of the olfactory receptors within the mucous epithelium travel within olfactory nerves to convey smell to the olfactory bulb. (b) Within the olfactory bulb, the olfactory receptor axons terminate in glomeruli on the dendrites of the mitral cells, which in turn send axons via olfactory tracts to the olfactory projection area in the cortex.

Clinical approach

In someone with a smell disorder, always ask about taste disturbance, and vice versa.

In a patient with a smell disorder you need to establish if it is due to nasal blockage preventing substances reaching the nasal epithelium, or to a disorder affecting the olfactory pathway, i.e. olfactory nerves, bulb, tract or cortex (Fig. 17 and Table 20) [1]. You then need to decide if the patient has:

• anosmia or hyposmia, i.e. loss or decreased sense of smell

• hyperosmia, i.e. hypersensitivity to smell, which is rare but may be seen in depression

• parosmia, i.e. perversion of smell, often associated with anosmia or hyposmia, and seen in traumatic olfactory bulb injury, temporal lobe seizure or depression.

For a taste disorder, you need to establish if the patient has:

• ageusia or hypogeusia, i.e. loss or decreased sense of taste, the causes of which are listed in Table 21

• hypergeusia, i.e. hypersensitivity to taste, which is uncommon but may be seen in cerebellar lesions

• parageusia, i.e. perversion of taste, seen in poor dental hygiene, ageing and in psychiatric disorders

• gustatory hallucinations, seen in temporal-lobe lesions or seizures [2] (see Section 2.7) but may also be psychogenic in origin.

Table 20 Causes of anosmia or hyposmia.

Nasal blockage	Rhinitis
	Upper respiratory tract infection
	Sinusitis
	Polyps
	Tumours
	Syphilis
Olfactory pathway	Olfactory groove meningioma
	Frontal lobe tumour
	Basal meningitis
	Ageing
	Head trauma
	Parkinson's disease
	Alzheimer's disease
	Kallman's syndrome

Table 21 Causes of ageusia or hypogeusia.

Mouth	Glossitis
	Periodontitis
	Sjögren's syndrome
	Smoking
	Penicillamine
	Captopril
Neural pathways	Bell's palsy
	Corda tympani lesions (e.g. ear surgery)
	Lingual nerve lesions (e.g. postlaryngoscopy)
	Glossopharyngeal nerve lesions (e.g. trauma)

Examination

Smell

Test smell by asking the patient to sniff aromatic substances (e.g. oil of cloves, coffee, peppermint) through each nostril separately, while the other nostril is occluded. The patient should have their eyes closed and should be told that there may or may not be anything in the bottle. Appreciation of an odour, despite not being able to name it, excludes anosmia. If a patient denies being able to detect ammonia, it is likely that they are either hysterical or malingering, since ammonia stimulates the trigeminal nerve.

Taste

Test taste by withdrawing the tongue from the mouth and placing sugar, salt, vinegar and quinine on it for sweet, salt, sour and bitter sensations, respectively. All four quadrants should be tested, with the mouth rinsed in between tests. Tastes should be identified by asking the patient to point to one of various cards, rather than by talking. Taste sensation from the anterior two-thirds of the tongue is carried by the facial nerve and the posterior third by the glossopharyngeal nerve.

Other

A full neurological examination may be required, but particularly close attention should be paid to the lower cranial nerves.

Approach to investigations and management

These will clearly be dictated by any clues derived from history and examination. Imaging with CT or MRI is likely to be needed if the cause of the problem is not obvious (Fig. 18).

1 Schiffman SF. Taste and smell in disease. *N Engl J Med* 1983; 308: 1275–1279 and 1337–1343.
2 Hausser-Hauw C, Bancaud J. Gustatory seizures in epileptic seizures. *Brain* 1987; 110: 339–359.

1.18 Facial pain

Case history

A 60-year-old woman complains of 'chronic' pain in her face. She is not acutely unwell.

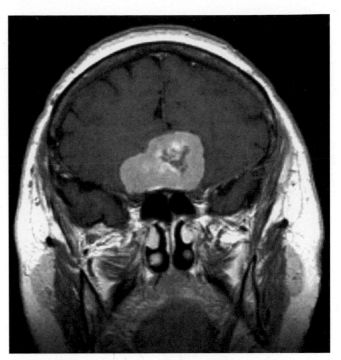

Fig. 18 Recurrent frontal glioma affecting the olfactory nerve.

Clinical approach

It will almost certainly be possible to make the diagnosis on the basis of history alone. Intermittent facial pain has a number of causes, and although the symptoms can be very distressing it is usually possible to help them as long as the correct diagnosis is made. Constant facial pain is less common, but trigeminal neuralgia and cluster headache can both leave the patient with a dull residual pain. Structural abnormalities of sinuses and nasopharynx must be excluded before the diagnosis of atypical facial pain is made, but this can occur in women of this age [1].

History of the presenting complaint

Characterize the pain

Ask the patient the following if the details are not volunteered:
- What is the pain like?
- Where do you feel the pain (Fig. 19)?
- Is it intermittent or constant?
- How long have you had it for?
- Are there any aggravating or relieving factors?

As you obtain the answers to these questions, consider the diagnoses shown below.

Trigeminal neuralgia

A unilateral, lancinating sharp pain, lasting for seconds, affecting the lower jaw and upper lip and set off by touch, chewing or talking (see Section 2.6.2, p. 81).

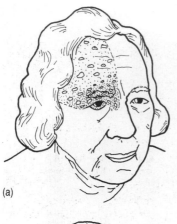
(a)

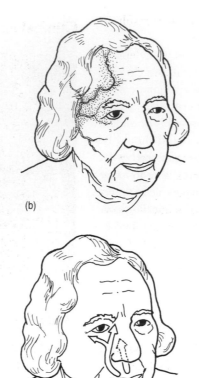
(b)

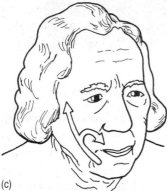
(c)

(d)

Fig. 19 Site of facial pain in different diagnoses. (a) Post-herpetic neuralgia. The whole area of the first division of the fifth nerve may have been involved but typically the most persistent and unpleasant pain is in the eye itself and the eyebrow. (b) Cranial arteritis. Although involvement of the superficial temporal artery has always been stressed, any artery in the head can be involved. There is a tendency for the pain to be worse nocturnally but present 24 hours a day and associated with systemic symptoms—weight loss and general ill-health. In most instances the ESR and CRP will be markedly elevated.(c) Trigeminal neuralgia. The commonest pattern is pain radiating from the lower jaw, particularly the canine tooth, up to a position deep in front of the ear. The less common variant (d) involves pain starting in the incisors or canines of the upper jaw, radiating up to and around the eye or, at its worst, up inside the nose.

Postherpetic neuralgia

The constant unilateral burning sensation (with occasional lancinating pains) comes on after 10% of herpes zoster ophthalmicus. Usually affects the upper face, especially the eyebrow.

Cluster headache

An episodic deep boring pain situated on or around one eye (see Section 2.6.3, p. 82).

Cranial arteritis

A diagnosis that should be considered in any patient over 60 with recent-onset headache. It may cause diffuse unilateral or bilateral headache, but the patient may concentrate on the symptom of temporal tenderness.

Costen's syndrome

Severe pain over the temperomandibular joint when eating.

Atypical facial pain

Described as a continuous unbearable pain, usually maxillary, and either unilateral or bilateral. This is a diagnosis of exclusion and is not to be made before other possibilities have been exhausted.

Are there any associated features?

Consider the following points.
• Have there been visual symptoms? These, together with jaw claudication, are important clues to the diagnosis of cranial arteritis, as would be the presence of constitutional symptoms (absent in this case).
• Has an eye gone red? Primary angle closure glaucoma often causes an intermittently painful red eye, but may cause non-specific headaches. In milder, less acute cases coloured haloes seen around lights may be the main diagnostic clue. (See *Ophthalmology*, Sections 1.1 and 1.2 for discussion of the patient presenting with a red eye.)
• Is pain around the eye associated with ophthalomoplegia? This would suggest ophthalmoplegic migraine (less likely to occur *de novo* at this age) or Tolosa–Hunt syndrome, which is caused by a granulomatous lesion of unknown cause in the cavernous sinus or superior orbital fissure.
• Has there been a rash or any spots? Postherpetic neuralgia will have been preceded by herpes zoster ophthalmicus.
• Cluster headache has a number of associated features (see Section 2.6.3).
• Has there been discharge or bleeding from the nose? These would suggest a sinus problem in this context.
• If facial pain is associated with signs or symptoms suggestive of cerebral ischaemia, look very closely for an ipsilateral Horner's syndrome, as there may have been a carotid artery dissection.

• Paget's disease affecting the skull base may result in symptoms similar to trigeminal neuralgia.
• Atypical facial pain is said to be associated with depressive symptoms, but this may be a feature of any chronic pain syndrome.

Examination

A full neurological assessment is very important, with particular reference to the cranial nerves as this may betray the presence of a mass lesion. Careful examination of the eyes, ears, nose and throat are also essential whenever the diagnosis is uncertain.

Approach to investigations and management

Investigations

These will be dictated by the likely diagnosis, but if a confident clinical diagnosis cannot be made the following tests or advice should be obtained:
• inflammatory markers (CRP and ESR)—if these are normal, then the diagnosis of cranial arteritis can be excluded with almost complete certainty
• CT scan of head
• ophthalmological opinion
• ENT opinion.

Management

This will clearly depend on the diagnosis.
• Trigeminal neuralgia—see Section 2.6.2.
• Postherpetic neuralgia—amitriptyline provides relief in 50%; topical capsaicin cream may help; consider TENS.
• Cranial arteritis—the response to steroids is characteristic. See *Medicine for the elderly*, Section 1.5; *Rheumatology and clinical immunology*, Section 2.5.1.
• Cluster headache—see Section 2.6.3.
• Atypical facial pain—may be limited response to amitriptyline.

 1 Solomon S, Lipton RB. Atypical facial pain: a review. *Semin Neurol* 1988; 8(4): 332–338.

1.19 Recurrent severe headache

Case history

A 29-year-old woman presents with recurrent severe headaches.

Clinical approach

> Severity of pain is not an indicator of whether a headache is life threatening or not.
> Your approach will be in two stages:
> • are these headaches benign?
> • if so, then what is their cause?
> In this patient the worry is that her headaches are related to raised intracranial pressure—secondary to a space-occupying lesion, hydrocephalus or to idiopathic intracranial hypertension—or that they are caused by a systemic condition. It is far more likely, however, that these headaches are benign and that the cause is migraine, tension-type headache (perhaps being exacerbated by analgesic overuse or depression) or even cluster headache. It is important to make the correct diagnosis of benign headache as different conditions have their own management strategy.

History of the presenting problem

The diagnosis, as with facial pain (see Section 1.18, p. 39), can virtually always be made on the history alone. It is certainly worth taking time over this: the commonest cause of an incorrect diagnosis is an incorrect history [1]. The following are a list of points that it is useful to establish:
• How long have you had these headaches? Long-standing (over 1 year) headaches are almost always benign, so establish when headaches truly began, not just when they got worse.
• How often do they occur and for how long? Determine whether the patient is describing episodic discrete headaches or exacerbations with a constant background which may also be described as recurrent, so ask specifically about the period in between headaches (Fig. 20).
• Where do you get the pain? Bilateral, strictly unilateral, alternating unilateral, frontal, temporal or occipital? The use of a finger or hand to indicate position will give some clue as to the quality of the pain (Fig. 21).
• What is the pain like? Throbbing (migraine), a deep, boring, intense unilateral pain (cluster headache), or band-like tightness/pressure around the head (tension-type headache)? The pain of a raised intracranial pressure headache is non-specific.
• What do you do with yourself during an attack? Most patients with severe headache prefer to remain still, but agitation during an attack is characteristic of cluster headache.
• Are there any precipitating or aggravating factors? Light, noise, movement and stress aggravate most headaches and so are not helpful in differentiating one type of headache from another. Exacerbation by coughing, sneezing or straining is also relatively non-specific. Alcohol can precipitate migraine and cluster headache (during a bout) but may alleviate tension-type headaches.
• Are there any associated features? 'Classical migraine' may be associated with visual phenomena such as seeing

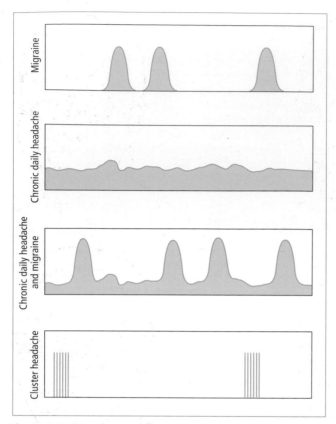

Fig. 20 Periodicity of pain in different headache syndromes.

dazzling zigzag lines (fortification spectra) and most patients feel intensely nauseated. Additional features such as weakness, parasthesiae, aphasia, diplopia and visual loss are often worrying but can all happen as part of migraine aura. Establish how closely these symptoms are associated with the headache. Any residual deficit should be taken seriously and investigated further. This young woman could not have cranial arteritis, but the diagnosis should be considered in anyone over the age of 60 years with severe headache: visual symptoms, jaw claudication, proximal muscle pain and constitutional symptoms would all support this diagnosis (see *Medicine for the elderly*, Section 1.5; *Rheumatology and clinical immunology*, Section 2.5.1).
• What medication are you on now? Either it is not working and needs to be changed, or it is contributing significantly to the headache and so should be stopped.

> **Warning symptoms or signs in the patient with a headache**
>
> • Headaches of subacute onset with steady progression over days or weeks.
> • A recent change in pattern or character of established headache.
> • Association with fever or other systemic features.
> • Association with focal neurological signs, papilloedema, personality change or seizures could all indicate a space-occupying lesion as the underlying cause.

> **Consider idiopathic intracranial hypertension** [2]
>
> Occurs characteristically in overweight young women who present with gradual-onset headache associated with features of raised intracranial pressure. They may also complain of visual obscurations (transient bilateral visual loss occurring with changes in posture) and occasionally tinnitus. The headache itself has no specific features.

Relevant past history

Ask about the following:
• A previous history of depression, anxiety or neck trauma will be relevant if considering tension-type headache.
• Current or previous use of tetracyclines or vitamin A derivatives may be associated with idiopathic intracranial hypertension.
• Previous head injury, subarachnoid haemorrhage or meningitis may predispose to communicating hydrocephalus.

Examination

Patients with benign headaches rarely have any abnormalities on examination. One is therefore looking to exclude serious conditions that may be associated with headache, and a full general examination should be performed.
• Is there evidence of raised intracranial pressure, such as papilloedema, or sixth nerve palsies?
• Are there any signs that may point to a focal intracerebral lesion?
• Is the patient overweight, as this is a strong association of idiopathic intracranial hypertension?

Approach to investigations and management

Investigation

In a patient with headache, this often boils down to whether or not a CT scan is performed. The yield will be very low and not infrequently an incidental finding will cause some difficulty, but if a clear diagnosis cannot be made and there are uncertainties as to whether the headache is benign, then it may be appropriate to perform the scan in order to exclude a space-occupying lesion or hydrocephalus. In a patient with idiopathic intracranial hypertension the CT may demonstrate slit-like ventricles, and diagnosis is confirmed by measuring an elevated opening pressure on lumbar puncture. Any systemic features should lead to the appropriate tests being performed.

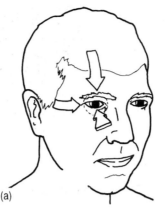
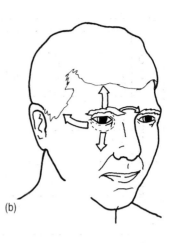
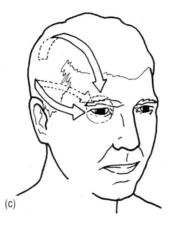
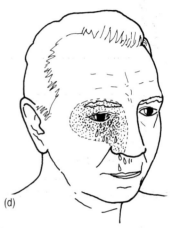

Fig. 21 Site of pain in different headache diagnoses. (a) Classical migraine. Pain is centred in and around the eye, forehead on one or other side and usually extends to involve the whole half head. (b) Orbital onset migraine. The pain tends to start in and around the orbit and may extend across to the opposite eye and to the adjacent facial, frontal and temporal areas but the main pain remains in the orbit itself. (c) Occipital onset migraine. The pain may start as a tightness in the occipital area, rather like tension headache, but will typically extend forward around the temporal area or over the top of the head. The ultimate location of the headache is in and around the eye. (d) Cluster headache. The pain is located in the eye and nostril. It is strictly unilateral and rarely changes sides. Lacrimation, nasal blockage and discharge are common. (e) Tension headache. The pain has a quality like a tight band around the head, coming forwards to the forehead.

Management

Management depends on the particular cause:
- migraine—see Section 2.6.1
- cluster headache—see Section 2.6.3
- tension-type headache with exacerbations—see Section 2.6.4
- idiopathic intracranial hypertension:
  dietary advice to lose weight
  repeat lumbar puncture
  acetazolamide 750–1000 mg daily
  any deterioration in vision is likely to need optic nerve sheath fenestration [2].

Idiopathic intracranial hypertension is no longer called 'benign' because of the danger of progressive visual loss. The sight must be monitored by regular formal visual field testing (see *Ophthalmology*, Section 3.1) and intraocular pressure measurement, not simply by testing of acuity.

1 Lance JW, Goadsby PJ. *Mechanism and Management of Headache* (6th edn). Oxford: Butterworth Heineman, 1998.
2 Wall M, George D. Idiopathic intracranial hypertension. A prospective study of 50 patients. *Brain* 1991; 114: 155–180.

1.20 Funny turns

Case history

A 76-year-old man is referred to the outpatient clinic complaining of a 3-month history of funny turns.

Clinical approach

'Funny turn' is a vague term that can be used to describe a multitude of different symptoms ranging from light-headedness to loss of consciousness. Making the diagnosis depends critically on the history. This can be difficult to obtain since the patient may have poor recollection of events, and ideally a witness account of at least one attack needs to be obtained. The key points to establish are whether or not the patient is experiencing vertigo, and whether there has been loss of consciousness. The differential diagnosis will vary accordingly (Table 22).

History of the presenting problem

'Funny turns'—the history is critical:
• the patient may not be able to give a clear account
• take a careful history from both the patient and from a witness.

Is he describing vertigo or not?

It can sometimes be difficult to be certain—ask about the following:
• A sensation of rotation of self or environment by definition is vertigo.

However, many patients will not be this explicit and will describe to-and-fro or up-and-down movement of the body or head, or that the wall/floor moves, or that they veer to one side during symptoms, 'as if being pulled down by a magnet'. These symptoms, which merge into the very non-specific compliant of 'unsteadiness', are difficult to sort out. Further probing is required.
• Are the symptoms aggravated by moving, closing the eyes or riding in a car? Is he disinclined to walk during an attack? All suggest that the symptom should be regarded as vertigo.
• The duration of attacks is crucial: benign positional vertigo (BPV) [1] lasts only minutes, whereas the vertigo of Ménière's disease can last for hours.
• The role of posture in the generation of vertiginous symptoms is often over-played: most cases of vertigo will be worse on movement. BPV is diagnosed using Hallpike's manoeuvre (see Examination, p. 45). If movement of the neck, e.g. twisting to look when reversing the car, precipitates vertigo then vertebrobasilar ischaemia is possible, but only if other symptoms suggesting brain ischaemia also occur.

Not uncommonly, the patient cannot describe their symptoms in any more detail than lightheadedness, giddiness, dizziness or intermittent unsteadiness. In these cases the wide differential diagnosis listed in Table 22 needs to be considered.

Is he describing presyncope?

Does he describe early visual symptoms, muffled sounds, feelings of hot or cold or feeling lightheaded? These features would be suggestive of a transient fall in cerebral blood flow. Symptoms on standing suggest postural hypotension, and those associated with effort, chest pain,

Symptom	Common causes	Other causes
Vertigo	Ménière's disease, Benign positional vertigo Cerebello-pontine angle lesion	Vertebrobasilar TIA Drugs, e.g. aminoglycosides
Giddy/dizzy/unsteady	Anxiety Drugs (various) Multiple deficits of sensory input	Cervical spondylosis TIA Anaemia or polycythaemia Hypoglycaemia
Presyncope or syncope	Postural hypotension Cardiac dysrhythmia Vasovagal Ventricular outflow obstruction, e.g. aortic stenosis, Hypertrophic obstructive cardiomyopathy Specific precipitant, e.g. carotid sinus syncope	Specific precipitant, e.g. cough or micturition syncope Myocardial ischaemia
Transient loss of awareness/consciousness	Epilepsy Causes of syncope	Transient global amnesia

TIA, transient ischaemic attack

Table 22 Common or important causes of recurrent 'funny turns'.

shortness of breath or palpitations are more likely to have a cardiac cause (see *Cardiology*, Section 1.2). Was it preceded by coughing vigorously or by micturition, suggesting a specific syncopal syndrome?

New onset of vasovagal presyncope or syncope would not be expected to occur at the age of 76 years, but such episodes typically occur when standing up in hot and stuffy rooms, have quite a long prodrome of 'feeling faint' and culminate in a dizzy feeling where noises seem to become loud before the patient collapses. Consciousness is restored almost as soon as the patient falls to the ground or is encouraged to lie down by someone who recognizes what is happening. In those susceptible, vasovagal syncope can also be induced by painful or unpleasant stimuli.

Was there loss of consciousness in these attacks (syncope)?

If syncope has occurred, was it preceded by presyncopal symptoms that could give a clue to the diagnosis? A witness account of pallor followed by flushing would be very suggestive of a Stokes–Adams attack (due to the intermittent development of complete heart block) but does not occur in all patients (see *Cardiology*, Section 1.3) [2].

Could the cause be epilepsy?

The presence of jerking limbs and incontinence does not prove epilepsy as the primary cause. Anoxic fits can occur following prolonged cerebral anoxia, such as when propped up after passing out. A helpful differentiating factor can be the length of time to come round after an episode, which may be prolonged in a postictal state and short after an anoxic fit.

If he was awake but unresponsive during an attack, ask specifically about any warnings that he or any witness may have noticed. Features such as lip smacking, fiddling with clothes or stereotyped movements would be suggestive of a complex partial seizure.

Are there any additional features in the history to help?

Consider the following points:
• A history of tinnitus and deafness in the context of episodic vertigo points towards Ménière's disease, or even a cerebello-pontine angle lesion, e.g. acoustic neuroma, if ataxia and/or facial weakness is also present.
• Do other neurological symptoms occur? In their absence, transient ischaemic attacks of either the anterior or posterior circulation are unlikely.
• If the patient mentions feeling unsteady, then ask about walking, particularly over uneven ground, or tripping on paving stones, and also about numbness in the feet and hands. Those with peripheral neuropathy (see Sections 1.1, p. 3 and 2.1, p. 57) may be susceptible to bouts of unsteadiness, especially when other sensory modalities such as vision are simultaneously impaired.
• Does he have any biological features of depression? It is not uncommon for this to present with somatic symptoms.
• Do not forget alcohol. Many are familiar with the 'funny turns' that can be precipitated by drinking!

> **Could the cause of a funny turn be transient global amnesia?**
>
> Did the patient have an episode of amnesia and confusion lasting hours? Consider the diagnosis of transient global amnesia, in which self-identity is preserved. The degree of retrograde amnesia shrinks significantly after the attack. The significance of recognizing this not uncommon condition is that it is benign, recurs only very infrequently, and does not require investigation [3].

Relevant past history

Has the patient ever suffered from stroke, myocardial infarction, angina, heart valve disease, cardiac dysrhythmia or epilepsy? A full history of current and recently prescribed drugs is clearly important, especially those likely to cause or exacerbate postural hypotension, e.g. diuretics, antihypertensives. Ask about risk factors for atheromatous vascular disease: smoking, hypertension, diabetes mellitus, family history of stroke, ischaemic heart disease, hyperlipidaemia.

Examination

There is often very little to find on examination, and this is particularly likely to be true of those in whom the history does not point to the diagnosis. Consider the diagnoses listed in Table 22 as you examine the patient.

Cardiovascular

Take careful note of pulse rate, rhythm, character; jugular venous pressure; apex; heart sounds; supine blood pressure compared to blood pressure 3 min after standing.

Neurological

A full neurological examination should be carried out with particular attention to:
• visual acuity
• fundal changes of hypertension or diabetes mellitus
• hearing
• nystagmus
• ataxia
• proprioceptive loss
• loss of reflexes and distal sensation

• auscultation over the carotid arteries
• Hallpike's manoeuvre: the patient is rapidly moved from the sitting position to recumbency with the head tilted 30 degrees over the end of the bed and 30 degrees to one side. A positive result is indicated by the onset, after a latency of some seconds, of torsional nystagmus associated with vertigo. The result will fatigue on repeat testing. For a diagnosis of benign positional vertigo to be made, both latency and fatiguability must be present
• effect of putting the neck through a full range of movement.

Approach to investigations and management

Investigations

In many cases a diagnosis can be made on the basis of the history, when selected confirmatory investigations may be required. When no clear diagnosis can be made, then consider the following:
• Are the 'funny turns' a marker of ill health? Check full blood count, electrolytes, renal and liver function tests, glucose, inflammatory markers and chest radiograph. In some cases other tests, e.g. thyroid function, vitamin B_{12} levels, may be indicated.
• Are the episodes cardiac? Check resting 12-lead ECG, 24-h ambulatory ECG and echocardiogram (if clinical suspicion of valvular or other structural abnormality). Some small studies have suggested that an ambulatory ECG is no more use than the standard ECG [4], but in the patient with frequent, troublesome, and potentially life-threatening syncope, repeated monitoring or even inpatient observation may be required.
• Are the episodes neurological? Any patient with focal neurological features or new-onset seizures must have a CT scan of the brain. An EEG is usually unhelpful and is unnecessary.
• If there is vertigo, then specialist otological referral should be considered.

Management

Management will depend on the precise diagnosis, but note in particular the following:
• Vestibular retraining may be useful for BPV.
• Vestibular suppressants can help in other forms of vertigo.
• Cardiac dysrhythmias may require permanent pacemakers and/or drug therapy and structural cardiac lesions, e.g. aortic stenosis, may warrant surgery.
• A clear history of seizures warrants treatment with antiepileptics, but these should not be given as a 'therapeutic trial'.

In many patients, particularly the elderly, it is likely that several factors will be identified without any one of them being clearly responsible for the 'funny turns'. It is always difficult to know how far to pursue investigation, the severity of symptoms and the patient's wishes being important considerations. In any case of 'funny turns, cause unknown' it is important to adopt a sensible approach to symptomatic treatment, e.g. giving advice regarding postural symptoms, provision of a stick to provide extra sensory input, control of hypertension, diabetes, etc.

See *Medicine for the elderly*, Sections 1.1, 2.3, 2.8 and 2.9.
See *Cardiology*, Sections 1.2, 1.3 and 2.2.
1 Baloh R *et al.* Benign positional vertigo: clinical and oculographic features. *Neurology* 1987; 37: 371–378.
2 de Bono D. Funny turns, cardiac. *B J Hosp Med* 1982; 27(3): 212–223.
3 Hodges J, Ward C. Observations in transient global amnesia. *Brain* 1989; 112: 595–620.
4 Taylor I, Stout R. Is ambulatory ECG a useful investigation? *Age Ageing* 1983; 12(3): 211–216.

1.21 Hemiplegia

Case history

A woman returns home from shopping to find that her 55-year-old husband has fallen. He has a right hemiplegia and difficulty expressing himself.

Clinical approach

This man has a lesion affecting his left cerebral hemisphere. The important decision to make is whether he has had a stroke or not, as therapeutic options for stroke will increasingly rely on rapid diagnosis [1]. The differential diagnosis initially lies between ischaemic or haemorrhagic stroke; space-occupying lesion, including subdural haematoma; focal cerebral infection, particularly herpes simplex encephalitis or a cerebral abscess; or postictal Todd's paresis. Hypoglycaemia is worth bearing in mind in a diabetic patient, especially as this is both easily missed and easily treated. If this is a stroke, then two uncommon but specific causes to consider, even if only to exclude immediately, are giant cell arteritis and carotid artery dissection [2].

History of the presenting problem

It is important to obtain as complete a history as possible, especially regarding onset of symptoms, even though this

Table 23 'Atypical presentations' of stroke.

Slower onset (sometimes)	Gradually occluding internal carotid artery
	Intracerebral haemorrhage on anticoagulants
	Lacunar strokes
Seizures	Lobar haemorrhage
Coma	Massive stroke/oedema
	Brain-stem stroke

man is likely, from the brief account given above, to find it difficult to speak or to comprehend and/or reply to questions. In this case the patient's wife is likely to be available and to be the most useful informant, but in other cases it may be necessary to track down relatives or neighbours, and at the very least to obtain the past medical history from his general practitioner.

Is this a stroke?

Stroke is by far the most likely diagnosis, the typical history being of focal neurological symptoms and signs:
• of sudden onset
• becoming maximal rapidly, i.e. within minutes to hours rather than hours to days
• consisting of predominantly negative features, e.g. loss of power, loss of sensation, rather than positive ones, e.g. involuntary movements of the limbs, pins and needles.

Atypical presentations of stroke can occur (Table 23), but if the picture varies significantly from that described above, then other diagnoses must be seriously entertained. If the picture is typical, then were there any preceding symptoms that might give a clue to the aetiology of stroke?
• Headache, nausea or vomiting—might indicate intracranial haemorrhage, including subarachnoid haemorrhage, or brain-stem stroke in this context.
• Unilateral headache or facial pain—might suggest carotid artery dissection.
• Muscle aches and pains, visual symptoms, temporal tenderness or jaw claudication could all indicate cranial arteritis.

Were the symptoms of more gradual onset?

Symptoms of gradual onset should lead you to consider a space-occupying lesion and to enquire further about the following.
• Subdural haematoma—is there a history of head injury, however innocuous? Does he take an anticoagulant?
• Primary or secondary brain tumours—is there anything that might suggest malignancy, e.g. known previous malignancy, history of recent weight loss, bony pain, rectal bleeding, new pigmented skin lesions?

• Focal cerebral infection—this needs to be considered if there are systemic features or seizures, when possible diagnoses would include herpes simplex encephalitis and brain abscess.

Relevant past history

Enquire about the presence of vascular risk factors such as hypertension, diabetes mellitus and smoking, also about previous strokes, but remember that a history of these does not exclude the possibility of another, non-vascular, diagnosis. Similarly, a diagnosis of epilepsy does not mean that this presentation is necessarily that of a Todd's paresis. Stroke should be diagnosed on the basis of presenting symptoms. However, if no history is available concerning the acute event, then all other available information is needed to try to piece together the most plausible picture.

What medication is he taking?

A patient's medication is a marker for their pre-existing disease and often a very useful source of information when the patient cannot communicate and previous medical records are unavailable, as is often the case on initial assessment in hospital. The following would be of particular note in someone presenting with hemiparesis:
• aspirin
• anticoagulants—this increases the chances of intracerebral haemorrhage
• antihypertensives
• lipid-lowering drugs
• antiepileptics
• digoxin/anti-arrhythmic drugs.

Pre-morbid health

What was his previous level of functioning? This is relevant when planning care: see *Medicine for the elderly*, Section 1.4.

Examination

General

How ill is the patient? Are they critically ill? Do they have a rapidly resolving deficit? Your subsequent management is dependent on this assessment.
• Check airway, breathing, circulation—is the patient protecting their airway? If not, nurse in recovery position, insert oropharyngeal tube (if tolerated) and give high-flow oxygen.
• Check Glasgow Coma Score—see *Emergency medicine*, Section 1.26. Ischaemic stroke does not cause coma or

impaired conscious level unless there is a very large infarct with mass effect, or there is significant brain-stem damage. Coma therefore should lead you to consider intracerebral haemorrhage or infection, ongoing seizure activity or hypoxia.

• Check vital signs: temperature, pulse, respiratory rate, blood pressure. High fever makes focal intracerebral infection more likely.

• Is the neck stiff? Nuchal rigidity raises the possibility of intracranial haemorrhage or infection.

For further discussion of the assessment and management of an acute stroke see *Emergency medicine*, Section 1.25.

Neurological

If the diagnosis is stroke, then what type is it? Note the following:

• It is possible to get a good idea about the anatomical site of the lesion by using a bedside clinical classification such as the Oxfordshire Community Stroke Study classification (see Section 2.8.1, p. 92). However, the most important distinction to make is whether there is intracerebral haemorrhage or not, and this cannot reliably be done at the bedside.

• The presence of a Horner's syndrome (see Section 1.16, p. 36) could represent brain-stem involvement, but in the context of unilateral headache one should consider a carotid artery dissection, even at the age of 55.

Are there any features to suggest that the diagnosis is not stroke? The presence of papilloedema would indicate raised intracranial pressure and suggest a space-occupying lesion; malignant phase hypertension complicated by haemorrhagic or ischaemic stroke would be another consideration.

Cardiovascular

Look for signs of atrial fibrillation, cardiac failure, heart valve abnormality, carotid bruits, hypertension and asymmetrical pulses, which might indicate aortic dissection complicated by stroke (see *Cardiology*, Sections 1.4 and 1.5).

Approach to investigations and management

Investigations

If this man has had a stroke, the diagnosis should be arrived at on clinical grounds, and quickly [3], as acute treatments will need to be given quickly. Early investigations may help plan management and should include the following:

• CT scan of head—to exclude haemorrhage and space-

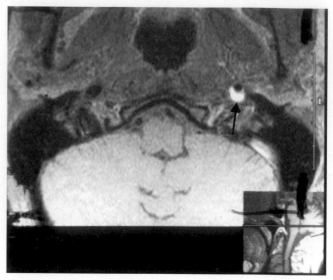

Fig. 22 Axial T-1 weighted MRI through the neck. Arrow indicates crescentic shape of blood in the wall of the left internal carotid artery.

occupying lesion, as soon as possible (within 48 h, but may need to be done urgently in some cases).

• Full blood count, electrolytes, renal function, glucose and inflammatory markers.

• Chest radiograph—to look at the lungs for tumour or signs of aspiration, at heart size for evidence of left atrial dilatation or cardiac failure and at the mediastinum: 'is it widened?'

• ECG—is the patient in atrial fibrillation? Is there evidence of recent myocardial infarction?

Also consider the following.

• Axial T1-weighted MRI scan from skull base to C4 to look for carotid artery dissection if this is a diagnostic possibility (Fig. 22).

• Lumbar puncture to examine the cerebrospinal fluid if intracranial infection is considered possible, but only if there is no mass effect or marked cerebral oedema on the CT scan.

Management

This will depend on the precise diagnosis.

• Stroke—see Section 2.8.1, also *Medicine for the elderly*, Section 1.4 and *Emergency medicine*, Section 1.25.

• Intracerebral haemorrhage—see Section 2.8.3, p. 96.

• Herpes simplex encephalitis—see *Infectious diseases*, Sections 1.15 and 2.10.1.

• Epilepsy—see Section 2.7, p. 85.

1 Vuadens P, Bogousslavsky J. Diagnosis as a guide to stroke therapy. *Lancet* 1998; 352 (Suppl III): 5–9.
2 Norris JW, Hachinski VC. Misdiagnosis of stroke. *Lancet* 1982; i: 328–331.
3 Lees KL. If I had a stroke…. *Lancet* 1998; 352 (Suppl III): 28–30.

1.22 Speech disturbance

Case history

A 57-year-old woman consults her doctor because her 'speech has become difficult'.

Clinical approach

The differential diagnosis of speech disturbance is determined by the type of disorder present: is it dysarthria, dysphasia or dysphonia?

• Dysarthria is a disorder of articulation in which the content of the speech is unaffected, the underlying diagnosis almost always being determined by eliciting other physical signs (Table 24).

• Dysphasia is a disorder of language that is caused by a cortical lesion of the dominant hemisphere [1] (Table 25).

• In dysphonia, articulation and language content are normal but voice production is defective (Table 26).

Table 24 Causes of dysarthria.

Cerebellar dysarthria	Any cause of a cerebellar syndrome
Bulbar palsy	Myopathy, myositis Myasthenia gravis Motor neurone disease Bulbar poliomyelitis Guillain–Barré syndrome
Pseudobulbar palsy	Small-vessel cerebral ischaemic damage Motor neurone disease Multiple sclerosis
Hypokinetic dysarthria	Extrapyramidal disease, especially Parkinson's disease
Hyperkinetic dysarthria	Chorea, myoclonus
Isolated cranial nerve palsies	CN V, VII, X, XII
Other	Hypothyroidism

Table 25 Causes of dysphasia.

Stroke	Dominant middle cerebral artery territory
Tumour	Dominant hemisphere
Trauma	
Cerebral abscess	
Herpes simplex encephalitis	
Degenerative CNS disease	Alzheimer's disease Fronto-temporal dementia Progressive non-fluent aphasia

Table 26 Causes of dysphonia.

Paralysis of both vocal cords	Post thyroidectomy Neck malignancy Poliomyelitis Guillain–Barré syndrome Brain-stem stroke Multiple sclerosis Syringobulbia
Paralysis of one vocal cord/recurrent laryngeal nerve palsy	Post thyroidectomy Carcinoma (bronchial, thyroid, lymphoma) Cervical node enlargement Aortic aneurysm Pulmonary tuberculosis
Neuromuscular respiratory failure	Guillain–Barré syndrome Myasthenia gravis Polymyositis
Spasmodic dysphonia	Associated with dystonia

The most important step in making the correct diagnosis of speech disturbance is to accurately characterize the abnormality: is it dysarthria, dysphasia or dysphonia?

History of the presenting problem

A great deal can be learnt simply by listening to the patient give their history: the way that they do this, as much as what they actually say, may give you the diagnosis. As they speak, listen carefully, and think about the aspects of speech and language production and comprehension described below (see Examination, p. 50). If the following information is not volunteered, then ask for it specifically.

• How long has she had this problem? A long history is against any malignant process. A sudden onset may have a vascular cause.

• Do the symptoms vary? Fatigability suggests a muscle disease and in particular myasthenia gravis.

• Are there associated features that suggest a particular diagnosis? Is the woman unsteady? In cerebellar problems gait ataxia almost always precedes dysarthria. Has she got weakness or clumsiness of her right arm/hand or right leg? This would suggest a left hemisphere lesion. Is there difficulty swallowing, indicating that the problem is one of the bulbar muscles (bulbar or pseudobulbar palsy, see Section 1.10, p. 20)?

Relevant past history

Any history of conditions listed in Tables 24, 25 or 26 is relevant. Are there any vascular risk factors (see Section 2.8.1, p. 90)?

Examination

Assessment of speech

Assessment of speech should include all the following elements:
- phonation
- articulation
- fluency
- verbal comprehension
- naming
- repetition
- reading
- writing.

Phonation and articulation

When the patient talks, listen for dysphonia (whispering, hoarse or otherwise abnormal voice) or disturbances of articulation characteristic of dysarthria. It may be possible to exaggerate dysarthria by asking the patient to repeat phrases such as 'biblical criticism' or 'West Register Street'. Repetition of particular letters can be used to assess individual parts of the articulatory process: lips ('pa'), tongue ('ta'), soft palate and posterior tongue ('ka'). Putting them all together rapidly ('pa-ta-ka') will uncover mild dysarthric speech. It is often difficult to characterize dysarthric speech purely on the basis of the way it sounds. It is frequently of mixed type, and the type(s) present can usually be deduced from the associated signs.
- Cerebellar speech is scanning or staccato, e.g. artillery pronounced 'art-til-ler-y', and associated with ataxic gait.
- Pseudobulbar or spastic dysarthria, caused by bilateral lesions in the upper motor neurone projections onto the bulbar nuclei in the brain stem (Fig. 5, p. 22), is associated with dysphagia, small spastic tongue and a brisk jaw jerk. There may also be signs of small vessel ischaemic damage such as '*marche à petit pas*', brisk reflexes and extensor plantars (see Section 1.4, p. 10).
- Bulbar dysarthria is due a deficit in the bulbar cranial nerves (lower motor neurone type) or the bulbar muscles, hence there may be wasting and fasciculation of the tongue, proximal muscle weakness or fatiguability.
- Check carefully for isolated cranial nerve palsies.

Fluency

If articulation is normal, consider that the speech disorder may be a dysphasia. Listen to the fluency of speech and in particular for the patient to substitute alternative words or phrases for words they may have forgotten (paraphasias), or to use nonsense words (neologisms).

Comprehension

Early in the assessment it is wise to check that the patient understands what you are asking; indeed, it may be appropriate to do this right at the beginning if initial attempts at conversation with the patient are not rewarding. Comprehension is not an all-or-nothing skill, the level of comprehension being gauged by the complexity of the task that can be performed: one-, two- or three-step commands. You might approach testing, starting with simple instructions and gradually increasing the complexity, as follows:
- 'I wonder if you are having some difficulty in understanding what I say … ?'
- 'I would like to test this …'
- 'Is that alright … ?'
- 'Can you open your mouth, please—open your mouth?'

If the patient does not do this, then open your own mouth and see if they copy you.
- 'Can you show me your left hand?'
- 'Can you put your right hand on top of your head?'
- 'Can you touch your left ear with your right hand, and put your left hand on your nose?'

Naming

The patient may not be able to do this at all, may seem to have forgotten how to pronounce a word, or may describe something without naming it (circumlocution). Start with simple objects, e.g. pen, watch, and then move on to more complex, e.g. stethoscope.

Repetition

Start with simple words, then use longer words or phrases.

Reading

This should be performed silently so as to test only visual comprehension. Ask the patient to read and follow a written command such as 'close your eyes'. Reading aloud is just another way of examining speech patterns, which by this stage in proceedings are already known.

Writing

Use verbal and written requests to write something.

Types of dysphasia

Classification of language disorders has been based on various theoretical models, none of which show a consistent correlation with anatomical lesions. Many consider it appropriate to think in terms of anterior or posterior dysphasia.

Anterior dysphasia

This is characterized by:
- non-fluent, hesitant speech, i.e. 'agrammatic' or 'telegraphic' speech, missing out words such as 'and'
- substitution of words or syllables
- poor writing, with errors similar to speech
- naming may be impaired
- comprehension, repetition (except for some word or syllabic substitution) and reading are preserved.

Posterior dysphasia

This is characterized by the following:
- Fluent speech with normal rhythm. However, because of poor comprehension the patient is unable to monitor their speech and so it contains neologisms and paraphrasias as well as substitutions (ultimately ending up as incomprehensible jargon—jargon aphasia [2]), and the patient talks incessantly.
- Poor comprehension, repetition and reading.

Approach to investigations and management

Investigations

This is dictated by the clinical judgement: dysphonia, dysarthria or dysphasia?

Dysphonia

It is essential that the vocal cords are viewed either directly or indirectly as a first step. Subsequent investigations may include chest radiograph, CT chest or thyroid ultrasound.

Dysarthria

The associated features will identify the most important investigations, e.g. cerebellar (MRI brain), bulbar (EMG and nerve conduction studies) or pseudobulbar (CT or MRI brain, EMG).

Dysphasia

CT or MRI brain are required, along with formal neuropsychological and cognitive assessment.

Management

Clearly depends on the underlying cause, but may range from ENT referral for dysphonia to neurosurgery for some lesions causing dysphasia. In addition it is likely that specialized speech and language therapy input will be required [3].

1 Margolin DI. Cognitive neuropsychology. Resolving enigmas about Wernicke's aphasia and other higher cortical disorders. *Arch Neurol* 1991; 48(7): 751–765.
2 Semenza C, Cipolotti L, Denes G. Reading aloud in jargonaphasia: an unusual dissociation in speech output. *J Neurol Neurosurg Psychiatry* 1992; 55(3): 205–208.
3 Thulborn KR, Carpenter PA, Just MA. Plasticity of language-related brain function during recovery from stroke. *Stroke* 1999; 30(4): 749–754.

1.23 Visual hallucinations

Case history

A middle-aged woman presents to the outpatient clinic complaining of visual hallucinations. She is not acutely unwell.

Clinical approach

There are many causes of visual hallucinations, which can usefully be classified as described in Table 27 [1]. Some cases present in the context of identifiable pre-existing disease—e.g. dementia, Parkinson's disease or diffuse Lewy body disease, psychoses, migraine—but in those occurring *de novo* you must decide which patients are likely to have an intracranial structural lesion.

History of the presenting problem

Keep the working classification shown in Table 27 in mind as you establish the features of the hallucination:
- Does the patient think it is real or not?
- What form does it take: simple or complex?
- Does it affect the whole visual field, or just a hemifield?
- Is it affected by closing or moving the eye(s)?
- How long does it last?
- If more than one, are they always the same?
- Are any other senses involved?

A full drug history is essential, including prescribed and non-prescribed drugs, as is a careful history of alcohol consumption (see *Gastroenterology and hepatology*, Sections 1.4 and 1.7; *Psychiatry*, Section 1.7). Medication for Parkinson's disease is particularly likely to induce visual hallucinations.

Relevant past history

Is the patient known to have a history of:
- stroke?
- Parkinson's disease?

Perceived by the patient as real	Psychiatric disorders
	Dementia
	Parkinson's disease—usually associated with anti-parkinsonian drugs
	Acute confusional states—occurs in addition to systemic features
	Delirium tremens—typically small moving objects or animals
	Some epileptic phenomena (see below)
	Some drugs
Recognized as unreal by the patient (pseudohallucinations)	Purely visual:
	Visual hallucinations secondary to eye disease, occurring in the whole visual field, disappearing with eye closure. May be simple or complex:
	Cataracts
	Macular degeneration
	Glaucoma
	Choroidal neovascularization
	Hemianopic hallucinations, i.e. occipital lobe lesions (infarct, haemorrhage, tumour) causing unilateral (usually complex) visual hallucinations, which disappear with saccadic eye movements.
	May involve hallucinations in other sensory modalities:
	Those associated with epileptic aura or seizures, stereotyped and usually short lived (<30 s), may be simple or complex occurring in a hemifield and not affected by saccadic eye movements. May be perceived as real by some patients
	Those associated with migraine aura, usually simple images, lines fortification spectra, flashing lights.
	Peduncular hallucinosis, a rare syndrome of often complex visual hallucinations, sleep disturbance and agitation, secondary to a lesion in the midbrain or thalamus.
	Some drugs

Table 27 Working classification of visual hallucinations.

- dementia?
- psychiatric disease?
- visual disturbance?
- epilepsy?
- alcohol abuse?
- drug abuse?

Examination

A full examination should be performed with particular reference to the following:
- neuropsychometry—see Section 3.1, p. 111, also *Medicine for the Elderly*, Sections 3.2 and 3.3
- the visual system (acuity, fields, fundoscopy—see *Ophthalmology*, Section 3.1)
- other neurological signs, in particular brain-stem signs ('peduncular hallucinosis') or evidence of Parkinson's disease.

Approach to investigations and management

Investigations

Any patient with complex visual hallucinations in the absence of known neurological disease (Parkinson's disease, dementia, delirium tremens, acute confusional state) should have a brain scan. In addition, simple visual hallucinations that are stereotyped may well be ictal and patients with these should also be scanned.

In addition, the following may be useful:
- 'Screening tests': full blood count, electrolytes, renal and liver function tests (including γGT), glucose, inflammatory markers and chest radiograph.
- EEG only if frequent suspected ictal events.

Management

This will depend on the diagnosis.
- Epileptic visual hallucinations usually respond to antiepileptics.
- Occipital lobe lesions—the hallucinations are often self limiting and outcome will depend on the nature of the lesion, e.g. stroke, tumour.
- Parkinson's disease—reduce anticholinergic therapy, then dopamine agonists, if the patient is disturbed by the hallucinations. May need to reduce dose of levodopa, but this is unfortunately not tolerated well by patients.
- Delirium tremens—not the diagnosis in a patient who is not acutely unwell, but see *Gastroenterology and hepatology*, Section 1.7.

1 Barodalawa S, Mulley GP. Visual hallucinations. *J R Coll Physicians Lond* 1997; 31(1): 42–48.

1.24 Conversion disorders

Case history

A 25-year-old man is referred to the outpatient clinic by his general practitioner. He complains of weakness and difficulty walking, but his general practitioner cannot find any abnormal signs and writes that 'this may be a case of hysteria'.

Clinical approach

The question of hysteria arises from time to time: your first obligation is not to miss a treatable condition. However, with experience it is possible to recognize some cases in whom extensive investigation is unlikely to provide any clear diagnosis. The following discussion should not be seen as a checklist for 'catching patients out', but may enable most of those with hysterical problems to be diagnosed early so that the appropriate treatment can be offered.

It is worth bearing in mind the often quoted but still controversial differences between a conversion disorder and malingering:
• the malingerer intends to deceive: the patient with a conversion disorder does not
• the patient with a conversion disorder can to some degree be persuaded: the malingerer cannot
• the malingerer seems less ill and more evasive.

History of the presenting problem

You should not take the history intent on making a diagnosis of conversion disorder or malingering, and issues discussed in Sections 1.4 and 1.11, should be explored. However, the following features may arouse your suspicions:
• The patient has been seen by several specialists, no diagnosis has been made and he is seeking a repeat opinion.
• A history of multiple symptomatology involving more than one organ system.
• A history of non-attendance or self-discharge from hospital without good reason.
• He seems overly aggressive.
• A history of recent psychosocial stresses or traumas.
It should be emphasized, however, that none of these can back up a diagnosis of conversion disorder or malingering on their own, especially in the face of abnormal neurological signs. You should ask specifically if the patient has any particular diagnoses that they are worried about, or any friends or relatives in whom serious diagnoses have recently been made. If this man's girlfriend has recently been diagnosed as having multiple sclerosis, then this could explain a great deal.

Examination

Suspicions are much more likely to be aroused by the examination than history. However, patients may display differing degrees of sophistication in their clinical presentation: gross cases are easy for most to diagnose, but some may be extremely difficult.

Hysterical gait

The following are features of an hysterical gait:
• It doesn't fit a recognized pattern but is 'a gait of his own invention'.
• It is hesitant, jerky and lurching in all directions. In doing so it often demonstrates normal power and balance, and if falls occur they are either slowly to the ground or into the arms of an observer.
• The abnormal leg is advanced in a hesitant, tremulous or ataxic manner that appears to be exaggerated. The abnormal foot is often pushed or dragged along on the ground, rather than any attempt being made to lift it.
• Characteristic circumduction of the leg is absent.
• If both legs are affected, the gait may be bizarre, or the patient may not walk at all.

Hysterical paralysis

The following are features of an hysterical paralysis.
• Pronator drift is not seen if arms are involved.
• In unilateral leg weakness, if there is an attempt to deceive, then on attempted hip flexion there will be no counter extension of the contralateral leg, which is seen normally or in genuine weakness (Hoover's sign).
• Testing power results in a slow tentative response, sometimes with activation of agonists and antagonists together: this does not happen when movement is genuinely attempted.
• There may be 'give way weakness', when the maximal response is generated only for some of the time. The power attributed to a muscle is that which is maximally generated, for however short a period of time. Pain will cause the same findings.
• An ability to walk relatively normally, when no movement was present whilst lying on the bed, may be a feature of a conversion disorder or malingering, but can also be seen in midline ataxia or frontal gait apraxia.

Sensory signs

These are often difficult to interpret at the best of times, but the following features are unlikely to be organic.

53

• Non-anatomical loss—but just be sure your anatomy is correct (see Section 2.1.1, p. 57 and *Anatomy*, Section 9).
• Loss of all modalities of sensation in one limb finishing at the top of the limb in a well-circumscribed ring.
• Whole-body hemisensory loss may occur on its own as a result of a small thalamic lesion, but is otherwise an unusual sign. The patient in whom vibration sense is different on one side of the sternum to the other is not likely to have genuine sensory loss.

> The following cases are particularly difficult to interpret, and may be misinterpreted as a conversion disorder.
> • Frontal lobe lesions, e.g. as seen in multiple sclerosis, may produce signs that are different on the bed and whilst standing and patients may also exhibit 'la belle indifference'.
> • Patients with severe loss of proprioception, e.g. some acute demyelinating neuropathies, sensory ganglionitides, may appear to have wildly fluctuating muscle power and control, but their main problem is one of proprioception. Always check joint position sense, and try testing power with the patient looking at the limb.

Approaches to investigations and management

Investigation

> **In suspected malingering or conversion disorder, investigate thoroughly—once!**

If there is any doubt, which there usually is, then it is reasonable to investigate the patient thoroughly on one occasion—but not repeatedly. The appropriate investigations depend on the symptoms: for gait disturbance see Section 1.4 (p. 10); for weak legs see Section 1.11 (p. 23). In brief, the following would help:
• Blood tests including full blood count, electrolytes, renal and liver function tests, glucose, inflammatory/vasculitic screen, vitamin B_{12} levels, creatinine kinase.
• If upper motor neurone features: MRI brain, cervical and thoracic spine; somatosensory evoked potentials and central motor conduction times.
• If lower motor neurone features: EMG and nerve conduction studies.
• CSF.
Whilst this list may seem like 'overdoing it', you are trying to avoid this patient having to undergo any investigations in the future in a 'no stone unturned' exercise as a result of incomplete work-up being performed at the time of presentation. Repeat investigations at different times are most unhelpful in the management.

Management

See *Psychiatry*, Section 1.6.

Outcome

In one study 73 patients with unexplained motor symptoms were followed up for 6 years [1], when 20% were better, 14% unchanged and 38% worse. In 28% the symptoms had changed to something else altogether. The most significant finding was that only three patients turned out to have new organic neurological disorders.

Good prognostic indicators were:
• short duration of illness
• changed marital status during the follow-up period
• coexistent anxiety or depression.

The diagnosis of conversion disorder should be made early, and the study described should help physicians to be more confident in drawing a line under the investigative process, which if repetitive and ongoing will impair the chances of a good outcome.

1 Crimlisk HL, Bhatia K, Cope H, David A, Marsden CD, Ron M. Slater revisited: 6 years follow up study of patients with medically unexplained motor symptoms. *Br Med J* 1998; 316: 582–586.

1.25 Multiple sclerosis

Case history

A young woman with unilateral visual disturbance and a previous episode of spastic paraparesis (now fully resolved) asks you about multiple sclerosis (MS). What should you say to her?

Clinical approach

If this woman's current problem sounds like optic neuritis, then clinically she probably has MS. Section 2.5 (p. 77) discusses the investigation and management of MS; this section will consider an appropriate approach to the initial consultation between patient and neurologist.

Patient concerns

'If it looks as though I've got MS, is there any point in investigating?'

The answer is yes. The patient has now had two episodes

separated in anatomical space and in time. Other illnesses, however, can mimic MS and so investigations are necessary to confirm the diagnosis before further discussion of the implications of such a diagnosis is appropriate:

• 'I'm afraid that it does look as though you've got MS ...'
• 'but that's not 100% certain ...'
• 'and we really need to be absolutely sure what we're dealing with to be able to give you the best advice and treatment'.

A dilemma arises if a patient presents with what sounds like a first episode of demyelination. In this scenario, by definition the patient does not have MS regardless of what the MRI shows. A patient presenting with a single episode of optic neuritis with widespread white matter lesions on MRI has a 70% chance of going on to develop MS. It may be inappropriate to spell this out to the patient. Trials have shown that multiple high signal lesions on MRI do not necessarily correlate with multiple relapses and the radiological burden of disease cannot be used to predict the severity of disease in an individual. If a patient presents having recovered from a probable episode of demyelination, many neurologists would choose not to investigate. If, however, the patient presents at the height of a neurological episode and imaging shows widespread lesions, many would choose to explain that the symptoms have been caused by an area of inflammation and that it is too early to say whether the patient is prone to further episodes. This may have been the case with this woman when she presented with a spastic paraparesis. Discussion of MS at this stage usually only occurs if initiated by the patient.

'Am I going to end up in a wheelchair?'

MS encompasses a whole spectrum of clinical outcomes. High-profile patients are often those with more severe disability requiring support: less vocal are the many MS patients getting on with a reasonably normal life, raising families and holding down jobs. The disease tends to follow one of three patterns: benign; relapsing–remitting becoming secondary progressive; and primary progressive (Fig. 23). The course of early years of a patient's illness will aid prognosis. Those with little or no permanent disability at 10–15 years can expect a benign course, whereas those with frequent early relapses and early accumulation of disability are, unfortunately, likely to have more aggressive disease:

• 'I don't know whether you're going to end up in a wheel chair ...'
• 'I'm not hiding anything: there's simply no way of telling at the moment ...'
• 'only time will tell ...'
• 'If you read the newspapers or watch the TV it's easy to

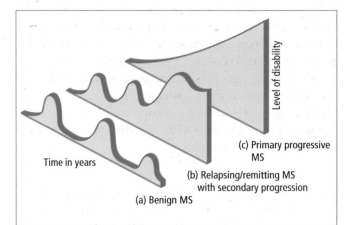

Fig. 23 Diagrammatic representation of the different clinical courses seen in multiple sclerosis (MS). (a) Benign MS. No accumulation of disability between relapses for more than 10 years. (b) Relapsing–remitting MS becoming secondary progressive. At first, complete recovery is made between relapses. Then, failure to recover fully from relapses leads to gradual accumulation of residual disability. Finally, the disability accumulates without clear relapses. (c) Primary progressive MS. Gradual accumulation of disability without relapses.

get the impression that everyone with MS is in a wheelchair ...'
• 'but that's not true ...'
• 'most patients with MS are not in wheelchairs and are getting on with a pretty normal life'.

'When do you want to see me again?'

MS is a common neurological disease that people have heard of and dread. Diagnosis often confirms patients' fears and results in an initial period of shock. After discussing the disease itself and the issues described above, it is helpful to give the patient a further follow-up in 4–6 weeks. This allows them time to let the news 'sink in' and to discuss it with family and friends.

The patient is likely to return with a long list of questions, many of which will probably be based on misconceptions, each of which should be quietly but definitely corrected. After further discussion they must be encouraged to get on with their lives as normally as possible and not to dwell on their diagnosis. This can be aided by an 'open appointment' system rather than a routine review: relapses seldom conveniently occur to coincide with clinic appointments and coming to see a doctor when one is well can reinforce illness behaviour. The neurology unit should be designed to accommodate MS patients at times of relapses.

Regular review is appropriate for primary progressive MS and relapsing–remitting patients entering a secondary progressive phase. If possible, review should be in a dedicated MS clinic with access to physiotherapists and an incontinence advisor.

Other issues

Patients with MS should be aware of treatments, both disease modifying and symptomatic, that are available. It is important that they do not live with distressing symptoms under the impression that 'nothing can be done'. Patients and clinicians must also be alert to the fact that those with MS can get other medical or neurological conditions like anyone else and must not be quick to blame everything on MS.

See *General clinical issues*, Sections 2 and 3.

2 Diseases and treatments

2.1 Peripheral neuropathies and diseases of the lower motor neurone

2.1.1 PERIPHERAL NEUROPATHIES

Pathophysiology

Peripheral nerves contain bundles of nerve fibres, both large-diameter myelinated fibres and small-diameter non-myelinated fibres. The large myelinated fibres carry both efferent motor signals and afferent sensory signals (proprioception and vibration sense). The small non-myelinated fibres carry afferent pain and temperature as well as autonomic signals. The peripheral nerve can react to injury or insult in one of four ways: axonal degeneration, demyelination, Wallerian degeneration and neuronal cell body disease (neuroneopathy).

Axonal degeneration

This is the commonest pathological process encountered in peripheral neuropathies, particularly those associated with systemic, toxic, nutritional and metabolic disorders. The commonest aetiology is diabetes mellitus (Table 28) which is the commonest cause of neuropathy in the UK (three-quarters of these being a distal symmetrical sensory or sensorimotor polyneuropathy). Large-diameter fibres are predominantly involved, and the longest fibres are affected first by this dying back process.

Demyelination

Destruction of the myelin sheath, leaving the axon intact,

Table 28 Classification of diabetic neuropathies.

Symmetrical polyneuropathies	Distal sensory or sensorimotor polyneuropathy Large-fibre neuropathy ('diabetic pseudotabes') Small-fibre neuropathy Autonomic neuropathy
Asymmetrical polyneuropathies	Cranial neuropathy (single or multiple) Limb mononeuropathy (single or multiple) Trunk mononeuropathy (single or multiple) Proximal diabetic neuropathy/diabetic amyotrophy

leads to segmental demyelination, commonly secondary to an immune mediated disorder (see Table 29). Demyelination may occur distally or proximally and is patchy.

Wallerian degeneration

This is the name given to the degenerative process of the distal stump seen after nerve transection (or equivalent insult). Regeneration from the proximal stump is slow and variable.

Neuroneopathy

Neuroneopathy describes a disease process that specifically attacks the neuronal cell bodies. In the case of motor nerves, within the anterior horn of the spinal cord, and in the case of sensory nerves, within the dorsal root ganglion. Examples of motor neuroneopathies include motor neurone disease, spinal muscular atrophies and poliomyelitis. The sensory ganglion cell may be the primary site of injury in paraneoplastic neuropathies (see Section 2.11.1, p. 104) or in Sjögren's syndrome.

Clinical presentation

The commonest type of neuropathy is the distal symmetrical sensorimotor axonal type [1]. Patients will first complain of tingling, burning or band-like sensations in the toes or soles of the feet. As symptoms progress, the sensory disturbance will extend onto the dorsum of the foot, the ankle reflexes will be lost, and there may be weakness of dorsiflexion of the toes and ankle and possibly muscle wasting. Patients may complain of a feeling of walking on cotton wool or on stumps. Progression may lead to foot drop and a high steppage gait; knee reflexes will be lost. Sensory symptoms in the fingertips do not develop until those in the leg have ascended at least to the knee. The gait may become unsteady due to proprioceptive loss. Progression continues smoothly, moving centrally up the arms and legs in a symmetrical fashion, eventually affecting the anterior torso. In extreme cases involvement of the intercostal and diaphragmatic muscles leads to ventilatory disturbance.

Variations from this clinical picture are discussed below.

Axonal vs demyelinating neuropathies

Although the pathological process cannot be reliably distinguished clinically, the following may act as pointers:

Table 29 Causes of peripheral neuropathy.

Motor	GBS/CIDP
	MMN
	Diphtheria
	Lymphoma
	Porphyria
	Lead
	HMSN
	DM
Sensory	Paraproteinaemic
	Sjögren's syndrome
	Amyloid
	HIV
	Leprosy
	Paraneoplastic
	B_{12} deficiency
	Alcohol/toxins
Painful	GBS
	Vascultis
	Amyloid
	HIV
	Leprosy
	Malignant infiltration
	DM
	Uraemia
Multifocal (mononeuritis multiplex)	Vasculitis
	MMN
	Sarcoidosis
	HIV
	Leprosy
	HNLPP
	DM
	Fabry's disease
Demyelinating	GBS/CIDP
	MMN
	Paraproteinaemic
	HIV
	Drugs (amiodarone)
	HMSN 1
Axonal (small fibre)	Amyloid
	Leprosy
	HIV
	DM (rare)
	HSAN
	Fabry's disease
	Tangier disease
Axonal (large fibre)	Vasculitic
	Paraneoplastic
	Toxins
	DM
	Porphyria
	Uraemia
	B_{12} deficiency
	HMSN 2
	Freidreich's ataxia

Table 29 (*continued*)

Autonomic	GBS/CIDP*
	Amyloid
	HIV
	Paraneoplastic*
	Porphyria*
	DM
	Toxins*
	HSAN

Notes: To aid memory each column is constructed using the following 'surgical sieve': inflammatory/immune, infective, malignant, toxic, metabolic, hereditary, other.

DM, diabetes mellitus; GBS, Guillain–Barré syndrome; CIDP, chronic inflammatory demyelinating polyneuropathy; HIV, human immunodeficiency virus; HMSN, hereditary motor and sensory neuropathy; HSAN, hereditary sensory and autonomic neuropathy; HNLPP, hereditary neuropathy with liability to pressure palsies; MMN, multifocal motor neuropathy with conduction block.

*Predominantly acute.

- Concurrent proximal and distal involvement suggests a demyelinating process. Remember that axonal degeneration is a distal dying back process, and demyelination can occur anywhere on the nerve.
- Loss of all reflexes early in the process, rather than sequential loss as described above, might suggest demyelination.

Asymmetry

Asymmetry of clinical findings suggests a multifocal process affecting individual nerve trunks or roots.

Large fibre vs small fibre neuropathies

In small fibre neuropathies, the following are more likely:
- No significant weakness (motor fibres are large myelinated axons).
- Preserved reflexes (the fibres subserving the afferent limb of the muscle stretch reflex arc are large myelinated axons, as are the efferent motor fibres).
- Preserved balance (proprioceptive information is conducted in large myelinated axons).
- Reduced pinprick and temperature sensation.
- Sometimes autonomic disturbance.

Arms vs legs

It is unusual for the first symptoms of a peripheral neuropathy to be in the arms, and this should bring diagnoses suggested in Table 30 to mind.

Investigation

Peripheral neuropathies are often investigated with a blanket screening process [2]. It is hoped that the preceding

Table 30 Neuropathies that can present in the arms before legs.

CIDP/GBS
Porphyria
Spinal muscular atrophy
HMSN
B_{12} deficiency (sensory symptoms)

Carpal tunnel syndrome

Bilateral carpal tunnel syndrome may initially be mistaken for a peripheral neuropathy. Patients complain of nocturnal parasthesia, numbness or burning sensations, often describing how they shake their hands or hang them over the side of the bed for relief [3]. Symptoms may be confined to the thumb, index, middle and lateral half of the ring finger, but often are more diffuse, extending to the elbow and sometimes to the shoulder. Look for reduced sensation on the lateral part of the palm, splitting the ring finger, and in more severe cases wasting of the thenar eminence and weakness of abductor pollicis brevis. In mild cases the diagnosis is made on the history and confirmed electrophysiologically.

Other upper limb entrapment neuropathies (Fig. 24)

Lower trunk of brachial plexus
Mainly affected by cervical rib syndrome, altered anatomy, cervical outlet syndrome, brachial neuritis or Pancoast tumour of lung apex.

Axillary nerve
Damaged by fracture of humeral neck, dislocation of shoulder, deep intramuscular injections (Fig. 24).

Radial nerve
May be damaged at the following sites:
• axilla—damaged by weight bearing on a crutch or resting the arm over back of chair while asleep or intoxicated
• spiral groove of humerus—vunerable to direct blow laterally (during anaethesia or while drunk), medially or midshaft humeral fracture (which may be either immediate or delayed as callus forms)
• supinator muscle—radial nerve (posterior interosseous nerve) passes through supinator and may be damaged by occupational over-use or acute haemorrhage into muscle during trauma.

Ulnar nerve
May be damaged at the following sites:
• elbow—often damaged by repeated minor trauma, prolonged bed-rest (patient resting on elbows) or delayed following fractures in childhood leading to minor anatomical abnormality (tardy ulnar palsy)
• palm—deep branch damaged by trauma to the heel of the hand or idiopathically due to a ganglion. Confusing clinically as often there is no sensory loss and is often mistaken for MND (Fig. 25).

Median nerve
May be damaged at the following sites:
• elbow—rarely damaged by direct trauma but may be involved in elbow fracture as deeply placed
• forearm—the anterior interosseous branch of the median nerve is a rarely damaged nerve, lies very deep, flexors of index finger and thumb affected (i.e. pinch grip).Haemorrhage into the muscle during physical exertion most common cause
• wrist—see carpal tunnel syndrome above (Fig. 25).

description of different types of neuropathy makes it clear that in some circumstances investigations can be targeted. Where this is not the case, blood screening is performed to consider the common or treatable causes of peripheral neuropathy.

Blood tests

• FBC, ESR, vitamin B_{12}/folate, U+E, glucose, LFTs, TFTs, CRP.
• Special blood tests: ANA, ENAs, ANCA, antineuronal antibodies, heavy metals, porphyrins, genetic testing.

Nerve conduction studies and electromyography

These tests should be able to inform you about whether the neuropathy is:
• generalized or multifocal
• motor and/or sensory
• axonal or demyelinating.

Standard nerve conduction studies (NCS) (see Section 3.3, p. 113) only detect abnormalities of large fibres. Hence a patient presenting with distal reduction in pain and temperature and preserved proprioception and reflexes may have normal nerve conduction studies. A more specialized test, detection of thermal thresholds, is required to detect an isolated small fibre neuropathy.

If relevant, limited NCS of affected family members.

CSF examination

This is not usually required for diagnosis. May be helpful in inflammatory neuropathies with proximal involvement (elevated protein).

Paraneoplastic neuropathies may also be associated with elevated protein.

Elevated white cell count in a patient with suspected Guillain–Barré syndrome (GBS) should raise the possibility of HIV-associated inflammatory neuropathy.

Hunt for underlying malignancy

Often unrewarding, but be guided by other symptoms, e.g. chest abdomen, blood film.

Nerve biopsy

Nerve biopsy is an invasive procedure and not without complication [4]. It should only be carried out in a specialist centre. You need to consider whether management is being helped, as diagnostic yields are often low. It is usual to biopsy either the superficial radial or sural nerve: readily accessible pure sensory nerves. If the process is exclusively motor, another nerve must be used. As

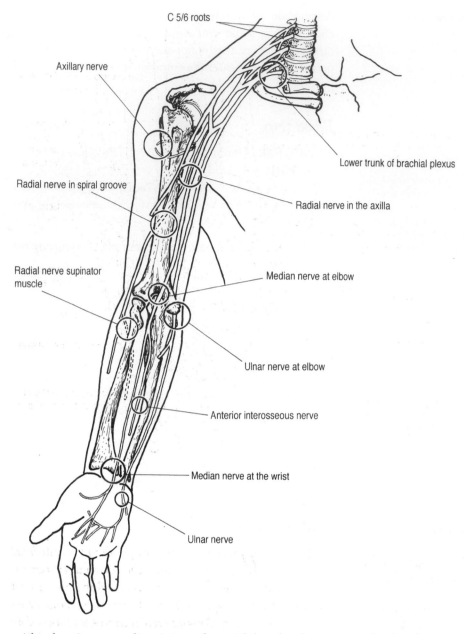

C 5/6 roots

Axillary nerve

Lower trunk of brachial plexus

Radial nerve in spiral groove

Radial nerve in the axilla

Radial nerve supinator muscle

Median nerve at elbow

Ulnar nerve at elbow

Anterior interosseous nerve

Median nerve at the wrist

Ulnar nerve

Fig. 24 Neurological anatomy of the arm showing main locations of damage.

with other tissue sampling, it is preferential that the chosen nerve is involved clinically, but not severely affected, in which case only end-stage disease process may be seen with little or no diagnostic value. Biopsies may show diagnostic abnormalities in vasculitis or amyloidosis. In the case of hereditary neuropathies, the availability of genetic testing is making the role of nerve biopsies less important.

Management

Depends on the underlying cause.

Remove insult or correct metabolic/endocrine abnormality as appropriate. While this may prevent further nerve damage, axonal recovery in particular is slow.

Inflammatory

Unlike GBS, chronic inflammatory demyelinating poly-

radiculopolyneuropathy (CIDP) may respond to steroids. Like GBS, both plasma exchange and intravenous immunoglobulin (IvIg) have equal efficacy. Some clinicians will try a 6–8-week course of high-dose oral prednisolone and reserve IvIg for steroid non-responsive cases [5]. Others use IvIg as a first-line treatment. Treatment courses may need to be repeated if the condition relapses and some become treatment dependant, requiring regular IvIg to maintain well being.

Vasculitic neuropathy

Initial treatment with high-dose oral prednisolone or if severe, a short course of intravenous methyl prednisolone followed by maintenance oral steroids. The use of IvIg is anecdotal but would appear sensible and is becoming more widely used. Systemic, necrotizing vasculitides may require cyclophosphamide.

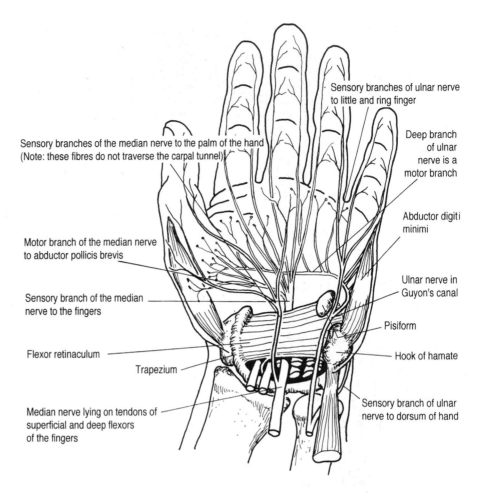

Sensory branches of ulnar nerve to little and ring finger

Deep branch of ulnar nerve is a motor branch

Abductor digiti minimi

Ulnar nerve in Guyon's canal

Pisiform

Hook of hamate

Sensory branch of ulnar nerve to dorsum of hand

Sensory branches of the median nerve to the palm of the hand (Note: these fibres do not traverse the carpal tunnel)

Motor branch of the median nerve to abductor pollicis brevis

Sensory branch of the median nerve to the fingers

Flexor retinaculum

Trapezium

Median nerve lying on tendons of superficial and deep flexors of the fingers

Fig. 25 The anatomy of the median and ulnar nerves in the hand.

Paraneoplastic neuropathy (see Section 2.11.1, p. 104)

1 Asbury AK, Thomas PK. The clinical approach to neuropathy. In: Asbury AK, Thomas PK, eds. *Peripheral Nerve Disorders 2*. Oxford: Butterworth-Heinemann Ltd, 1995.
2 McLeod JG. Investigation of peripheral neuropathy. *J Neurol Neurosurg Psychiatry* 1995; 58: 274–283.
3 Dawson DM. Entrapment neuropathies of the upper extremities. *N Engl J Med*. 1993; 329: 2013–2018.
4 Chia L, Fernandez A, Lacroix C, Adams D, Plante V, Said G. Contribution of nerve biopsy findings to the diagnosis of disabling neuropathy in the elderly. A retrospective review of 100 consecutive patients. *Brain* 1996; 119: 1091–1098.
5 Hadden RD, Lunn MP, Hughes RA. Autoimmune inflammatory neuropathy. *J R Coll Physicians Lond* 1999; 33: 219–224.

2.1.2 GUILLAIN–BARRÉ SYNDROME

Disease

This is defined as an acute (postinfectious) inflammatory demyelinating polyneuropathy, affecting 2 : 100 000 per annum. It is usually monophasic but relapses have been described.

Pathology

This is an inflammatory condition, leading to multifocal demyelination of spinal roots and peripheral nerves. Demyelination may occur anywhere along the lower motor nerve pathway, but the ventral (motor) roots, proximal spinal nerves and lower cranial nerves are most often affected, which accounts for the pattern of clinical features. Much evidence suggests that Guillain–Barré syndrome (GBS) is an organ-specific autoimmune disorder mediated by autoreactive T-cells and humoral antibodies to peripheral nerve antigens. Preceding infections, particularly *Campylobacter jejuni*, may trigger this response through molecular mimicry [1].

Clinical presentation

Approximately 60–70% report an illness in the preceding weeks (often 1–4 weeks prior to the onset). This is usually an upper respiratory tract illness or diarrhoea and many pathogens have been implicated (Table 31).

The onset is subacute, usually over a few days, but can be rapid with complete paralysis in hours. The progression of symptoms, however, may continue for up to 4 weeks (but no longer, by definition).

Table 31 Common pathogens implicated in Guillain–Barré syndrome.

Viral	CMV
	EBV
	HIV
	HepA
Bacterial	Mycoplasma
	Campylobacter jejuni
Immunization	Tetanus toxoid
	?Rabies
	?Swine influenza

The main complaints are of ascending sensory symptoms (symptoms are more prominent than sensory signs) and ascending, or occasionally proximal, weakness. In most cases the legs are affected first and to a greater degree than the arms, but occasionally the arms can be worst affected. Muscle pain is common, as deep intrascapular or lower back pain, or even initiating bilateral sciatica.

Physical signs

The main signs are of symmetrically reduced tone, areflexia, varying degree of glove and stocking sensory disturbance (often mild) and lower motor neurone weakness. Facial involvement and ophthalmoplegia may be present.

Autonomic features occur in approximately half the patients (fluctuations in blood pressure, heart rate, ileus, and urinary retention) [3].

 The clinician must be aware that fixed pupils can occur with autonomic involvement and this must not be confused with brain-stem pathology.

Other clinical variants of GBS are described in Table 32.

Investigations

If the condition is suspected clinically, your priorities are to monitor for potential complications, particularly respiratory and cardiac. Further investigations may confirm the diagnosis but are unlikely to be available immediately.

Table 32 Clinical variants of Guillain–Barré syndrome.

Miller–Fisher syndrome (ataxia, areflexia and ophthalmoplegia)
Cranial nerve variant (polyneuritis cranialis)
Pure sensory variant
Pharyngeal-cervical-brachial variant
Acute autonomic variant
Axonal variant (motor and sensory)
Acute motor axonal variant

Initial management therefore has to be based on clinical suspicion.

Measurement of respiratory function

Monitor forced vital capacity (not peak flow) at regular intervals, the frequency depending on the severity of the weakness or rate of change.

Cardiac monitor

Doctors are aware of the respiratory complications of GBS but neglect the autonomic complications. Dysrhythmias can be fatal without intervention.

CSF

May be normal in the first few days. Later protein rises as a consequence of inflammation in the proximal roots (within the subarachnoid space). If pleocytosis is present, consider other diagnosis (see Differential diagnosis, below).

Nerve conduction studies

In GBS peripheral nerve demyelination starts proximally at the nerve roots. Distal conduction velocities and distal motor latencies are therefore normal early in the illness, even in the face of profound weakness. The earliest electrophysiological abnormality is prolongation, impersistence or absence of the F wave (see Section 3.3.4, p. 115). EMG will show denervation in later stages.

Antiganglioside antibodies

Gangliosides are sialyated glycosphingolipids found on nerves. Anti GQ1b antibodies appear to be present in all cases of GBS with associated ophthalmoplegia, particularly the Miller–Fisher variant (triad of ataxia, areflexia and ophthalmoplegia).

Identification of the infective agent

- Often negative, but may help with prognosis if positive [1].
- Stool culture for *Campylobacter jejuni*.
- Serology for atypical pneumonias.
- CSF viral analysis.

Differential diagnosis

The differential diagnosis of acute/subacute weakness is broad but important. Given a good history together with examination features that are clear, GBS is the commonest cause, but consider the following.

- Other acute neuropathies including porphyria.
- Metabolic disturbances (severe hypophosphataemia, hypokalaemia, hypermagnesaemia) should be excluded.
- Myasthenia gravis may cause subacute onset weakness. Look for fatigability.
- Occasionally CNS disease, such as acute brain-stem stroke, spinal cord compression or transverse myelitis, may cause confusion, but a careful history and examination should prevent this mistake from being made.
- Poliomyelitis is now a less common differential. The presentation is usually strikingly asymmetrical, which helps differentiate it from the symmetrical picture of GBS.
- Typical features of GBS associated with CSF pleocytosis (over 50 cells/µL) raise the possibility of meningoradiculitis caused by HIV, Lyme disease, tuberculosis or cytomegalovirus infection.

Treatment

The following points need to be considered:
- Patients who are deteriorating should be transferred to a unit that is able to deal with neuromuscular respiratory failure and autonomic dysfunction.
- Consider elective ventilation early if the patient is tiring.
- Cardiac arrhythmias should be treated as appropriate (see *Cardiology*, Section 2.2).
- Antihypertensive drugs must be used with extreme caution in the presence of autonomic dysfunction.
- Note that tracheal suction may trigger hypotension or bradycardia in the presence of autonomic dysfunction.
- Treat pain with non-steroidal anti-inflammatory drugs or opiates.
- Feed patients via nasogastric tube or PEG if necessary.
- Prophylactic subcutaneous heparin and TED stockings for immobile patients.
- Regular chest physiotherapy.
- Regular turning.
- Early physiotherapy.
- Psychological support for the patient and their family.

Specific treatment

Prior to 1997, plasma exchange (PE) was the favoured treatment. In January 1997 the results of an international, multicentre randomized trial comparing PE with intravenous immunoglobulin (IvIg) alone, or with both PE and IvIg were reported in the *Lancet*. This study showed that a 5-day course of IvIg (0.4 g/kg/day) was as efficacious as PE but with fewer side effects. PE followed by IvIg did not confer a significant advantage. The entrance criteria were patients within 14 days of the onset of symptoms and who were unable to walk unaided. Patients with mild GBS do not require treatment [4].

IvIg is easily administered. This should not dissuade the clinician from early transfer of the patient to a centre with a good ITU. If a patient requires treatment, they require transfer!

Prognosis

GBS begins with a period of deterioration, then a plateau phase, followed by a period of recovery. In series, up to 30% of patients require ventilation. Mortality remains about 4.5% despite treatment. On the whole this is a self-limiting disease. In very broad terms, one-third make a full recovery (although may remain areflexic), one-third are left with mild disability and one-third have moderate to severe disability.

Preceding illness with *Campylobacter jejuni* can result in a severe axonal variant with a poor prognosis.

1 Rees JH, Soudain SE, Gregson NA, Hughes RAC. *Campylobacter jejuni* infection and Guillain–Barré syndrome. *N Engl J Med* 1995; 333: 1374–1379.
2 Desforges JF. The Guillain–Barré syndrome. *N Engl J Med* 1992; 326: 1130–1136.
3 Pascuzzi RM, Fleck JD. Acute peripheral neuropathies in adults. *Neurol Clinics* 1997; 15(3): 529–547.
4 Plasma Exchange/Sandoglobulin Guillain–Barré Syndrome Trial Group. Randomised trial of plasma exchange, intravenous immunoglobulin, and combined treatments in Guillain–Barré syndrome. *Lancet* 1997; 349: 225–230.

2.1.3 MOTOR NEURONE DISEASE

Aetiology

The causes of motor neurone disease (MND) are unknown, but many hypotheses have been suggested [1]. Mutations in the cytosolic Cu/Zn superoxide dismutase gene on chromosome 21 accounts for 20% of cases of familial amyotrophic lateral sclerosis and 2% of all cases of amyotrophic lateral sclerosis (ALS). Glutamate is a major excitatory neurotransmitter, and overstimulation of glutamate receptors is associated with neurotoxicity in MND. Oxidative stress with free radical damage is also implicated in the pathogenesis of MND. Other proposed causes of MND are environmental agents (e.g. heavy metals), viral infections and autoimmunity, although none of these is substantiated.

Epidemiology

The incidence of MND is 1–3 per 100 000, with the mean age of onset being 55 years. The male to female ratio is 3 : 2. Ten per cent of cases are familial, usually of an autosomal dominant inheritance. Most cases of MND are of the ALS type that has both upper motor neurone (UMN) and lower motor neurone (LMN) involvement. The other clinical variants, progressive muscular atrophy (PMA) with its purely LMN involvement and primary lateral sclerosis (PLS) with its purely UMN involvement, may just represent ends of the spectrum of ALS.

Clinical presentation

Muscle weakness is the most common presenting complaint, with onset in the arms more common than in the legs. Occasionally, one limb may become involved on its own.

Some patients notice muscle twitching or fasciculations, muscle cramps and easy fatigability.

 Fasciculations are virtually never the sole presenting feature of MND.

In 20% of patients, bulbar symptoms are the initial problem, e.g. dysarthria, dysphagia, difficulty chewing or coughing, and eventually sialorrhoea. Weight loss may occur. Rarely, respiratory muscle weakness causing breathlessness is the first symptom.

Physical signs

Cranial nerve examination may reveal lower cranial nerve involvement, e.g. facial weakness (VIIth), depressed gag reflex (IXth/Xth), poor palatal movement (Xth) and a wasted, fasciculating tongue (XIIth, bulbar palsy). A brisk jaw jerk (Vth), increased gag reflex or a spastic tongue indicates pseudobulbar palsy.

In the limbs, UMN involvement produces spasticity, weakness, hyperreflexia and Babinski sign, while LMN involvement produces atrophy (Fig. 26) fasciculations, flaccidity, weakness and hyporeflexia.

In MND there is no extraocular or sphincter disturbance, and sensory examination is normal.
You should never examine for fasciculations when the tongue is protruded, as you will often see 'abnormalities' that are not really present.

Investigation

See Section 1.10, p. 20.
Further points on investigation are as follows:
• Anti-GM1 ganglioside antibodies and EMG are important in ruling out multifocal motor neuropathy (MMN).
• MRI excludes cervical spine and foramen magnum lesions, e.g. syringomyelia, syringobulbia and cervical spondylosis.

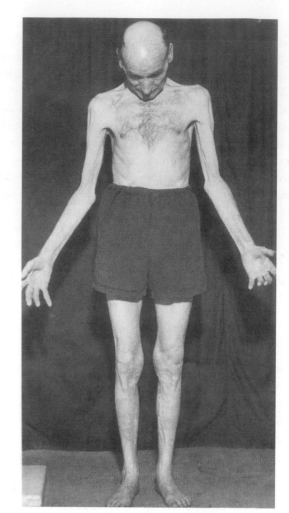

Fig. 26 Wasted muscles in motor neurone disease.

Differential diagnosis

Misdiagnosis of MND is a common clinical problem with serious implications. Certain differentials should always be considered.
• Spondylotic cervical myelopathy should always be considered. Although this is a potentially treatable condition, there is increasing doubt as to whether it can actually mimic MND as it almost always causes only spastic paraparesis [3].
• It is important to diagnose MMN because it is potentially treatable with intravenous immunoglobulin or cyclophosphamide. It is associated with LMN signs only and anti-GM1 ganglioside antibodies, although these are not specific [4].
• X-linked bulbospinal neuronopathy (Kennedy's disease): associated with perioral fasciculation, LMN signs only, gynaecomastia, testicular atrophy, diabetes mellitus and a CAG expansion in the androgen receptor locus.
• Benign fasciculations, hexosaminidase A deficiency (Tay–Sachs disease), lymphoproliferative disorders and thyrotoxicosis may all mimic MND and should be excluded in atypical cases.

Treatment

Symptomatic treatment and supportive care are the mainstays of management in MND. The patient's right to self-determination should be respected at all times.

Riluzole, a sodium channel blocker that inhibits glutamate release, has only modest effects on disease progression but is expensive. Liver function needs to be monitored when it is used [5].

Neurotrophic factors, e.g. brain-derived neurotrophic factor (BDNF), are undergoing clinical trials to assess their effectiveness.

Prognosis

Death usually ensues in 3–5 years from aspiration pneumonia and respiratory failure.

Poor prognosis factors include:
- older patients
- shorter duration between onset and diagnosis
- ALS (rather than PLS or PMA)
- low amplitude muscle action potentials
- low serum chloride.

1 Shaw PJ. Motor neurone disease. *Br Med J* 1999; 318: 1118–1121.
2 Traynor BJ, Codd MB, Corr RN, Forde C, Frost E, Hardiman O. Amyotrophic lateral sclerosis mimic syndromes: a population based study. *Arch Neurol* 2000; 57: 109–113.
3 Rowland LP. Diagnosis of amyotrophic lateral sclerosis. *J Neurol Sci* 1998; 160 (Suppl 1); S6–S24.
4 Bentes C, de Carvalho M, Evangelista T, Selas Luis ML. Multifocal motor neuropathy mimicking motor neurone disease: nine cases. *J Neurol Sci* 1999; 169: 76–79.
5 Riluzole for amyotrophic lateral sclerosis. *Drug Ther Bull* 1997; 35(2): 11–12.

2.2 Diseases of muscle

A wide range of sporadic and hereditary insults can affect muscle. These include:
- systemic disorders of metabolism
- local and systemic inflammatory conditions
- hereditary disorders of muscle itself
- abnormalities of membrane ion channels.

Presentation may be with weakness, cramps, pain or a combination of these. The age of onset, presence or otherwise of a positive family history, nature of presentation and distribution of muscle involvement are all instructive pointers to the aetiology [1]. A classification of muscle disorders is given in Table 33.

Table 33 Classification of muscle disease.

Metabolic	Disorders of carbohydrate metabolism
	Disorders of lipid metabolism
	Mitochondrial myopathies
Inflammatory	Polymyositis
	Dermatomyositis
	Inclusion body myositis
Inherited myopathies	Disorders of dystrophin
	Limb girdle muscular dystrophies
	Fascioscapulohumeral dystrophy
	Emery–Dreifuss muscular dystrophy
	Myotonic dystrophy
	Others
Channelopathies	Periodic paralysis
	Myotonia

2.2.1 METABOLIC MUSCLE DISEASE

Disorders of carbohydrate metabolism (glycogen storage diseases)

Pathophysiology

Figure 27 describes the biochemical pathway by which

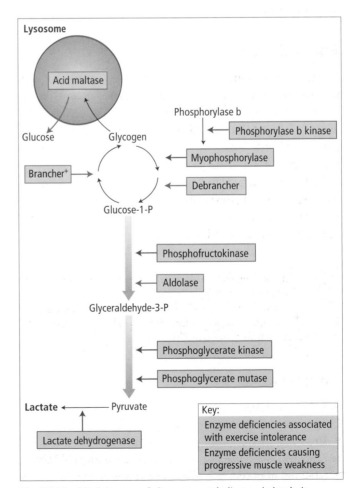

Fig. 27 Simplified diagram of glycogen metabolism and glycolysis.

glycogen metabolism and glycolysis occurs within muscle cells (see *Biochemistry and metabolism*, Section 2). Deficiency of enzymes shown have all been associated with disease. Clinically, enzyme deficiencies can be divided into those associated with exercise intolerance and those causing progressive muscle weakness. The most important disease of each group is described below.

McArdle's disease

Also called myophosphorylase deficiency or type V glycogenosis. The same clinical picture is seen with phosphorylase b kinase deficiency (Fig. 27). First described by McArdle in 1952.

Genetics

Myophosphorylase gene encoded on 11q.13. Usually autosomal recessive (AR) but autosomal dominant (AD) inheritance described.

Clinical presentation

Carbohydrate stores within muscle are necessary in the early stages of exercise prior to added energy supply being provided by lipid metabolism. Disorders of carbohydrate metabolism therefore present with exercise intolerance after minimal exercise. A 'second wind' phenomenon may be described if the patient exercises gently through the initial barrier allowing diversion of blood flow to muscle and onset of fatty acid metabolism.

Symptoms

Often presents in the second and third decade, although in retrospect there may have been poor exercise tolerance as a child. Symptoms include:
• muscle pain after minutes of exercise
• painful muscle contractures
• episodes of dark urine (myoglobinuria secondary to rhabdomyolysis).

Physical signs

Usually no abnormal signs when resting. Patients may develop a mild myopathy late in the disease.

Investigation

Consider the following:
• Provocative exercise tests to demonstrate increased creatinine kinase (CK) or failure to increase lactate (ischaemic lactate test) may precipitate muscle necrosis and are potentially harmful.

• EMG: may be normal. Painful contractures are electrically silent.
• Muscle biopsy: routine histology may be normal or may show some necrosis. May show increased glycogen. Specific muscle biochemistry confirms enzyme deficiency.

Acid maltase deficiency

Also called Pompe's disease or type II glycogenosis. First described by Pompe in 1932.

Clinical presentation

There are four types: infantile, late infantile, juvenile and adult, the severity decreasing with the increased age of onset. Cardiac involvement is almost invariable in the severe infantile type but is less frequent in the adult form.

Symptoms

Progressive weakness. There may be respiratory involvement, often as the prominent feature.

Physical signs

Muscle weakness ± signs of cardiac or respiratory involvement.

Investigation

The following will confirm the diagnosis:
• Creatinine kinase (CK) may be normal or moderately raised.
• EMG is usually myopathic with neurogenic changes and complex repetitive discharges late in the disease.
• Muscle biopsy demonstrates evidence of increased glycogen storage.
• Enzyme analysis: from muscle, leucocyte or fibroblast culture.

Treatment

Supportive only.

Disorders of lipid metabolism

Carnitine palmitoyl transferase (CPT) deficiency

Pathophysiology

Lipid metabolism, in particular oxidation of fatty acids, takes over from carbohydrate metabolism on sustained exercise. The enzyme CPT catalyses the coupling of carnitine to long-chain fatty acids, a reaction that must occur for the transfer of fatty acids across the mitochondrial membrane (see *Biochemistry and metabolism*, Section 3).

Clinical presentation

Presents in young adults.

Symptoms

Suspect this diagnosis if the following are features.
• Bouts of weakness after prolonged exercise.
• Myoglobinuria (more severe than in the glycogenoses).
• Respiratory involvement may be associated with severe attacks.

The patient may subconsciously adapt to his circumstances, preferring sprinting to long distance running and snacking on sweet food to improve stamina.

Physical signs

Examination may be normal.

Investigations

• CK is normal unless soon after an attack.
• Muscle biopsy shows increased lipid storage.
• Biochemical analysis of muscle will show the enzyme defect.

Treatment

Avoid precipitating factors.

Mitochondrial disorders

The respiratory chain of mitochondria is responsible for oxidative metabolism within cells. Diseases of mitochondrial function tip the cell towards anaerobic mechanisms and lactic acidosis [2]. Mitochondrial myopathies are one group in a range of diseases of mitochondrial dysfunction, the mitochondrial cytopathies.

Mitochondria and their disorders are inherited through the maternal line. Some aspects of their function, however, are under nuclear control, therefore some mitochondrial disorders may have a defect of nuclear rather than mitochondrial DNA.

2.2.2 INFLAMMATORY MUSCLE DISEASE

Polymyositis and dermatomyositis have been covered elsewhere (see *Rheumatology and clinical immunology*, Section 2.3.5) and will not be repeated here.

Inclusion body myositis

This can be sporadic or hereditary.

Sporadic IBM

Clinical presentation

• Inclusion body myositis (IBM) affects men more than women. More common over the age of 50.
• Painless weakness and wasting, with selective involvement of long finger flexors and anterior thigh muscles (quadriceps). May be asymmetrical.
• Relentless progression.

Investigation

• CK mildly elevated.
• Imaging: MRI can show the pattern of wasting and therefore distinguish sporadic from hereditary IBM (see below).
• EMG as in polymyositis, with spontaneous activity and myopathic features.
• Muscle biopsy shows myopathic changes with endomysial CD8+ T-cell infiltrate. Rimmed vacuoles and characteristic tubulofilamentous inclusions. Interestingly, there is an abnormal accumulation of proteins within the diseased muscle fibres including β amyloid, amgloid precursor protein (APP) and prion protein.

Treatment

IBM does not respond to steroids, despite the inflammatory changes. This may suggest that the inflammation is a secondary phenomenon.

Hereditary IBM

This is far less common than the sporadic type, and can be differentiated as follows:
• Usually AR and linked to chromosome 9.
• Dramatic sparing of quadriceps.
• No inflammation on biopsy.

2.2.3 INHERITED DYSTROPHIES (MYOPATHIES)

These are a diverse group of hereditary muscle disorders.

Disorders of dystrophin

Pathophysiology

The key to understanding why a defect in dystrophin, or

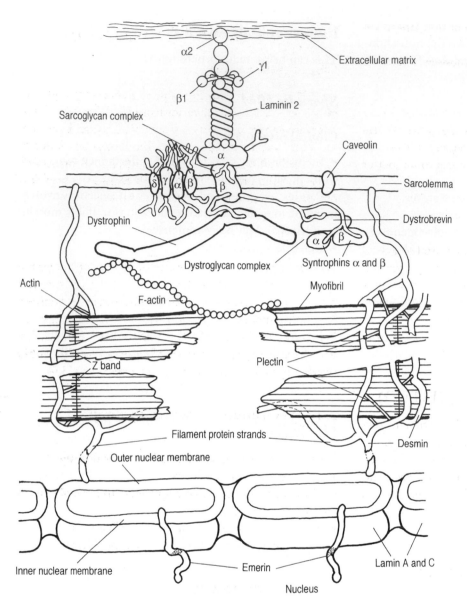

Fig. 28 The dystrophin-associated glycoprotein complex (DGC) is found in the muscle fibre membrane and is connected to the supporting and contractile apparatus of the muscle fibre.

certain other proteins (see AR limb girdle muscular dystrophy (LGMD) C-F below) can have such a devastating effect on muscle is the dystrophin–glycoprotein complex (DGC) shown in Fig. 28. This is a protein complex found within the sarcolemma that couples the contractile apparatus of the cell to the extracellular matrix through laminin 2. Each member of the DGC is an integral component, with deficiency of any one leading to disease.

Duchenne's muscular dystrophy (DMD)

Clinical presentation

X-linked. Presents in early childhood, often in second year, with clumsiness. Proximal weakness and falls develop over the next few years, and pseudohypertrophy of the calf muscles is noticed.

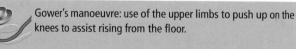

Gower's manoeuvre: use of the upper limbs to push up on the knees to assist rising from the floor.

The patient is wheelchair bound by the early teens, with the loss of mobility contributing to contractures and scoliosis. Cardiac involvement usually occurs and is characterized by cardiomyopathy. Death is from respiratory or cardiac involvement.

Investigations

- CK (often >10 000 mU/mL).
- EMG: myopathic.
- Muscle biopsy: severe dystrophic changes with

characteristic hyaline fibres. Absence of dystrophin on immunocytochemistry.
- DNA analysis: Xp21, molecular diagnosis available.

Treatment

The use of corticosteroids is controversial, but some feel they are beneficial. Other than this, treatment is primarily supportive, although gene therapy may offer better outcomes in the future.

Becker's muscular dystrophy

X-linked. This is a milder form of DMD caused by a deficiency or defect in, rather than absence of, dystrophin. It presents late in the first decade of life and patients may not be wheelchair bound until their third decade. Cardiomyopathy may be severe. Female carriers of an abnormal dystrophin gene may have a raised CK and cardiomyopathy.

Limb girdle muscular dystrophy (LGMD)

LGMDs have historically been lumped together to distinguish them from the X-linked muscular dystrophies (above) and facioscapulohumeral dystrophy (below). Recent developments have allowed molecular classification of these disorders. Only the briefest of synopsis will be given here, but the reader is referred to two excellent reviews [3,4].

Autosomal dominant limb girdle muscular dystrophy (AD LGMD or LGMD1)

Features are as follows:
- Less severe than autosomal recessive LGMD (AR LGMD), often with adult onset.
- Most have been identified in single large families.
- In 2000, five different genetic loci had been identified, LGMD1A-E.

Autosomal recessive limb girdle muscular dystrophy (AR LGMD or LGMD2)

Features are as follows:
- Often presents in childhood and can be clinically similar to the dystrophinopathies.
- Eight types have been identified, LGMD2A-H.
- LGMD2A has a deficiency of the protein calpain.
- LGMD2B has a deficiency of the protein dysferlin.
- LGMD2C-F have deficiencies of the sarcoglycans (see Fig. 28).

Facioscapulohumeral dystrophy (FSH)

Clinical presentation

An AD condition with incomplete penetrance and sporadic cases. Clinically, it varies from mild facial weakness to severe generalized weakness involving particularly, face, scapular fixators, triceps, biceps, hip flexors and anterior thigh and calf muscles. Deltoid is often well preserved. Typically it commences around early teens with only slow progression, but this is extremely variable.

Genetics

Tandem repeat deletion identified at 4q35. The longer the deletion, the more severe the illness with earlier onset and more rapid progression. Anticipation is seen in families, suggesting increasing deletion size with each generation. Penetrance varies, being 95% in males and 65% in females. The deletion appears to be located close by (possibly within regulatory DNA) but not within an actual gene [3,4].

Emery-Dreifuss muscular dystrophy (EDMD)

This rare disease is characterized by the following:
- Xq28, deficiency of emerin.
- Similar phenotype also recognized with normal emerin and AD inheritance.
- Early contractures and cardiac complications.
- Female carriers may develop cardiac problems.

Myotonic dystrophy

Clinical features

Myotonia is best demonstrated by getting the patient to open and close the fist rapidly, or by percussing the thenar eminence with a tendon hammer, which causes the thumb to flex across the palm. Myotonia is difficult to demonstrate in the tongue as the mouth is warm, and myotonia is best demonstrated in the cold.

Mild, progressive myopathy starting distally. Facial involvement with ptosis.

ASSOCIATED FEATURES

Look for the following:
- cardiac conduction abnormalities
- frontal balding
- cataracts
- gonadal atrophy
- glucose intolerance
- mental retardation.

Investigations

GENETICS

AD gene at 19q13.1 in which there is an abnormal large expansion of CTG trinucleotide repeats. The disorder shows anticipation (i.e. worse in successive generations) and may have been undiagnosed in older generations in whom signs may have been restricted to cataracts and mild ptosis.

OTHER INVESTIGATIONS

DNA analysis should be first line and it is no longer necessary to subject patients to EMG. EMG, however, will demonstrate characteristic myotonic discharges (likened to a dive-bomber or motorcycle revving up).

Treatment

Mainly supportive.

2.2.4 CHANNELOPATHIES

A group of disorders characterized by episodic paralysis or myotonia due to mutations of either the calcium or sodium channel gene [5].

1 Mastalgia FL, Laing NG. Investigation of muscle disease. *J Neurol Neurosurg Psychiatry* 1996; 60: 256–274.
2 Leonard JV, Schapira AH. Mitochondrial respiratory chain disorders I: mitochondrial DNA defects. *Lancet* 2000 22; 355(9200): 299–304.
3 Bushby KMD. Making sense of the limb-girdle muscular dystrophies. *Brain* 1999; 122: 1403–1420.
4 Beckmann JS, Brown RH, Muntoni F, Urtizberea A, Bonnemann C, Bushby KMD. 66th/67th ENMC sponsored international workshop: the limb-girdle muscular dystrophies 26–28 March 1999, Naarden, The Netherlands. *Neuromuscul Disord* 1999; 9: 436–445.
[These are two excellent, up-to-date reviews of the LGMDs.]
5 Lehmann-Horn F, Rudel R. Channelopathies: the non-dystrophic myotonias and periodic paralyses. *Semin Paediatr Neurol* 1996; 3(2): 122–139.

2.2.5 MYASTHENIA GRAVIS

Aetiology/pathophysiology

Myasthenia gravis (MG) is caused by an antibody-mediated autoimmune attack against acetylcholine receptors at neuromuscular junctions. This leads to a degradation of acetylcholine receptors and reduced neurotransmission to skeletal muscle. Anti-acetylcholine receptor antibody titres tend to be higher in more severe disease, but 20% of patients (50% in ocular myasthenia) are seronegative.

Seventy-five per cent of patients have thymic abnormalities, usually hyperplasia, but thymomas are seen in 10%. The thymus, with its antigen-presenting cells, T cells and B cells, is therefore thought to play a key role in the pathophysiology of MG [1].

Epidemiology

The prevalence of MG is estimated at approximately 10 cases per 100 000 population. It has a bimodal age distribution: the second and third decades in women and the seventh and eight decades in men. The female to male ratio is 2 : 1. MG is often associated with other autoimmune diseases, e.g. Graves' disease [2].

Clinical presentation

Patients most commonly present with ptosis and diplopia (70%), not with fatigue. Oropharyngeal weakness (difficulty chewing, swallowing and talking) is the initial symptom in 15%, and limb weakness in 10%. The severity of symptoms fluctuates during the day, being less severe in the morning and more severe as the day goes on. Exacerbation of symptoms may occur in intercurrent infections, pregnancy, menses and with certain drugs [3], e.g. aminoglycosides, β-blockers, calcium antagonists, procainamide, quinidine and neuromuscular blocking agents. D-penicillamine may induce MG.

 Since many drugs have been observed to worsen weakness, all patients with MG should be monitored when a new drug is started.

MG remains purely ocular in 10%, and the rest develop generalized weakness, usually within 2 years. After 10–15 years the weakness becomes fixed with little fluctuation.

Physical signs

In MG the weakness shows fatigability. Repetitive testing is therefore needed to fully appreciate this feature. The pattern of weakness does not conform to the distribution of any particular nerves. In the eyes there is ptosis and extraocular muscle weakness, particularly the medial rectus, with sparing of the pupillary reflexes. There may be facial weakness that characteristically gives a 'myasthenic snarl' on attempted smiling, dysarthria, hoarseness, nasal speech, dysphagia and difficulty chewing.

 Weakness of neck flexors is often a good indicator of weakness. However, any limb or trunk muscles may be weak. Deep tendon reflexes are normal. Patients are occasionally diagnosed as hysterical because of the odd distribution of weakness and the fatigability.

Investigation

The following may be useful:
• The edrophonium chloride (Tensilon) test is positive in about 90% of those with MG. It is performed as follows: first identify what it is that you are going to measure, best results being obtained with diplopia, ptosis and dysarthria. The patient is pretreated with 400 µg atropine i.v., then given edrophonium, in doses of 2 mg, 3 mg, 5 mg with at least 1–2 min between each injection. Observe for a transient response.
• Serum antiacetylcholine receptor antibodies are present in 80% of patients with generalized MG and 50% with ocular MG. Anti-striated muscle antibodies are associated with thymoma.
• An autoantibody screen and thyroid function tests should be done because of the association with other autoimmune diseases.
• Single-fibre electromyography (SFEMG) shows increased jitter in MG, but this also occurs in other neuromuscular transmission disorders (see clinical pointer box below).
• Electromyography shows decremental response to repetitive nerve stimulation in muscles.
• A chest radiograph (Fig. 29) and CT thorax should be done to look for a thymoma.

SFEMG is performed by simultaneously recording the evoked responses from two muscle fibres of the same motor unit. In a normal muscle, action potentials recorded from two such muscle fibres are not synchronous. This variation in interpotential interval is defined as 'jitter'. Because of the variable neuromuscular transmission, this jitter is increased in disorders of the neuromuscular junction.

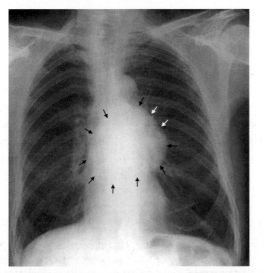

Fig. 29 Thymoma. (From Ray, Ryder, Wellings, *An Aid to Radiology for the MRCP.* Oxford: Blackwell Science 1999.)

Differential diagnosis

Genetic forms of myasthenia are not immune mediated, but are caused by mutations of the acetylcholine receptor. These need to be excluded. The Lambert–Eaton myasthenic syndrome (LEMS) usually occurs in association with malignancy, mostly small-cell lung cancers. Autoantibodies against voltage-gated calcium channels are thought to result in insufficient release of acetylcholine upon depolarization of the presynaptic membrane. Unlike MG, muscle strength increases after exercise (postexercise facilitation), deep tendon reflexes are depressed (but increase with exercise), extraocular muscles are usually spared, autonomic dysfunction may be prominent and there is incremental response to repetitive nerve stimulation. (See also Sections 1.10, p. 20 and 1.14, p. 31.)

Treatment

Drugs

Anticholinesterases produce temporary improvement. Immunosuppressives are effective but take weeks or months to work. Steroids should be started at low doses to prevent exacerbation of weakness after initiation. Plasma exchange or intravenous immunoglobulins are used for temporary but rapid benefit of sudden worsening of MG.

Thymectomy

Thymectomy should be considered for most patients [4].
• Maximum response is seen 2–5 years after surgery.
• Best response is seen in young patients, but benefit can occur in late disease, and older patients should certainly be considered.
• Is not generally recommended for patients with purely ocular disease, but occasionally dramatic benefit is also seen in this patient group.
• Occasionally, thymic tissue is left behind, so repeat surgery should be considered for chronic or relapsing disease if this is felt to be the case.

Complications

The most serious consequence of MG is neuromuscular respiratory failure.

Respiratory failure may be due to the disease itself and/or inadequate doses of anticholinesterases (myasthenic crisis) or overdose of anticholinesterases (cholinergic crisis). It ought to be simple to tell the two apart, but in practice it can be difficult. Therefore the safest option is to discontinue all anticholinesterases temporarily and ventilate the patient if necessary.

1 Boonyapisit K, Kaminski HJ, Ruff RL. Disorders of neuromuscular junction ion channels. *Am J Med* 1999; 106: 97–113.

2 Drachman DB. Myasthenia gravis. *N Engl J Med* 1994; 330: 1797–1810.

3 Wittbrodt ET. Drugs and myasthenia gravis. *Arch Intern Med* 1997; 157: 399–408.

4 Urschel JD, Grewal RP. Thymectomy for myasthenia gravis. *Postgrad Med J* 1998; 74: 139–144.

2.3 Extrapyramidal disorders

2.3.1 PARKINSON'S DISEASE

Pathophysiology

Idiopathic Parkinson's disease (IPD) is characterized by degeneration primarily of the striato-nigral pathway with loss of dopaminergic cells, and by the presence of Lewy bodies seen at *post mortem*.

Aetiology

This is unknown, but probably multifactorial. Some genes and loci (e.g. α-synuclein) are now identified in a few families. Many external factors have been suggested in the past, but no causative agents have been clearly implicated.

Epidemiology

• Prevalence increases with age: ~1% in over sixties (~0.1% in the general population).
• No geographical differences exist, and it is just as common in males as females.
• Previous epidemiological studies indicated a lower incidence in smokers, but it is unclear whether this is actually protective.

Clinical presentation

See also Section 1.3, p. 8.

Common presenting features

Common features are listed below:
• gait disturbance
• slowness/decreased dexterity
• pain and stiffness in limbs and back
• deterioration in handwriting
• tremor.

Non-motor features

These include:
• depression
• anosmia
• erectile and urinary dysfunction
• constipation.

Later problems

These features would not normally be part of the presenting or early clinical picture:
• loss of balance
• dementia
• swallowing difficulties, drooling and severe speech impairment.

Treatment complications

These may become the dominant clinical features later in the disease:
• 'wearing off' of medication between doses, and later
• 'motor fluctuations': sudden changes between 'on' state (medication working and symptom relief) and 'off' state (medication apparently ineffective)
• 'peak dose' and 'end of dose/beginning of dose' dyskinesias
• gait 'freezing', even when otherwise 'on'
• hallucinations (usually visual) and confusion, usually drug related.

Investigations

> IPD is a clinical diagnosis and in the context of a typical history and examination, no investigations are required.

If the diagnosis or response to dopaminergic therapy is unclear, a formal levodopa or apomorphine challenge can help, and if positive, point towards IPD, although a small proportion of patients with other syndromes may respond partially.

Where the diagnosis is still unclear, time will always tell. Functional imaging of the basal ganglia (using SPECT or PET) can be very helpful by showing greatly reduced striato-nigral dopaminergic activity. In some cases the correct diagnosis may not be made until *post mortem*.

In younger patients, serum copper studies should be performed to exclude Wilson's disease, and the Westphal variant of Huntington's disease (and, if indicated, genetic counselling and testing) should also be considered (see Section 1.5, p. 12).

Table 34 Common causes of parkinsonism.

Pseudoparkinsonism	Benign essential tremor
	Vascular parkinsonism
True parkinsonism	Idiopathic Parkinson's disease
	Drug-induced parkinsonism
	Steele–Richardson–Olszewski disease
	Multiple system atrophy

Table 35 Clinical 'red flags' in the diagnosis of idiopathic Parkinson's disease.

Early instability or falls
Poor response to L-DOPA
Absent L-DOPA-induced dyskinesias
Rapid progression
Pyramidal or cerebellar signs
Dementia
Downgaze palsy (upgaze palsy is non-specific)
Severe dysphonia, dysarthria, dysphagia
Respiratory stridor
Myoclonus

Differential diagnosis

The commoner causes of parkinsonism are listed in Table 34.

> Cerebrovascular disease is only very rarely a cause of true parkinsonism, and the 'lower body parkinsonism' caused by extensive small vessel ischaemic cerebrovascular disease should not be misdiagnosed as IPD (see Section 1.4, p. 10).

The most important differential diagnosis of IPD is drug-induced parkinsonism as this is treatable. The parkinson-plus syndromes are rarer, but certain clinical 'red-flags' should alert you to the possibility that IPD is not the correct diagnosis (Table 35) [1].

Treatment

See Section 2.12, p. 106, for background to neuropharmacology.

Levodopa

Levodopa remains the gold-standard treatment for Parkinson's disease (PD), being the most effective and well tolerated of the anti-parkinsonian drugs [2].

Mechanism of action

To understand the rationale for the various different treatment strategies in PD, it is necessary to consider levodopa metabolism (Fig. 30). Seventy per cent of peripheral levodopa

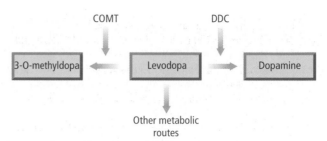

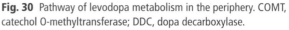

Fig. 30 Pathway of levodopa metabolism in the periphery. COMT, catechol O-methyltransferase; DDC, dopa decarboxylase.

is converted to dopamine via the dopa-decarboxylase (DDC) pathway. Stimulation of peripheral dopamine receptors causes nausea and vomiting. To prevent this, common levodopa preparations contain a DDC inhibitor (e.g. 'sinemet' = levodopa + cocareldopa; 'madopar' = levodopa + benseraside). This increases CNS bioavailability from 1% to 10%. Inhibition of DDC shifts peripheral metabolism of levodopa to previously minor pathways, such as metabolism by catechol O-methyltransferase (COMT).

Side effects

Peripheral dopaminergic side effects, such as nausea and postural hypotension (usually only a problem when starting treatment) can be controlled by coadministration of the peripheral dopaminergic antagonist; domperidone (the only safe antiemetic to give to parkinsonian patients).

Central effects such as hallucinations, confusion and dyskinesias can become a problem in later disease and may be dose limiting. Some experts advocate delaying levodopa therapy to try and delay the onset of long-term complications, but this area is controversial and there is no evidence that levodopa is toxic to human substantia nigra.

Dopamine agonists

These act directly on the postsynaptic receptors, thus mimicking the effect of endogenous dopamine. They can be effective 'levodopa-sparing' agents and have longer half-lives than levodopa, thus are extremely useful in the later stages of disease, when 'wearing-off' and motor fluctuations become a problem. There is some evidence to suggest that early use of dopamine agonists, rather than levodopa, delays the onset of dyskinesias; however, the question as to whether early agonist monotherapy has any real benefit in the long term remains controversial.

Examples are bromocriptine, pergolide, ropinirole, pramipexole and cabergoline. The side-effect profile is similar to levodopa, although the agonists tend to be less well tolerated, especially by the elderly, and need to be titrated up cautiously. There have been some reports of sudden onset of sleep at the wheel, which is relevant when prescribing for patients who are still driving.

Apomorphine is a very potent agonist, usually given subcutaneously (a very high first pass metabolism excludes the oral route) either by intermittent injections or, in severe disease, by a continuous infusion. It is extremely effective in improving motor fluctuations and, when used as monotherapy, dyskinesias [3].

Side effects

Consider the following:
• Domperidone is usually given from the start of treatment to avoid nausea and postural hypotension.
• Autoimmune haemolytic anaemia is a rare but serious complication, and thus 3-monthly full blood count and Coombs' tests should be performed on all patients on apomorphine.

Amantadine

This is an NMDA receptor antagonist, but its exact mechanism of action in IPD is unclear. Amantadine was previously used in early disease but fell out of favour. However, following new evidence to demonstrate an anti-dyskinetic effect, it is receiving renewed interest.

Side effects

These include confusion, hallucination and leg oedema.

Selegiline ('Deprenyl'/'Eldepryl')

This is an irreversible monoamine oxidase B inhibitor. Two interesting issues have arisen surrounding this drug.

First, experimental evidence that it is also 'neuroprotective', slowing disease progression, has not been substantiated in humans. The DATATOP study suggested a delay in the need to commence levodopa but interpretation of this trial has been questioned and long-term follow up showed no lasting benefit [4].

Second, does selegiline increase mortality? The UKP-DRG paper of 1995 [5] concluded that increased mortality was seen in patients taking a combination of selegiline and levodopa compared to levodopa alone. Further studies suggest that any true increase in mortality is likely to be less than the 60% reported, and no excess was seen in the long-term DATATOP follow up; however, it is prudent not to coprescribe selegiline and levodopa, unless severe symptoms dictate otherwise.

COMT inhibitors (see Levodopa, above)

These are used for wearing off and motor fluctuations to increase 'on' time.

Side effects

These include:
• potentiation of levodopa side effects
• gastrointestinal disturbance
• a reduction in levodopa dose may be necessary
• the first available COMT inhibitor 'Tolcapone' was withdrawn due to hepatic toxicity. Entacapone does not appear to affect the liver.

Anticholinergics (e.g. benzhexol ('Artane'))

This is used less nowadays. It was previously believed to be effective in tremor that was resistant to other therapies, although this is now questionable.

Side effects

These include:
• confusion (particularly in elderly patients)
• dry mouth
• constipation
• may *worsen* dyskinesias.
When stopping it may be very difficult to wean patients off.

Surgery

Stereotactic surgery, either by lesioning a specific target, or by implanting a high-frequency stimulator, is increasingly used. Lesioning is irreversible, can only be performed unilaterally and may be more hazardous. By contrast, stimulation is reversible and can be performed bilaterally, but is much more expensive and higher maintenance.

In simple terms, the targets are:
• thalamus for tremor
• globus pallidus for dyskineisas.
However, the vogue is now towards the subthalamic nucleus for dyskinesia and bradyskinesia relief.

General measures

The treatment of PD requires a multidisciplinary approach, with the specialist nurse, speech therapist, occupational therapist and physiotherapist often able to contribute more than the doctor to improving patients' quality of life.

Prognosis

Most patients with IPD have near-normal life expectancy. Disease progression is extremely variable and it is important to reassure patients that it can run quite a benign course. Some patients may become disabled after many years, or ifs hallucinations limit treatment, whilst others will lead a fairly normal life, ultimately succumbing to other medical problems.

1 Quinn N. Parkinsonism-recognition and differential diagnosis. *Br Med J* 1995; 310: 447–452.
2 Developments in the treatment of Parkinson's disease. *Drug Ther Bull* 1999; 37: 35–40.
3 Colzi A, Turner K, Lees AJ. Continuous subcutaneous waking day apomorphine in the long term treatment of levodopa induced interdose dyskinesias in Parkinson's disease. *J Neurol Neurosurg Psychiatry* 1998; 64: 573–576.
4 Parkinson Study Group. Effect of deprenyl on the progression of disease ability in early Parkinson's disease. *N Engl J Med* 1989; 321: 1364–1371.
5 Lees AJ, on behalf of the Parkinson's Disease Research group of the United Kingdom. Comparison of the therapeutic effects and mortality data of levodopa and levodopa combined with selegiline in patients with early mild Parkinson's disease. *Br Med J* 1995; 311: 1602–1607.

2.4 Dementias

2.4.1 ALZHEIMER'S DISEASE

Aetiology/pathology

In familial early-onset (usually between early forties and mid-fifties) Alzheimer's disease (AD), autosomal dominant mutations of three genes account for most cases: presenilin 1 on chromosome 14, presenilin 2 on chromosome 1 and amyloid precursor protein on chromosome 21. Over the age of 65 years, carrying the E4 allele of apolipoprotein E (encoded by a gene on chromosome 19) increases the risk of developing AD.

Neuropathological changes of AD are cerebral atrophy, senile plaques with a central core of β-amyloid, neurofibrillary tangles (Fig. 31) and amyloid in blood vessels. β-Amyloid deposition and loss of choline acetyltransferase activity in the cerebral cortex are thought to be important in the pathogenesis of AD.

Epidemiology

AD is the most common form of dementia. Familial AD accounts for less than 5% of cases. Increasing age is the most important risk factor, but patients with Down's syndrome (trisomy 21) are also susceptible to developing AD.

Clinical presentation

Guidelines for the diagnosis of probable, possible and definite AD have been developed [1].

The earliest feature of AD is usually forgetfulness of recent events. As the disease progresses, the patient develops disorientation (initially to time), impairment of verbal fluency, loss of computational ability, inattentiveness, agitation, personality change, depression and difficulty with activities of daily living.

Late features include severe memory impairment, loss of social graces, complete disorientation, psychosis, delusions and hallucinations. Rarely, patients may develop extrapyramidal signs (e.g. rigidity), pyramidal signs (e.g. hyperreflexia), seizures, myoclonus, mutism and incontinence. Progression of the disease is slow and gradual.

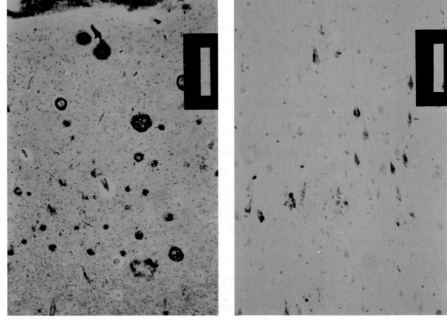

Fig. 31 β-Amyloid (a) and neurofibrillary tangles (b) in Alzheimer's disease.　(a)　　　　　(b)

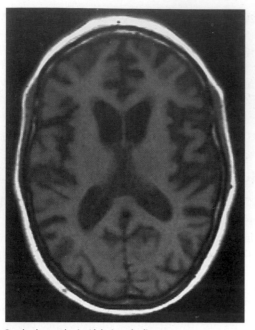

Fig. 32 Cerebral atrophy in Alzheimer's disease.

Investigation

MRI of the brain may show cerebral atrophy (Fig. 32). See also Section 1.9, p. 19.

Differential diagnosis

 You must rule out reversible causes of dementia [2], e.g. hypothyroidism, vitamin B_{12} deficiency and space-occupying lesions (see also Table 10, Section 1.9, p. 19).

Important irreversible causes of dementia, other than AD, should be considered.

Vascular dementia

Stepwise progression often associated with hypertension. Other features include impaired executive function, gait disturbance, emotional lability, urinary dysfunction, episodic neurological dysfunction and preservation of personality. MRI suggests cerebrovascular disease.

Frontotemporal dementia

Loss of social awareness, mental rigidity, loss of initiation and planning, shallow affect, disinhibition, apathy, hyperorality, perseverative behaviour and decreased speech output.

Dementia with Lewy bodies

Progressive cognitive deterioration, fluctuating symptoms, and visual hallucinations, extrapyramidal signs (rigidity and bradykinesia more common than tremor), sleep pattern reversal, recurrent falls, syncope and hypersensitivity to neuroleptics (dopamine-blockers).

Other irreversible causes

Also consider the following:
- Idiopathic Parkinson's disease.
- Progressive supranuclear palsy.
- Corticobasal ganglionic degeneration.
- Huntington's disease (see Section 1.5, p. 12).
- Creutzfeldt–Jakob disease (see Section 2.10, p. 103).

Treatment

AD is not a curable disease, but much can be done to ease some of the strain.

Supportive care is an integral part of managing AD. A familiar environment reduces confusion and it disorientation. Education and support of caregivers are important.

Depression commonly coexists with AD and it is important that it is recognized and treated.

 Tricyclic drugs have anticholinergic side effects that may worsen cognitive deficits. Selective serotonin reuptake inhibitors are a better choice.

Other behavioural disturbances, e.g. agitation and anxiety should also be treated.

Cholinesterase inhibitors, e.g. donepezil and rivastigmine, modestly improve cognitive function [3]. Recent studies suggest this class of agents may also improve non-cognitive functions, e.g. activities of daily living and behaviour. However, most of the trials are short (between 3 and 6 months) [4].

Selegiline, vitamin E and gingko biloba (a plant derivative) have been reported to benefit patients with AD, but there are no data to support this.

Prognosis

Mean survival is about 8 years after the onset of the disease. Pneumonia is the usual cause of death.

1 McKhann G, Drachman DA, Folstein M, Katzman R, Price DL, Stadlan EM. Clinical diagnosis of Alzheimer's disease—Report of the NINCDS-ADRDA Work Group under the auspices of Department of Health and Human Services Task Force on Alzheimer's Disease. *Neurology* 1984; 34: 939–944.
2 Geldmacher DS, Whitehouse PJ Jr. Differential diagnosis of Alzheimer's disease. *Neurology* 1997; 48 (Suppl 6): S2–S9.
3 Gauthier S. Do we have a treatment for Alzheimer's disease? Yes. *Arch Neurol* 1999; 56: 738–739.
4 Pryse-Phillips W. Do we have drugs for dementia? No. *Arch Neurol* 1999; 56: 735–737.

2.5 Multiple sclerosis

Aetiology/pathophysiology/pathology

Several infectious agents have been suggested as a cause for MS but none have been convincingly proven. Autoimmunity is another proposed cause of MS. Molecular mimicry of several viral and bacterial peptides with proteins of myelin may trigger an immune response. Myelin basic protein has been implicated as a target of attack.

 Demyelination with preservation of axons has long been considered the pathological hallmark of MS. However, there is increasing evidence that axonal loss and remyelination also occurs, with the axonal loss contributing to the progressive neurological impairments.
Loss of myelin makes it difficult to depolarize axons and interrupts conduction of an action potential.

Epidemiology

The prevalence of MS increases with increasing distance from the equator. People who migrate from a high-risk area to a low-risk one at or after the age of 15 retain the risk of their birthplace; below the age of 15 they do not. Mean age of onset is 30, being slightly earlier in women than in men and in relapsing–remitting MS than progressive MS. The female to male ratio is 3 : 2. Polygenic inheritance is suspected in MS.

Clinical presentation

Common symptoms are weakness, sensory disturbances, blurred vision or loss of vision (optic neuritis), unsteadiness, incoordination, dysarthria, sphincter or sexual dysfunction and fatigue. Lhermitte's sign (electric shock-like sensation down the spine on neck flexion) and Uhthoff's phenomenon (worsening of symptoms with increasing body temperature) may occur. The risk of developing MS after an acute episode of optic neuritis or transverse myelitis may be as high as 75% and 90%, respectively, if MRI appearances are compatible with MS.

Four disease courses are recognized: relapsing–remitting, primary progressive, secondary progressive (relapsing–remitting followed by continuous progression) and progressive–relapsing (progressive disease from the start with distinct episodes of acute relapses).

Physical signs

Cranial nerves

Pale optic discs, scotoma, relative afferent pupillary defect in optic neuritis, internuclear ophthalmoplegia and facial numbness.

Motor and sensory

UMN signs (e.g. spasticity, weakness, hyperreflexia), impaired pain, temperature, vibration and joint position sense.

Cerebellar

Nystagmus, dysmetria, incoordination, scanning dysarthria, dysdiadochokinesis and gait ataxia.

Investigation

CSF

Mild lymphocytosis and increased protein may be seen, but cell count and total protein are usually normal. Oligoclonal bands (bands in the IgG region) are found in CSF but not serum (indicating intrathecal synthesis) in 90% of cases with clinically definite MS. However, oligoclonal bands may also be detected in many inflammatory conditions affecting the CNS.

Visual, somatosensory and brain stem auditory evoked potentials

May be abnormal in 50–80% of patients, but these tests are usually only employed in difficult cases.

MRI

MRI is the investigation of choice to aid diagnosis, with good sensitivity but poor specificity [1]. MS lesions are typically located in the periventricular white matter (Fig. 33), corpus callosum, pons, mesenencephalon and cerebellar hemispheres. In chronic MS, there are confluent plaques, cortical atrophy and ventricular enlargement. Enhancement with contrast is a sign of an acute lesion and indicates disruption of the blood–brain barrier.

Unfortunately, lesion load on MRI correlates poorly with disability scores. This is probably due to the fact that some lesions may be silent and some may be in strategic areas. This is likely to be more clinically relevant than overall amount of inflammation at any given time.

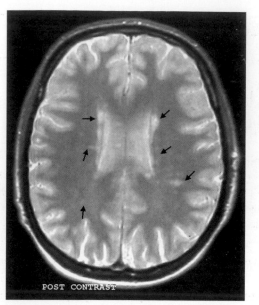

Fig. 33 Periventricular white matter lesions in MS. (From Ray, Ryder, Wellings, *An Aid to Radiology for the MRCP.* Oxford: Blackwell Science 1999).

Differential diagnosis

The diagnosis of MS in the context of a young adult with two or more episodes of CNS dysfunction is straightforward.

However, apparent monophasic illnesses may be caused by many pathologies including stroke, infections of the nervous system, inflammatory disease of the nervous system and tumours.

Progressive MS may be more difficult to diagnose clinically, but the most important diseases to exclude are potentially treatable causes of the symptoms, such as compressive spinal cord lesions, vitamin B_{12} deficiency, arteriovenous malformations and Arnold–Chiari malformation. The differential diagnosis in this category is broad and includes inflammatory and granulomatous CNS disease, CNS infections and hereditary disorders such as adrenoleukodystrophy and metachromatic leukodystrophy.

Treatment

Relief or modification of symptoms

Modification of troublesome symptoms is currently the most effective way of helping improve the patient's quality of life [2].

Spasticity

Spasticity impairs mobility and may cause painful spasms. The treatment options are as follows:
- baclofen (GABA agonist), oral or intrathecal
- tizanidine (α-2 agonist)
- benzodiazepines
- botulinum toxin
- intrathecal phenol injection (last resort).

Bladder disturbance

This occurs in 50–80% of patients. Assessment is as follows.
- Establish whether the bladder empties or not using pre- and post-micturition ultrasound (the patient will not reliably be able to tell whether the bladder empties or not).
- If the residual is less than 100 mL, then use oxybutynin 2.5 mg 2–3 times daily (anticholinergic side effects are less likely to be a problem at this dose). Consider also antidepressants with anticholinergic action. Desmopressin nasal spray used at night may be helpful for nocturnal symptoms.
- If the residual is greater than 100 mL, it is not advisable to use these drugs until outflow obstruction has been overcome. Intermittent self-catheterization is the best and simplest way to achieve this, but special training is needed.

Sexual dysfunction

This is common, but often not discussed with patients. You need to ask, as they are unlikely to volunteer the information. Viagra may be helpful for both men and women.

Fatigue

This is a common symptom, occurring in 70–80% of patients, which interferes with the patient's ability to perform activities of daily living. Amantadine is often used without success. It is important to look for correctable causes of fatigue, so check haemoglobin level and thyroid function tests.

Depression

This occurs in 50–60% of patients, so is important to identify and treat it.

Tremor

This may be severe enough to impair activities of daily living. Various drugs have been tried (antiepileptics, clonazepam, isoniazid) with only limited success. Thalamotomy may help in refractory disease.

Paroxysmal symptoms

These include trigeminal neuralgia, pain, paraesthesia, ataxia, dystonia, and weakness, and are thought to be due to ephaptic transmission of nerve impulses at sites of previous disease activity. Carbamazepine may be of some help.

Treatment of acute attacks

Bearing in mind that relapses are self limiting, the following options are available:
• For acute relapses, high-dose intravenous methylprednisolone with or without a follow-up short course of low-dose oral prednisolone is used. Steroids may shorten an acute attack, but have no effect on disease progression.
• Rest may be just as effective.
• Physiotherapy at the time of the relapse is often of benefit.

Treatment of the underlying disease

Beta-interferons are licensed for use in relapsing–remitting MS, and immunosuppressive agents have been used, but the results are not dramatic.

• In relapsing–remitting MS, interferons beta-1a and beta-1b both reduce the frequency of relapses and the number of new lesions appearing on MRI, although the effect on clinical disability is less convincingly [3]. There is emerging evidence that interferons may also be effective in progressive forms of MS.
• Glatiramer acetate (a synthetic polymer) has been shown to reduce relapses and benefit disability in relapsing-remitting MS.
• Immunosuppressives that have been tried include azathioprine, methotrexate, cyclophosphamide, cyclosporin, mitoxantrone and total lymphoid irradiation.

Side effects of immunosuppression are a major drawback.

Prognosis

The following factors may be associated with a better prognosis:
• diplopia, optic neuritis or sensory symptoms at onset
• women rather than men
• earlier age of onset
• long first remission.

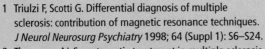
1 Triulzi F, Scotti G. Differential diagnosis of multiple sclerosis: contribution of magnetic resonance techniques. *J Neurol Neurosurg Psychiatry* 1998; 64 (Suppl 1): S6–S24.
2 Thompson AJ. Symptomatic treatment in multiple sclerosis. *Curr Opin Neurol* 1998; 11: 305–309.
3 Tselis AC, Lisak RP. Multiple sclerosis. Therapeutic update. *Arch Neurol* 1999; 56: 277–280.

2.6 Causes of headache

2.6.1 MIGRAINE

Pathophysiology

The cardinal features of migraine are headache in the distribution of the trigeminal nerve and upper cervical roots, in association with transient neurological symptoms.

The pain is mediated through trigeminal nerve fibres that innervate the large intracranial extracerebral vessels (mediated via 5HT 1B serotonin receptors). These fibres project into the trigeminal nucleus (5HT 1D serotonin receptors) where they may receive projections from high cervical nerve fibres. This interaction accounts for the characteristic distribution of pain.

The pain is likely to be related to episodic dysfunction of brain-stem or diencephalic systems that modulate the trigeminovascular system [1].

Epidemiology

• Lifetime prevalence is 5–10% for men, and 15–25% for women.
• The first attack is experienced in the first decade by 25%, and is less common after 50 years.

Clinical presentation

Common

• Migraine headache is episodic, with complete resolution between attacks, each attack lasting a few hours up to 3 days.
• Pain is often temporal and may be unilateral or bilateral. It may be descibed as throbbing or constant.
• Patients with migraine will often describe how they take to their beds with the curtains closed. Although this is in marked contrast to the patient with cluster headache (see Section 2.6.3, p. 82), aggravation by light, noise and movement is common to many other types of headaches. Stress (and relaxation from stress) and various foodstuffs are often considered by patients to precipitate their attacks.
• Headache may be accompanied by nausea (90%) and vomiting (75%).
• The aura occurs prior to, but occasionally with or after the headache, and is most often visual. Transient hemianopic disturbance, fortification spectra and spreading scintillating scotomata (but not blurring or nonspecific spots), are symptoms of a migrainous aura. In

addition, patients may describe unilateral parasthesia, or even mild weakness, of face and hand, and occasionally aphasia.

Migraine variants

Hemiplegic migraine

In true hemiplegic migraine the weakness is more marked than that ocassionally encountered in the common aura, and may long outlast the headache. For this diagnosis to be made, there needs to be a clear family history or a good history of preceding migraine with aura. It may be sporadic or familial, with some families carrying a dominant gene.

Vertebrobasilar migraine

Vertebrobasilar migraine is accompanied by an aura in which there is frequently visual disturbance that is characteristically bilateral, associated with vertigo, ataxia, dysarthria and bilateral sensorimotor features.

Ophthalmoplegic migraine

In ophthalmoplegic migraine, the headache is associated with extraocular muscle palsies, particularly the third and rarely the sixth, which develop as the headache subsides.

Retinal migraine

Retinal migraine is associated with monocular blindness, disc oedema and peripapillary haemorrhages. Vision may not recover for weeks or even months.

Migraine equivalents

Migraine equivalents cause diagnostic problems, in that the presence of a typical migrainous aura without headache can be mistaken for transient cerebral ischaemia. A previous history of migraine with aura makes the diagnosis easier, but migraine equivalents can occur *de novo* in older patients. Characteristically, the symptoms evolve over a few minutes or longer, compared to transient ischaemic attacks (TIAs) (see Section 2.8.2, p. 94).

Investigations

Investigations do not contribute to the diagnosis of migraine, but if a serious cause of headache needs to be excluded then investigation may be appropriate, (as discussed in Section 1.19, p. 41).

Differential diagnosis

The main differentials are:
• episodic tension type headache
• cluster headache
• chronic migraine (usually transformed by analgesic misuse) and other forms of chronic daily headache (see Section 2.6.4, p. 83) can be very difficult to distinguish.

The aura, if it involves prominent sensorimotor features, may be confused with stroke or TIA. Migraine auras typically spread over many minutes or longer, whereas TIA symptoms do not spread. Furthermore, migraine auras are more likely to be positive phenomena (flashing lights, coloured spots, tingling) than TIAs.

See Section 1.19, p. 41, for more information.

Treatment

Objectives and principles

• To minimize impact on the patients' lifestyle, as the tendency to headaches cannot be cured.
• To explain and reassure.
• To identify and avoid predisposing factors (stress, depression, anxiety) and triggers (alcohol, missed meals, change in sleeping habits) within reason. However, some of these may be unavoidable and so the patient should be encouraged to have regular habits.

Acute treatment

Step 1

Simple analgesia (aspirin 900 mg or paracetamol 1000 mg) or non-steroidal anti-inflammatory drugs, with or without an antiemetic such as metoclopramide 10 mg or domperidone 20 mg. Consider suppositories (especially diclofenac plus domperidone) if nausea and vomiting is a persistent problem.

Step 2

• Specific antimigraine drugs (triptans, 5HT 1B/1D agonists). Different drugs may suit different patients, so it may be worth trying each one.
• At 2 hours the response rates (headache improving from severe/moderate to mild/absent) are approximately 50–65%, and the proportion of patients who are headache free is approximately 20–35%.
• Recurrence of symptoms occurs within 24 h in 20–40% of patients for all triptans.
• Oral preparations are available, together with subcutaneous, nasal spray (sumatriptan), and rapidly dispersible wafer placed on tongue (rizatriptan). Subcutaneous or

wafer preparations can be used if vomiting affects oral administration.

• Naratriptan is of slower onset, but there may be lower recurrence rate with this drug [2].

Step 3

Before proceeding to step 3 review the diagnosis and then compliance. Consider dihydroergotamine nasal spray 1 mg. Potential for misuse and development of toxicity.

Emergency treatment

As a one-off treatment, intramuscular chlorpromazine 25–50 mg may improve headache that is not otherwise responding.

Prophylactic treatment

Patients are the best judge of when to commence a prophylactic agent. Continue with a prophylactic agent for 2–3 months, as long as it is tolerated, before deciding whether it has worked or not. Because migraine is cyclical, prophylactic agents that are effective should be continued for no more than 6 months.

These agents may be tried:
• atenolol 25–100 mg b.d. or propranolol LA 80–160 mg b.d.
• sodium valproate 600–2000 mg daily
• pizotifen 0.5–1.5 mg nocte
• amitriptyline 10–100 mg nocte
• methysergide 1–2 mg t.d.s. Often not considered because of associations with retroperitoneal fibrosis, but if used in short courses as suggested above, then this side effect can be avoided.

In pregnancy

Paracetamol is the safest option for acute headache and prochlorperazine is the safest option for nausea.

Most migraines improve, but should a prophylactic agent be required, then propranolol has the safest record.

Migraine and hormone replacement therapy

Hormone replacement therapy (HRT) is not contraindicated in the migraineur. Menopause may exacerbate migraine, so HRT may help symptoms. Worsening migraine on HRT occasionally happens but may be helped by changing dose or formulation of HRT.

Prognosis

If migraine starts in childhood

• 50% of males and 30% of females are migraine free at 30 years.
• Over 50% still get migraines at 50 years.
• In half these cases the migraine is less severe.

If migraine starts in adulthood

70% lose migraine or experience signifinant improvement over 15 years.

1 Weiller C, May A, Limmroth V, Juptner M *et al.* Brain stem activation in spontaneous human migraine attacks. *Nat Med* 1995; 1: 658–660.
2 Goadsby PJ. A triptan too far. *J Neurol Neurosurg Psychiatry* 1998; 64: 143–147.

2.6.2 TRIGEMINAL NEURALGIA

Disease

Trigeminal neuralgia (TN) occurs predominantly in patients over the age of 40 years. It is attributed to compression of the sensory root of the trigeminal nerve, either by an aberrant blood vessel (Fig. 34) or occasionally by tumours in the cerebello-pontine angle. In addition, TN may be seen in MS, with demyelination in the trigeminal sensory root.

Clinical presentation

• Patients characteristically describe a severe paroxysmal pain in the distribution of the trigeminal nerve (usually

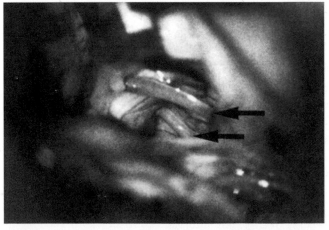

Fig. 34 Perioperative view of trigeminal nerve root entry zone in contact with two divisions of the superior cerebellar artery (black arrows) in a patient with trigeminal neuralgia. The arteries can be seen to indent the nerve. (Reprinted from [2] with kind permission of Mr P.J. Hamlyn and Elsevier Science.)

mandibular or maxillary: the ophthalmic branch is affected only rarely).
• The pain is described as lancinating or electric-shock-like, and lasts only for seconds.
• Occasionally, the paroxysms are so frequent that they blur into one, giving the impression of lasting longer. There may also be a residual ache in between bouts.
• Attacks may occur in clusters, but are clearly differentiated from cluster headache by the quality of the pain.
• Triggers are common, with almost any stimulus setting off an attack. Consequently, many patients are unable to wash, shave, chew or even talk during an attack.
• Pain is unilateral in over 95% of cases, and bilateral TN should raise the possibility of multiple sclerosis.

Physical signs

There are usually no physical signs. However:
• the presence of a reduced corneal response, reduced sensation in the affected distribution or ipsilateral hearing loss should raise the possibility of a structural lesion
• a larger compressive lesion may lead to weakness of the muscles of mastication, ipsilateral ataxia, or other cranial nerve palsies.

TN in a patient under 40 years should raise the possibility of MS or a structural lesion.

Investigation

In the event of a structural lesion being suspected, MRI should be performed, as this will detect demyelination as well as extra-axial mass lesions.

Differential diagnosis

When the patient describes the classical history of TN, the diagnosis is easy to make. If there is a chronic element to the pain then the differential broadens (see Section 1.18, p. 39).

Treatment

Medical

• Carbamazepine is the drug of choice, with a response rate of 75%. Start with 100 mg daily and increase at weekly or 2-weekly intervals, up to a dose of 1600 mg in divided doses. Lower doses usually suffice.
• If carbamazepine does not work, consider baclofen, phenytoin or clonazepam, but the chances of success are much lower with these drugs.

The chances of medical treatment succeeding if carbamazepine fails are relatively small, so consider surgical options early.

Surgical

For patients with medically intractable TN neurosurgical intervention should be considered [1]. The options are as follows.
• Peripheral nerve block with alcohol or phenol injections, which causes facial numbness, but is temporary, lasting 18–24 months.
• Percutaneous denervation, either by glycerol injection or radiofrequency thermocoagulation of the trigeminal ganglion. This may cause facial and corneal numbness. Anaesthesia dolorosa, a severe dysaesthesia which is generally unresponsive to therapy, occurs as a complication in 5–10% of cases.
• Microvascular decompression via a posterior fossa approach. The surgeon separates the trigeminal sensory root from the compressing aberrant blood vessel using a non-absorbable sponge. This approach is more likely to cause death, stroke, facial weakness, or hearing loss, but is less likely to be associated with recurrence, dysaesthesias or anaesthesia dolorosa.

1 Brisman R. Surgical treatment of trigeminal neuralgia. *Semin Neurol* 1997; 17(4): 367–372.
2 Hamlyn PJ. *Neuromuscular Compression of the Lower Cranial Nerves.* Amsterdam: Elsevier Science, 1999.

2.6.3 CLUSTER HEADACHE

Pathophysiology

• The mechanism of the pain is similar to migraine, in that the trigeminovascular system is involved.
• The central disorder is likely to involve the pacemaker regions of the posterior hypothalamus [1].

Epidemiolgy

Migraine is 20 times more common. Cluster headache occurs predominantly in males (male to female ratio 6 : 1) over the age of 20 years.

Clinical presentation

The following features are characteristic.
• Severe unilateral orbital, supraorbital and/or temporal headache described as an intense, constant, boring pain.
• Typically, each attack lasts 15–180 min, occurs 1–3 times daily for 4–8 weeks, with each cluster occurring once or twice a year. There is, however, considerable variation.

Table 36 Associated features of cluster headache. Patients should have one of more of these features to be diagnosed as having cluster headache.

Conjunctival injection
Lacrimation
Nasal congestion
Rhinorrhoea
Ptosis
Meiosis
Eyelid oedema

- 80–90% of patients will have recurrent attacks at the same time each day, particularly in the early hours of the morning ('alarm clock headache').
- There are several important associated features (see Table 36).
- During a bout, alcohol seems to be a potent trigger.
- A chronic form of cluster headache may develop from episodic cluster or may occur *de novo*, in which the patient experiences recurrent attacks for more than a year with little or no remissions.

Physical signs

In chronic cluster headaches a permanent Horner's syndrome may develop, but examination is usually normal between attacks.

Differential diagnosis

- Episodic cluster headache is simple to diagnose, but the chronic form may be more difficult (see Section 1.18, p. 39).
- Attacks with the features of cluster headache, but of shorter duration (3–45 min) and occurring more frequently (20–40 times per day) have been termed chronic paroxysmal hemicrania, and are almost invariably responsive to indomethacin [2].

In a patient with unilateral facial pain and a Horner's syndrome, any contralateral focal neurological signs should make you consider a carotid artery dissection (see Section 1.18, p. 39).

Treatment

Acute

Try the following:
- 100% oxygen relieves approximately 80% of attacks within 15 min.
- Sumatriptan 50–100 mg orally is as effective as oxygen.
- Ergotamine tablets or suppositories may be used the night before alarm clock headaches.

- Verapamil 80 mg q.d.s. is effective in stopping a bout.
- Corticosteroids are also effective in stopping a bout, but recurrence is a problem.

Prophylaxis

The following agents may be helpful.
- Verapamil 240–600 mg daily has been used in the prevention of both episodic and chronic cluster headache, and is the drug of choice as a prophylactic agent. High doses need to be used [3].
- Lithium carbonate is efficacious in the suppression of chronic, but less so episodic, cluster headache in doses of 300–600 mg daily (maintaining serum levels at less than 1.2 mEq/L).
- Sodium valproate has also been used with some benefit.

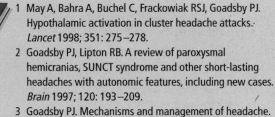

1 May A, Bahra A, Buchel C, Frackowiak RSJ, Goadsby PJ. Hypothalamic activation in cluster headache attacks. *Lancet* 1998; 351: 275–278.
2 Goadsby PJ, Lipton RB. A review of paroxysmal hemicranias, SUNCT syndrome and other short-lasting headaches with autonomic features, including new cases. *Brain* 1997; 120: 193–209.
3 Goadsby PJ. Mechanisms and management of headache. *J R Coll Physicians Lond* 1999; 33: 228–234.

2.6.4 TENSION-TYPE HEADACHE

Tension-type headache (TTH) is described as a constant tight or band-like sensation (non-pulsatile) around the head, which is usually bilateral (80–90%), and which is not aggravated by physical activity. It may be episodic (occurring on less than 15 days each month) or chronic (more than 15 days each month).

The term 'chronic daily headache' is often used for this type of headache, but is a descriptive, not diagnostic, term. Varieties of primary chronic daily headache are described in Table 37 [1]. Secondary causes are discussed in the differential diagnosis.

Pathophysiology

The pain of TTH is probably generated by activation and sensitization of second-order trigeminal neurones. The current phenotypic classification is likely to be reorganized

Table 37 Varieties of primary chronic daily or near-daily headache.

Chronic tension-type headache
Transformed or chronic migraine (analgesic overuse)
Chronic cluster headache
Chronic paroxysmal hemicrania
New persistent daily headache

once the underlying biological and genetic processes are better understood [2].

Epidemiology

Daily headache is common, with a lifetime prevalence of approximately 5% of the population.

Clinical presentation

Characteristic features include the following:
• The quality of the headache, as described above, may be of band-like, bifronto-temporal pressure, or a weight pressing down on top of the head.
• Occasional unilateral stabbing sensations may occur.
• Mild nausea (but not vomiting) and photophobia are common.
• Chronic forms are worsened by anxiety and stress, but pain is not limited to these occasions.
• Alcohol may relieve TTH, unlike migraine.
• There are no abnormal features on examination.

Investigations

Many patients are anxious to have a brain scan, but if there are no abnormal physical signs and the headache has characteristic features as described above, then it is not indicated, and reassurance is appropriate.

Differential diagnosis

If the headache is of more recent subacute onset, then the following can present with generalized non-specific headaches, and so must always be considered in the appropriate age group.
• Expanding intracranial lesion (any age, but will produce symptoms more quickly in a young brain rather than atrophic one).
• Progressive hydrocephalus (any age, but as for intracranial lesion).
• Temporal arteritis (over 55 years old).
• Idiopathic intracranial hypertension (young females).
• Primary angle-closure glaucoma (headache and eye pain associated with coloured haloes around lights, but may cause bilateral pain. Rare before middle age).

> **Overdiagnosed causes of chronic headache**
>
> Headache should not be attributed to:
> • sinus disease unless there are other symptoms supporting this
> • disease of the ears, teeth or temperomandibular joint, unless there are other symptoms supporting this
> • errors of refraction, as this only occasionally causes a very mild frontal headache not present on waking.

Treatment

Principles

Reassurance is a key component of treatment.
It is essential to identify contributory factors such as:
• functional or structural cervical or cranial musculoskeletal abnormalities
• depression
• analgesic overuse.

> Analgesic overuse may be the commonest cause of chronic daily headache. Drugs implicated are aspirin, paracetamol (especially when combined with opiate derivatives), codeine, 5HT 1B/1D agonists (triptans) and, to a lesser extent, nonsteroidal anti inflammatories. Their continued use for most days over several weeks or months is associated with the development of chronic daily headaches (see Table 37). The mechanism is unclear.

Non-pharmacological

These approaches are also useful:
• encourage regular exercise in the sedentary
• suggest stress management if stress is prominent in the history
• physiotherapy may help to correct posture and to improve symptoms secondary to trauma such as whiplash, but may be less successful in degenerative disease of the neck.

Pharmacological

Simple analgesia

Regular simple analgesia is inappropriate as it may be implicated in the genesis of the headache, although a single course of naproxen 500 mg b.d. for 3 weeks occasionally breaks the cycle of frequently occurring headaches.

Amitriptyline

Amitriptyline is the drug of choice. It is important to explain that this drug is not being used as an antidepressant, otherwise the patient may stop taking it when they find out. Start with 10 mg nocte, increasing to 75–100 mg, by increasing at 25 mg every 1–2 weeks. If tolerated, continue with this drug for 6–8 weeks before assessing efficacy, as it may take this long to work. If it has a beneficial effect then continue for a further 6 months before withdrawing the drug.

Other agents

Also consider:
- other drugs such as prothiadin and sodium valproate
- selective serotonin reuptake inhibitors seem to have little effect on chronic TTH, but may help depression
- where chronic TTH and migraine coexist, in addition to the above measures the migraine may require symptomatic treatment (see Section 2.6.1, p. 79), but on no more than two days per week.

> Analgesic overuse requires that the appropriate drugs are withdrawn over 2–4 weeks if possible. It is wise to warn the patient that the headaches are likely to get worse before they get better, but unless the offending analgesics are withdrawn, the headache is unlikely to improve.

1 Silberstein SD, Lipton RB, Sliwiski M. Classification of daily and near daily headaches: a field study of revised IHS criteria. *Neurology* 1996; 47: 871–875.
2 Goadsby PJ. Chronic tension-type headache: where are we now? *Brain* 1999; 122: 1611–1612.

2.7 Epilepsy

Definition

Epilepsy is a condition characterized by recurrent (two or more) epileptic seizures, unprovoked by any immediate identified cause.

An epileptic seizure is a clinical manifestation presumed to result from an abnormal and excessive discharge from a set of neurones in the brain. The clinical manifestation consists of sudden and transitory abnormal phenomena which may include alterations in consciousness, motor, sensory, autonomic or psychic events perceived by the patient or an observer.

Pathophysiology

Pathological studies, increasingly from postoperative studies of resected foci, have shown a wide range of abnormalities, in particular the characteristic mesial temporal sclerosis seen in temporal lobe epilepsy, implying that these focal lesions may be epileptogenic. Diffuse cortical microdysgenesis may similarly play a part in the pathogenesis of idiopathic generalized epilepsy.

Aetiology

In childhood-onset seizures, there is a strong association with congenital, developmental and genetic abnormalities.

In elderly patients, stroke is the commonest association (in 50% of first-time seizures in the over-sixties). At any age, head trauma, CNS infection and tumours have strong associations with epilepsy.

In general, there are likely to be multifactorial aetiologies. Genetic predisposition could lower the susceptibility to other aetiological factors.

Epidemiology

- Incidence: 40–70/100 000 per year in developed countries.
- Prevalence: 0.5–1.0% of the general population have active epilepsy.
- Life-time prevalence: 2–5% of general population. See [1] for review.

Clinical presentation

> A witness account is essential, and a hand-held video recording of an attack would be extremely useful, as the diagnosis of epilepsy is a clinical one.

Epilepsy may be most usefully classified according to seizure types (Table 38). The classification of epilepsy as syndromes is less useful clinically at present, partly because future classifications will change as more is learned about their underlying, possibly genetic, aetiologies [2].

Generalized seizures

Tonic–clonic

- Sudden-onset loss of consciousness often associated with an audible cry, followed by a fall to the ground.
- Tonic stiffening phase lasts 10–30 s, during which time respiration may be impaired, leading to cyanosis.
- Followed by clonic phase, in which there is low-amplitude jerking of all four limbs. As the seizure progresses, frequency slows and amplitude increases. Lasts 30–60 s.
- Flaccidity of muscles with slow recovery of consciousness over 2–30 min.
- Associated with incontinence, tongue biting and autonomic features.
- May be more tonic or clonic.
- Does not imply pathological type, unless preceded by clear partial onset.

Typical absence

- Sudden loss of consciousness and motor activity without warning, resulting in a blank stare.

Table 38 Classification of epileptic seizures.

Partial seizures	Simple	
		Motor: either limb or adversive head turning (parietal)
		Sensory or special sensory, e.g. visual: Symptoms usually positive (pins and needles) rather than negative (numbness)
		Autonomic: rising epigastric sensation, changes in skin colour, blood pressure, heart rate, pupil size may all indicate a temporal lobe origin
		Psychic: dysphasia/speech arrest, déjà vu, sensations of unreality or depersonalization, fear, anger, elation, illusions or structured hallucinations, may all originate from a temporal lobe focus
	Complex	
		Simple partial onset followed by impairment of consciousness
		With impaired consciousness at onset
	Partial seizures evolving to secondary generalized seizures	
Generalized seizures	Absence seizures	
		Typical
		Atypical
	Myoclonic seizures	
	Clonic seizures	
	Tonic seizures	
	Atonic seizures	
	Tonic–clonic seizures	
Unclassifiable seizures		

• Sudden cessation, so that patient continues what they were doing, often unaware.
• Short attacks: <30 s.
• Automatisms, slight clonic movements or eyelid fluttering may occur in longer attacks.
• Occur as part of idiopathic generalized epilepsy.

Atypical absence

• Blank stare.
• Onset and cessation more gradual.
• Consciousness only partially impaired.
• Focal signs more prominent.
• Occurs in patients with diffuse cerebral damage.

Myoclonic

• Brief jerk either in single muscle or generalized, of rapid onset and cessation.
• No loss of consciousness.
• Often part of idiopathic generalized epilepsies [2].

Partial seizures

Simple

• No alteration in consciousness, no amnesia.
• Sudden onset and cessation.
• Symptoms depend on site of underlying cortical lesion (Table 38).
• Last only seconds.

Complex

• Preceded by simple partial seizure (aura).
• Alteration in consciousness associated with blank staring, and often with motor signs such as unilateral dystonic posturing (temporal lobe).
• Automatism. This is a 'more or less co-ordinated involuntary motor activity occurring during clouding of consciousness during or after an epileptic seizure, usually followed by amnesia'. They may take many forms (Table 39).
• Sixty per cent of complex partial seizures arise from the temporal lobes, 30% from the frontal lobes. Automatisms may occur as part of complex partial seizure from any location.

Table 39 Clinical features of automatisms.

Type	Feature
Oro-alimentary	Lip smacking
	Chewing
	Swallowing
Gestural	Fiddling with hands
	Picking at clothing
	Tidying
Ambulatory	Walking
	Running
	Circling
	Purposeless complex movement
Verbal	Humming
	Whistling
	Grunting
Mimicry	Displays of laughter, fear, anger, excitement

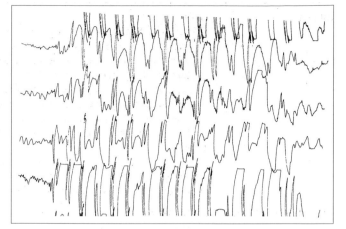

Fig. 35 3 Hz spike-and-wave.

Physical signs

• Uncommon unless seizures are due to underlying cortical structural lesion.
• Epilepsy may occur as part of a wider phenotype in some neurodegenerative diseases.
• Consider the neurocutaneous syndromes (see Section 2.9, Table 53).

Investigation

• Routine biochemical and haematological profiles
• EEG
• MRI
• Hand-held video is very useful, especially if the diagnosis is not clearly epilepsy.

EEG

In practice, most patients require an EEG as part of their initial evaluation. However:
• a normal interictal EEG does not exclude epilepsy. An abnormal EEG may support a primary idiopathic process and provide evidence of photosensitivity
• EEG is a poor guide to seizure control, with the exception of 3 Hz spike-and-wave changes which are sensitive to treatment (Fig. 35)
• minor asymmetries are not diagnostic.

MRI

Structural imaging is indicated as follows:
• partial seizures on history (Fig. 36)
• deficit revealed on neurological or psychological examination that is not transient
• difficult seizure control with antiepileptics
• generalized seizures, onset before 1 or after 20 years of age.

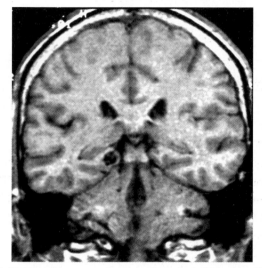

Fig. 36 Right parahippocampal angioma in patient with temporal lobe epilepsy seen on coronal MRI scan.

The last point is debated. The reason for suggesting it is that a generalized seizure with no suggestion of partial onset is extremely likely to be a primary idiopathic type of epilepsy in this age range. Some specialists will scan all new presentations.

Differential diagnosis

Fifty per cent of new epilepsy referrals may have an alternative diagnosis [3] (see Sections 1.20, p. 44 and 2.8.2, p. 94).

The distinction between an epileptic attack and a non-epileptic attack is discussed in Table 40, but it should be remembered that they may coexist.

Treatment

Emergency

For management of status epilepticus see *Emergency medicine*, Section 1.24.

Table 40 Differentiation between an epileptic attack and a non-epileptic attack.

	Epileptic attack	Non-epileptic attack
Precipitant	Rare	Commonly stress related
Onset	Short	May be short or prolonged
Movement	Synchronous small amplitude jerks if clonic	Asynchronous flailing of limbs, pelvic thrusting, opisthotonus
Injury	Tongue biting, fall, but directed violence rare	May bite tongue, cheeks, lip, hands, throw themselves to ground, directed violence occurs
Consciousness	Complete or incomplete depending on type	Variable, but may be inconsistent with seizure type
Response to stimuli	None unless complex partial seizure	May terminate the attack. Suggestible
Incontinence	Common	Sometimes
Duration	Minutes	May be prolonged
Recovery	Few minutes, but may be prolonged confusion	Rapid or very prolonged

When should antiepileptic medication be commenced?

To answer this, one needs an appreciation of the risks of seizure recurrence to balance against the risk of antiepileptic medication.
- The risk of recurrence is highest in the first few days and weeks, then falls with time.
- 30% will have a recurrent seizure by 3 months, 67% by 12 months and 78% by 36 months [1]. Antiepileptic medication reduces but does not abolish this risk.
- At 12 months the risk of recurrence in those with a partial seizure is 94%. In those with seizures precipitated by an acute illness it is much lower at 40%.

On the basis of these figures you can see that it might be desirable to treat some patients after one seizure, rather than wait for the customary two seizures, as the risk of recurrence may be high (about 80% with time overall). If a patient presents having had a single seizure 12 months before, then the subsequent risk of recurrence may be lower, and one may choose to wait.

The decision to initiate antiepileptic treatment is based on the risk of recurrent seizures vs the risks of the drug itself, not on arbitrarily waiting for two seizures to occur.

Natural history of epilepsy on treatment

- Reassure the patient that 70–80% of newly diagnosed patients treated with a single antiepileptic drug will eventually be seizure free.
- If remission is defined as 5 years seizure free, then about 40% enter remission in the first year, 20% in the next 9 years and 10% in the next 10 years.

Once the decision to initiate treatment has been made, follow these general principles [2].
- Start the drug at low dose, titrate up slowly until seizures are abolished or the maximum tolerated dose has been reached.
- First-line drugs are usually carbamazepine for partial seizures or secondary generalized seizures (start at 100 mg daily, increasing by 200 mg every 2 weeks, up to 600–1800 mg total daily dose), and sodium valproate for most generalized or idiopathic epilepsies (start at 500 mg daily, increasing by 500 mg every 2 weeks, up to 1000–2500 mg total daily dose).
- If seizures continue, reconsider the diagnosis, check compliance, review or obtain neuroimaging.
- If epilepsy is still thought to be the diagnosis, then introduce another first-line agent, probably whichever of carbamazepine or sodium valproate has not been used, as detailed above. When a reasonable dose is achieved then the first drug can be withdrawn slowly.
- Adjust the dose of the second drug to optimum.
- If seizures continue, try both first-line drugs together. Thereafter add in a second-line drug at the expense of the least well tolerated first-line drug. Consider other second-line drugs in a similar manner.
- Three drugs are rarely better than two.

For further discussion of individual antiepileptic drugs see [4] and [2].

'When can I come off my tablets, doctor?'

This question is likely to be asked by the patient when in some form of remission. The first two points that need to be highlighted are:
- no guarantees can be made that seizures will not recur
- think about driving: if the loss of a driving licence would be a devastating blow to the patient, they may decide to stay on medication.

The decision is up to the patient, but you must provide them with the information:
- In patients in remission for 2 years or more, the chance of a seizure in the next 2 years are 43% if the drug is withdrawn, compared to 10% in those maintaining therapy.
- This figure may alter with the presence or absence of certain risk factors (Table 41) [2].
- Within 10–15 years after onset of epilepsy at least 70% are in 5 years remission and 50% are off all drugs, so the prognosis is actually quite good.

Surgical treatment

Focal resections

- Consider surgical options in patients with seizures of partial onset, refractory to intensive medical therapy over at least 2–3 years.

Table 41 Factors affecting risk of recurrent seizure following drug withdrawal.

Increased risk
Age over 16
Taking more than one antiepileptic drug
A history of seizures after starting antiepileptic drugs
A history of tonic–clonic seizures
A history of myoclonic seizures
An abnormal EEG in the previous year

Decreased risk
Risk of seizures declines the longer the seizure-free period

• Presurgical evaluation includes detailed clinical assessment, EEG and video telemetry to obtain ictal EEG, high-resolution structural MRI (epilepsy protocol), PET scan if structural imaging is unclear, neuropsychological and neuropsychiatric evaluation.
• One is looking for convergence of data, implying one epileptogenic area. Data suggesting multifocal foci indicates less chance of success.
• The commonest site of resection is the temporal lobe [2].

Other operations

• Corpus callosal resection is reserved for patients with severe intractable seizures and drop attacks. The operation is aimed at reducing the number and severity of attacks, especially the drop attacks.
• Hemispherectomy is reserved for children or adolescents with medically intracable seizures due to severe unilateral hemisphere damage.

Management of the pregnant patient with epilepsy

General information

Preconception counselling is very important.
• The background risk of fetal malformations in developed countries is 3%, and this is thought to rise to rise to 7% with one antiepileptic drug, and 15% with two or more.
• The background risk of neural-tube defects is 0.2–0.5%, being increased to 1% by carbamazepine and 1–2% by sodium valproate.

Principles of drug management

• If possible, maintain the patient on as few drugs and at as low a dose as possible.
• Consider withdrawing drugs prior to pregnancy if the patient has been seizure free for 2 years.
• Advise folic acid 4–5 mg daily for 12 weeks before and after conception, to reduce the risk of neural-tube defects.

• Serum alphafetoprotein measurement and fetal ultrasound should be carried out at 16–18 weeks to screen for neural-tube defects, especially in those taking sodium valproate or carbamazepine.
• Oral vitamin K (20 mg/day) should be given to the mother if she is taking an enzyme-inducing drug (pheytoin, carbamazepine, phenobarbitone or mysoline) in the last month of pregnancy to protect the baby from haemorrhagic disease of the newborn. The risk lasts for a week or so post partum and so some suggest that oral vitamin K be given to the baby for a further week to cover this period. Vitamin K is still usually given by intramuscular injection to the newborn baby. Fears still exist over the risk of childhood neoplasia with the injectable form, although more recent trials have failed to find this link.

Prognosis

Epilepsy carries an increased risk of death, mainly attributable to the underlying disease, accidents or suicide.

Patients with epilepsy are at risk of SUDEP (sudden unexplained deaths in epilepsy) at a rate of one per 200–1000/year. Young patients and those with frequent generalized seizures and mental retardation have higher risk. The cause and strategies for prevention are not clear [5].

Occupational aspects

Driving

Patients may apply for a driving licence if they have been seizure free for 1 year, or if they have an established pattern of seizures occurring only during sleep for the previous 3 years. Stricter rules apply to drivers of heavy goods vehicles (HGVs) and passenger-carrying vehicles (PCVs).

It is recommended, but not covered by legislation, that driving be suspended from the start of antiepileptic drug withdrawal until 6 months afterwards.

Employment

Recruitment is barred in the armed forces, the fire brigade, London Regional Transport, the merchant navy and diving. For many other occupations no specific legislation exists but employment is unlikely.

Leisure

To a large extent, this depends on the individual's particular seizure pattern, but in general adequate supervision for activities such as swimming, cycling and rock climbing is needed, together with an acceptance that risk is not something that can be eliminated from all activities.

1 Sander JWAS, Shorvon SD. Epidemiology of the epilepsies. *J Neurol Neurosurg Psychiatry* 1996; 61: 433–443.
2 Duncan JS, Shorvon SD, Fish DR. *Clinical Epilepsy*. London: Churchill Livingstone, 1995.
3 Sander JWAS, Hart YM, Johnson AL, Shorvon SD. The National General Practice study of epilepsy: newly diagnosed seizures in a general population. *Lancet* 1990; 336: 1267–1271.
4 Chadwick D. The use of new antiepileptic drugs. *J R Coll Physicians Lond* 1999; 33: 328–332.
5 Nashef L. From mystery to prevention: sudden unexplained death in epilepsy, time to move on. *J Neurol Neurosurg Psychiatry* 1999; 67: 427.

Table 43 Main modifiable risk factors for stroke.

Hypertension
Atrial fibrillation
Cigarette smoking
Previous transient ischaemic attack
Heart failure
Ischaemic heart disease
Diabetes mellitus
Excess alcohol
Hyperlipidaemia
Elevated haematocrit

2.8 Cerebrovascular disease

2.8.1 STROKE

Stroke is a clinically defined syndrome of rapidly developing cerebral dysfunction with no cause other than that of vascular origin. Although it is often thought of as causing purely focal symptoms, the loss of function can at times be global (coma, subarachnoid haemorrhage).

The classification of stroke is broadly into ischaemic and haemorrhagic (Table 42). Ischaemic stroke is dealt with in this section, and intracerebral haemorrhage (see Section 2.8.3, p. 96) and subarachnoid haemorrhage (see Section 2.8.4, p. 98 and *Emergency medicine*, Section 1.22) are discussed elsewhere.

Aetiology

Ischaemic stroke can be caused by thromboembolism from the heart or major vessels, or by occlusion of small penetrating vessels, found predominantly in the basal ganglia, internal capsule or pons (lacunar stroke) (Fig. 37).

Occlusion of vessels may occur as a result of thrombosis and local occlusion, or subsequent to embolization and distal occlusion.

Thrombosis is attributable to any element of Virchow's triad:

- abnormality of the vessel wall (atherosclerosis (especially if ulcerated), dissection or vasculitis in large vessels, and lipohyalinosis in the small perforating vessels)
- abnormality of the blood (e.g. polycythaemia)
- disturbances of blood flow (e.g. atrial fibrillation).

The main constituents of thrombi are:
- platelets (forming in fast-flow areas such as the internal carotid artery as a result of atheromatous plaque)
- fibrin and red blood cells (forming in slow-flow areas such as the cardiac atria in atrial fibrillation).

This explains the theoretical rationale for the use of secondary preventative agents; antiplatelet drugs in atherothrombosis and warfarin in atrial fibrillation and heart failure.

Risk factors for vascular disease (Table 43), e.g. hypertension, are responsible for the underlying pathological disease of blood vessels, particularly atherosclerosis [1].

Table 42 Classification of stroke types.

Ischaemic (85%)	Large vessel atherothrombotic disease
	Small vessel thrombotic disease/lacunar infarcts
	Embolic disease from cardiac source
Haemorrhagic (15%)	Primary intracerebral haemorrhage
	Subarachnoid haemorrhage

Pathophysiology

Reduction in cerebral blood flow (CBF) below the normal of over 50 mL/100 g/min, sets off a cascade of events which will ultimately lead to cell death if not reversed.

As CBF falls below about 20 mL/100 g/min, there is loss of electrical neuronal function, a potentially reversible stage. Below 10 mL/100 g/min irreversible damage starts to occur. Increased energy demands of the cell cannot be met and ATP becomes depleted. Consequently, energy-dependent ion homeostasis fails, leading to equilibration of all ions across the cell membrane (anoxic depolarization), and the release of potentially toxic levels of glutamate and calcium inflax. Several processes interact leading to an ischaemic cascade and, ultimately, cell death [2].

Epidemiology

- The annual incidence is 312 per 100 000 in 45–84-year-olds (200 per 100 000 overall).

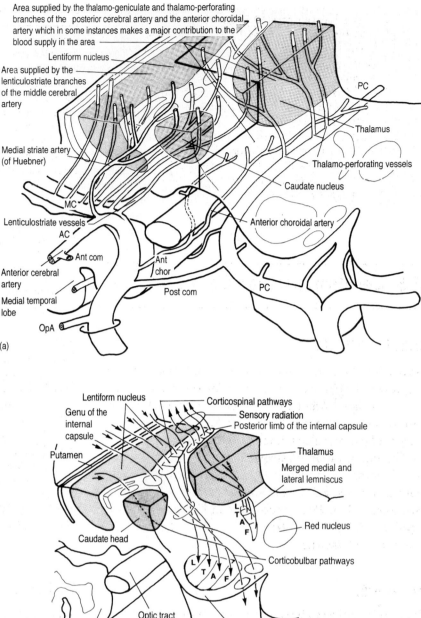

Area supplied by the thalamo-geniculate and thalamo-perforating branches of the posterior cerebral artery and the anterior choroidal artery which in some instances makes a major contribution to the blood supply in the area

Lentiform nucleus

Area supplied by the lenticulostriate branches of the middle cerebral artery

Medial striate artery (of Huebner)

MC

Lenticulostriate vessels

AC

Ant com

Anterior cerebral artery

Medial temporal lobe

OpA

(a)

PC

Thalamus

Thalamo-perforating vessels

Caudate nucleus

Anterior choroidal artery

Ant chor

Post com

PC

Fig. 37 (a) Schematic representation of the blood supply to the region of the internal capsule. Note that main motor pathways at capsular level are supplied by the middle cerebral branches and the main sensory pathways are mainly supplied by the posterior cerebral-derived vessels. This explains why capsular strokes tend to be primarily motor or sensory. The blood supply of the sublenticular visual pathways, the optic tract and the lateral geniculate body is derived from anterior choroidal or posterior cerebral derived vessels. (b) Key diagram of pathway anatomy in the internal capsule. The right internal capsule is shown from above and anteriorly to indicate the motor and sensory rotations between the internal capsule and upper mid-brain. A, arm; F, face; L, leg; T, trunk.

Lentiform nucleus

Genu of the internal capsule

Putamen

Caudate head

Corticospinal pathways

Sensory radiation

Posterior limb of the internal capsule

Thalamus

Merged medial and lateral lemniscus

Red nucleus

Corticobulbar pathways

Optic tract

(b) Medial temporal lobe

Right cerebral peduncle

• 12% of all deaths in industrialized countries are due to stroke.

• Stroke is the commonest cause of severe physical disability and accounts for 5% of NHS hospital costs.

Physical signs

The neurological examination should allow one to identify the site of the lesion accurately, but in routine clinical practice this degree of accuracy has no value over and above a bedside system of classification, such as the Oxfordshire Community Stroke Study classification (Table 44). In the case of evolving signs, this simple analysis is more likely to be incorrect, but it is used in some units, and is worth being aware of. The immediate assessment of an acute stroke patient is discussed fully in Section 1.21, p. 46 and *Emergency medicine*, Section 1.25.

Investigations

The most important specific investigation is a CT scan to exclude haemorrhage and allow early treatment with antiplatelet agents, and to exclude other possible diagnoses such as space-occupying lesions. In ischaemic stroke scans may initially appear normal, but remember that early signs of ischaemia are subtle and easily missed (see Fig. 38).

Table 44 The Oxfordshire community stroke subclassification system. From [3] with permission.

Total anterior circulation syndrome (TACS) Implies large cortical stroke in middle cerebral artery, or middle and anterior cerebral artery territories	A combination of: New higher cerebral dysfunction (e.g. dysphasia, dyscalculia, visuospatial disorder) **and** Homonymous visual field defect **and** An ipsilateral motor and/or sensory deficit involving at least two out of three areas of the face, arm or leg
Partial anterior circulation syndrome (PACS) Implies cortical stroke in middle or anterior cerebral artery territories	Patients with 2 out of 3 components of TACS, **or** new higher cerebral dysfunction alone **or** a motor/sensory deficit more restricted than those classified as LACS (e.g. isolated hand movement)
Lacunar syndrome (LACS) Implies a subcortical stroke due to small vessel disease	Pure motor stroke Pure sensory stroke Ataxic hemiparesis Dysarthria and clumsy hand NB evidence of higher cortical involvement or disturbance of consciousness excludes a lacunar syndrome
Posterior circulation syndrome (POCS)	Ipsilateral cranial nerve palsy with contralateral motor/sensory deficit Bilateral motor and/or sensory deficit Disorder of conjugate eye movement Cerebellar dysfunction without ipsilateral pyramidal involvement (which would be ataxic hemiparesis—see LACS) Isolated homonymous visual field defect

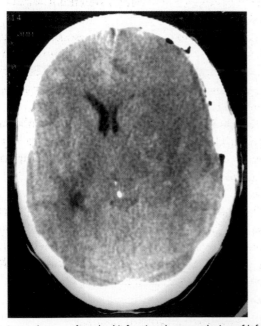

Fig. 38 Acute changes of cerebral infarction due to occlusion of left middle cerebral artery shown on CT scan.

At presentation patients should also have:
- ECG
- Chest radiograph
- FBC, ESR, U+Es, glucose.

Differential diagnosis

Misdiagnosis of ischaemic stroke occurs in up to a quarter of cases, usually when a clear history is not available (see Section 1.21, p. 46). Intracerebral haemorrhage is the most important differential diagnosis, and can only reliably be differentiated on CT scan. Other alternatives include brain tumour, subdural haematoma, cerebral venous thrombosis, focal cerebral infection, hypoglycaemia and postictal Todd's paresis. In a young person, consider MS.

> Stroke is a clinical diagnosis, but the most important distinction, between ischaemia and haemorrhage, requires special investigation, i.e. CT scan. This has an impact on subsequent management, and with the advent of acute therapies for ischaemic stroke, will become ever more important.

Treatment

Short term

General care

Important points to consider in the acute investigation management are as follows:
- Early treatment is supportive in order to prevent complications.
- Careful monitoring of neurological status, blood pressure, oxygenation, glycaemic control, hydration, nutrition, swallowing function, temperature control and bladder function are all crucial, and proper management in these areas will have an enormous impact on the

mortality and morbidity of stroke patients. This is fully discussed in [4], and see *Emergency medicine*, Section 1.25 and *Medicine for the elderly*, Section 1.4.
• Management of stroke patients in a designated stroke unit reduces mortality and long-term dependency. Much planning needs to go into the ongoing care of an often elderly patient, whose stroke has left them dependant (see *Medicine for the elderly*, Section 1.4).

Acute therapies designed to minimize the size of infarct

Specific early treatments designed to reduce the size of infarct include thrombolysis and neuroprotective agents.

THROMBOLYSIS

The NINDS trial [4] demonstrated that patients treated within 3 h of onset of their stroke had a favourable outcome at 3 months. There was a significant increase in the number of treated patients suffering from symptomatic intracranial haemorrhage, but importantly there was no overall increase in mortality at 3 months. Subsequent trials using rtPA have failed to show significant benefit in terms of functional outcome. However, a meta-analysis of 12 thrombolysis trials demonstrated significant improvements in functional outcome in those patients treated with thrombolysis up to 6 h after stroke, but there was an increase in overall mortality in this group. Patients treated up to 3 h after stroke also gained benefit in functional outcome, without the increase mortality seen in the 0–6 h treatment group [5]. Hence it appears that rtPA given up to 3 h post stroke seems to have some benefit, but it is not clear how many patients will present within 3 h in order to be eligible for such treatment.

NEUROPROTECTION

Neuroprotective agents have been disappointing to date, but it is likely that they will need to be given in combination with thrombolysis so that cerebral tissue preserved in this manner will benefit from reperfusion.

Agents used to reduce stroke recurrence in the acute setting

ANTIPLATELET AGENTS

Aspirin prevents 10 deaths or recurrent strokes per 1000 patients treated in the first 2 weeks following acute ischaemic stroke and should be commenced once haemorrhage has been excluded at a dose of 300 mg daily.

ANTICOAGULANTS

Warfarin and heparin are not associated with any overall benefit because of an increase in haemorrhagic complications and so cannot be recommended for acute treatment. Heparin is occasionally used for 'stroke in evolution' and basilar artery thrombosis, and is frequently used in carotid or vertebral artery dissection [4].

Long term

The diagnosis has been made and treatment initiated. Subsequent management is directed at establishing the underlying cause of the stroke and initiating secondary preventative measures.

Further investigations

In appropriate circumstances the following are likely to be helpful in determining cause, and identifying factors important in secondary preventative treatment.
• Electrocardiography should have been performed acutely but it is critical to ensure that it is reviewed. The diagnosis of atrial fibrillation will have a significant impact on further management.
• Carotid dopplers and magnetic resonance angiography (MRA) to look for symptomatic ICA stenosis, in a case of carotid territory ischaemia. If these two investigations are in agreement, they should avoid the need for intra-arterial angiography.
• Transthoracic echocardiogram if an embolic source is suspected. In a young stroke patient in whom an embolic source is considered, transoesophageal echocardiography should be performed.
• Serum cholesterol.
• Thrombophilia screen—at present the significance of these tests is not clear, so reserve for cases with no other clear aetiological risk factors, young patients and those with a strong family history. Similarly, a sickle cell screen is crucial when appropriate.

Secondary preventative treatment

RISK FACTOR REDUCTION

Most of the evidence is from primary prevention studies [1], but removal of as many risk factors as possible is sensible.

ANTIPLATELET THERAPY

Aspirin is beneficial in secondary prevention of all vascular events, as demonstrated by the Antiplatelet Trialists' Collaboration, and seems to reduce subsequent vascular events by about 23%. The time to commence it is established to be as soon as possible (i.e. after haemorrhage excluded), both by the International Stroke Trial (IST) and the Chinese Acute Stroke Trial (CAST) [6].

Dipyridamole mr 200 mg b.d. should be added if further events occur on aspirin monotherapy.

If the patient has multiple vascular risk factors, start with combination therapy (aspirin plus dipyridamole mr).

If the patient is genuinely aspirin intolerant, use clopidogrel. Alternatively, dipyridamole mr monotherapy could be considered in patients with low vascular risk factors, but not in those with high vascular risk factors, as dipyridamole mr alone seems to have no effect on non-stroke vascular events [6].

ANTICOAGULANTS

Warfarin should be prescribed for most patients having had an ischaemic stroke with atrial fibrillation. It is not clear exactly when to start this, but after major stroke wait at least 2 weeks, possibly less in minor strokes, to reduce the chances of haemorrhagic conversion.

CAROTID SURGERY

Two trials, the North American Symptomatic Carotid Endarterectomy Trial (NASCET), and the European Carotid Surgery Trial (ECST), studied patients with recent TIA or minor stroke, and found a beneficial effect of carotid endarterectomy in those with a greater than 70% stenosis. If risk of recurrent stroke in those with high-grade stenosis is 20% in first-year data from the control group, and risk of death or stroke as a result of surgery and cerebral angiography is 10%, then for every 10 patients treated, 1 stroke will be caused and 2 prevented [7]. To improve this figure, one would need to select patients with higher risk of recurrence (tighter stenosis, ulcerated plaque, intraluminal thrombus) and reduce the risk of surgery and in particular angiography, perhaps by considering the use of Doppler studies and MRA in conjunction.

CHOLESTEROL

Raised cholesterol is an important risk factor for coronary artery disease (CAD), but the association with cerebrovascular disease is less clear. CAD is a major cause of death in stroke patients, and so it seems reasonable to treat a cholesterol level over 5 mmol/L (and some would say even lower) after stroke or TIA with a statin.

Complications

Complications of acute stroke include the following:

- Cerebral oedema: commonest cause of death, usually at 4–5 days.
- Haemorrhagic transformation.
- Seizures complicate 10% of infarcts or haemorrhages, but do not influence mortality.
- Depression occurs in 50% of acute strokes, particularly with left anterior lesions.
- Deterioration in glycaemic control.
- Syndrome of inappropriate antidiuretic hormone secretion, peaking at 7–9 days.
- Pressure sores.
- Pulmonary embolism.
- Aspiration.

Prognosis

- 20% death in first month, 30% in first year.
- In those alive at 1 year annual death rate is 8.5%
- The annual risk of recurrence is 13% in the first year, 5% thereafter.
- The risk of stroke or cardiac event by 5 years is 40%.

It is very important to remember not only risk of recurrent stroke but also of cardiac events.

Occupational aspects

Following stroke, patients often report reduced exercise tolerance and increased fatigue levels, which may continue beyond good functional recovery. This has implications for the timing of return to work when appropriate.

Driving is discouraged for 3 months.

1 Bronner LL, Kanter DS, Manson JE. Primary prevention of stroke. *N Engl J Med* 1995; 333: 1392–1400.
2 Pulsinelli W. Pathophysiology of acute ischaemic stroke. *Lancet* 1992; 339: 533–536.
3 Bamford J, Sandercock P, Dennis M *et al.* Classification and natural history of clinically identifiable subtypes of cerebral infarction. *Lancet* 1991; 337: 1521–1526.
4 Davenport R, Dennis M. Neurological emergencies: acute stroke. *J Neurol Neurosurg Psychiatry* 2000; 68: 277–288.
5 Wardlaw JM, Warlow CP, Counsell C. Systematic review of evidence on thrombolytic therapy for acute ischaemic stroke. *Lancet* 1997; 350: 607–614.
6 McCabe DJ, Brown MM. Prevention of ischaemic stroke— antiplatelets. *Br Med Bull* 2000; 56: 510–525.
7 Warlow CP. Can neurologists influence stroke incidence, and do they? *J R Coll Physicians Lond* 1998; 32: 466–472.

2.8.2 TRANSIENT ISCHAEMIC ATTACKS

A transient ischaemic attack (TIA) is an episode of acute loss of focal cerebral or monocular function with symptoms lasting less than 24 h, which is thought to be due to

Table 45 Symptoms raising the possibility of transient ischaemic attacks.

Carotid	Vertebrobasilar
Contralateral paresis, heaviness, or clumsiness in leg, arm/hand, face	Bilateral, unilateral, or alternating paresis (may be contra- and ipsilateral in face/limbs)
Contralateral, predominantly negative, sensory symptoms in leg, arm/hand, face	Sensory loss, unilateral or bilateral (may be contra- and ipsilateral in face/limbs)
Contralateral homonymous hemianopia	Diplopia
Unilateral monocular visual loss	Bilateral visual loss
Aphasia	Dysphagia
Dysarthria	Dysarthria
Combination of the above	Combination of the above

inadequate cerebral or ocular blood supply as a result of arterial, cardiac or haematological cause [1].

The clinical significance of a TIA is no different to that of a minor stroke. Both patients make a good recovery (TIAs usually recover within 30–60 min, despite the definition), and the challenge for the clinician is how to prevent a major stroke occurring. Investigation and secondary prevention is as detailed in Section 2.8.1. The distinct characteristics of TIAs are discussed below.

Clinical presentation

The diagnosis is made on a history of focal neurological symptoms (Table 45), as signs will almost certainly have disappeared by the time of assessment. The vascular territory involved, carotid or vertebrobasilar, is suspected on the same basis as for ischaemic strokes. Isolated dysarthria or homonymous hemianopia are more difficult to interpret, as they may be caused by TIAs in either territory.

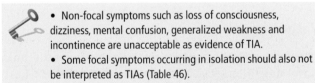

- Non-focal symptoms such as loss of consciousness, dizziness, mental confusion, generalized weakness and incontinence are unacceptable as evidence of TIA.
- Some focal symptoms occurring in isolation should also not be interpreted as TIAs (Table 46).

Physical signs

Examine for the following:
- There are usually no abnormalities, but a full cardiovascular examination for predisposing factors is warranted.

Table 46 Symptoms not acceptable as TIA if isolated.

Vertigo
Diplopia
Dysphagia
Loss of balance
Tinnitus
Scintillating scotomas
Amnesia
Drop attacks
Sensory symptoms confined to one part of limb or face

- It is essential to listen for a carotid bruit, although its absence may just as well indicate a very tight stenosis as a fully patent vessel.
- A cholesterol embolus visualized on fundoscopy indicates that the aetiology is atheromatous plaque in the aortic arch or internal carotid artery in a case of amaurosis fugax.

Consider subclavian steal syndrome

Vertebrobasilar symptoms brought on by exercise of the ipsilateral arm may be the result of the stenosis of the proximal subclavian artery, or aortic arch, leading to retrograde flow down the vertebral artery (Fig. 39). On examination there may be a bruit in the supraclavicular fossa with reduced blood pressure and pulse pressure in the ipsilateral arm.

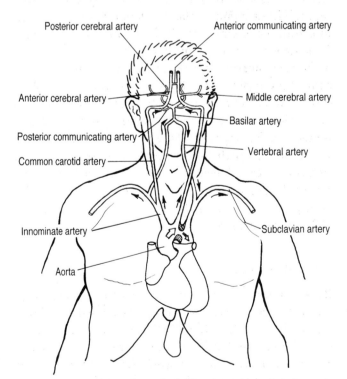

Fig. 39 Subclavian steal syndrome. The lesion is in the aortic arch between the take-off of the left common carotid artery and the left subclavian artery. The blood therefore tends to flow up both carotids and the right vertebral artery and then flows back down the left vertebral artery, ultimately rejoining the subclavian artery to supply the left arm.

Table 47 Differential diagnosis of TIA.

Partial epilepsy
Migraine with aura
Migraine equivalents
Multiple sclerosis
Intracranial space occupying lesions
Intracranial vascular malformations
Cardiac dysrhythmia
Vestibular disorders
Peripheral nerve or root lesions
Anxiety, hyperventilation
Hypoglycaemia
Transient global amnesia

Differential diagnosis

See Table 47.

Migraine and epilepsy are two of the commonest differential diagnoses encountered.

Migraine

The difficulty arises when considering migraine equivalents, i.e. migraine without headache. The following points are helpful.
• Migrainous symptoms are usually positive (tingling, scintillating scotoma), whereas TIA symptoms are usually negative (numbness, reduced vision, weakness).
• The spread of symptoms in migraine tends to be slow, i.e. over several minutes.
• After a migraine, patients often feel generally unwell for hours, which doesn't seem to happen after a TIA.

Partial epilepsy

• Symptoms are usually positive (shaking, tingling) and are brief, compared to TIA.
• Very frequent attacks are usually epileptic.
Note that occasionally focal lower limb shaking, occurring on standing, has been associated with severe contralateral carotid artery stenosis.

Prognosis

Risk of stroke following TIA

• The risk of stroke is increased 13 times in the first year following a TIA, and by 7 times for each subsequent year.
• 4% in the first month.
• 9% in the first 6 months.
• 12% in the first 12 months.
• 4% per annum thereafter.

Most strokes occur in the same territory as the previous TIA. Amaurosis fugax, possibly for this reason, has a much lower chance of leading to a stroke.

Patients with TIA have arterial disease, and as such have a higher risk of heart disease. In fact, the risk of

myocardial infarct and sudden cardiac death is about 4% per annum, which emphasizes the point that you must consider heart disease in TIA and stroke patients.

1 Warlow CP. Can neurologists influence stroke incidence, and do they? *J R Coll Physicians Lond* 1998; 32: 466–472.

2.8.3 INTRACEREBRAL HAEMORRHAGE

Aetiology

Almost all cases of intracerebral haemorrhage (ICH) are caused by one of the following.
• Primary hypertensive ICH (at least 50%).
• Ruptured saccular aneurysms and arteriovenous malformations (30%).
• ICH associated with bleeding disorders (10%).

In addition, cerebral amyloid angiopathy (CAA) is recognized as a common cause in the elderly.
Other causes include:
• tumours
• haemorrhagic infarction
• trauma
• sympathomimetic drugs
• cerebral vasculitis
and rarely:
• mycotic aneurysm (endocarditis)
• haemorrhagic leukoencephalopathy
• herpes simplex encephalitis.

Pathology

Chronic hypertension causes a vasculopathy in the small perforating arteries characterized by lipohyalinosis, fibrinoid necrosis and the formation of Charcot–Bouchard microaneurysms. Rupture of these results in haemorrhage in predominantly deep areas of the brain (Table 48).

Small haematomas dissect along white matter tracts, but large haematomas rupture into the parenchyma, causing destruction of tissue and elevation of intracranial pressure. Death occurs due to hemisphere and/or brainstem compression.

Table 48 Sites of hypertensive intracerebral haemorrhage.

Site	Percentage (%)
Putamen	35–50
Subcortical (lobar)	30
Cerebellum	16
Thalamus	10–15
Pons	5–12

Epidemiology

- 10–15% of all strokes.
- Twice as common as subarachnoid haemorrhage.

Clinical presentation

Clinically indistinguishable from ischaemic stroke, but headache, vomiting and seizures at onset are more likely in ICH. A large haemorrhage will cause death or coma within hours, no matter where the location. Onset may be rapid, but ICH associated with anticoagulant therapy may evolve slowly.

 ICH cannot reliably be distinguished from ischaemia on clinical grounds.

Physical signs

Smaller haematomas may have distinguishing physical signs depending on the site.

Supratentorial

- *Putamen*: predominantly hemiplegia, also aphasia, homonymous hemianopia, hemineglect and deviation of eyes away from the affected side.
- *Thalamic*: predominantly hemisensory deficit, also hemiparesis, aphasia (dominant side), neglect (non-dominant side). Ocular signs may be prominent with forced downward deviation of the eyes, skew deviation (vertical separation of gaze) and ipsilateral Horner's syndrome.
- *Lobar*: depends on the site of the lesion.

Infratentorial

- *Cerebellar*: may be slow to develop, so unlikely to be comatose at onset. Deviation of eyes away from haemorrhage, ipsilateral CNV-VII palsies, ipsilateral Horner's syndrome. Hemiplegia and aphasia are absent, as are cerebellar signs early on. Progresses to coma as a result of brain-stem compression.
- *Pontine*: total paralysis, decerebrate rigidity (extension to pain), pinpoint reactive pupils, absent doll's eyes response.

Investigation

CT scan will be diagnostic (Figs 40–42).

If the patient is under 40 years old with no history of hypertension, it may be wise to enhance the scan, to look for an underlying lesion.

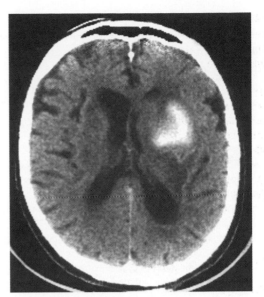

Fig. 40 Putaminal haemorrhage on CT scan.

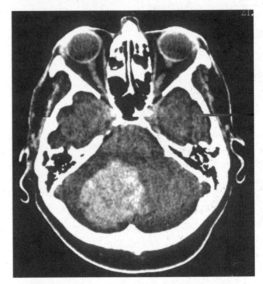

Fig. 41 Cerebellar hemisphere haemorrhage on CT scan. Courtesy of Professor M. Brown, Institute of Neurology, University of London.

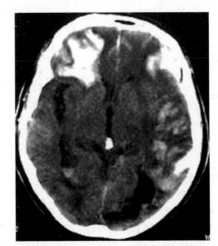

Fig. 42 Multiple surperficial haemorrhages of different ages seen on CT head scan. This patient was presumed to have cerebral amyloid angiopathy. Courtesy of Professor M. Brown, Institute of Neurology, University of London.

An angiogram is warranted when there is significant suspicion of an underlying lesion. Factors that increase the likelihood of finding an abnormality are:
- under 45 years old
- absence of hypertension
- lobar haemorrhage, unless the patient is over 65 years old as CAA would then be a more likely aetiology.

> **Cerebral amyloid angiopathy**
>
> - Common cause of ICH in the elderly; sporadic but a few autosomal dominant families.
> - Subcortical, often multiple, haemorrhage, particularly in occipital and parietal lobes [1].
> - Pathological changes found in 10% of septuagenarians and in 60% of those over 90.
> - Association between CAA and Alzheimer-type pathology.
> - 10–30% of those with CAA have a progressive dementia.

Differential diagnosis

See Section 2.8.1, p. 90.

Treatment

Medical management

See Table 49.

Surgical

Trials have not shown benefit for surgical intervention in ICH [2]. However, selected patients may benefit from surgery.

Surgery indicated

- Cerebellar haemorrhage over 3 cm, because of the risk

of hydrocephalus and brain-stem compression. Remember, these patients may deteriorate slowly. Don't wait for brain-stem signs to occur as it will be too late to reverse any deficit.
- Young patients who were initially stable but subsequently deteriorate may benefit from surgery, especially if there is superficial lobar haemorrhage.

Surgery not indicated

- Glasgow Coma Score (GCS) ≤4 (unless cerebellar).
- Small lesion, minimal deficit.

For other types surgery is probably not indicated at present, but this is not clear.

Complications

- Death
- Hydrocephalus
- Disability.

Prognosis

- 35–50% death by 1 month.
- 10% independent at 1 month, 20% by 6 months.

> 1 Miller JH, Wardlow JM, Lammie GA. Intracerebral haemorrhage and cerebral amyloid angiopathy: CT features with pathological correlation. *Clin Radiol* 1999; 54(7): 422–429.
> 2 Hankey GJ, Hon C. Surgery for primary intracerebral haemorrhage: is it safe and effective? A systematic review of case series and randomized trials. *Stroke* 1997; 28(11): 2126–2132.

2.8.4 SUBARACHNOID HAEMORRHAGE

Aetiology

Eighty per cent of non-traumatic subarachnoid haemorrhages (SAH) are caused by ruptured saccular (berry) aneurysms. These are usually found at bifurcations and branchings of the arteries of the circle of Willis or its major branches. The reason why some aneurysms rupture and others do not is not known. The risk is greater for larger aneurysms than for smaller.

Epidemiology

The incidence of SAH is between 8 and 12 per 100 000 per year and is the diagnosis in 1–4% of patients presenting to emergency departments with headache. Risk factors include hypertension, cigarette smoking, alcohol consumption (particularly binge drinking), adult polycystic kidney disease and some connective tissue disorders.

Table 49 Principles of medical management of patients with ICH.

Immediate priorities (first few hours)
Protect and maintain airway
Prevent hypoxia—give oxygen if saturation <95% on pulse oximetry
Regular monitoring and neurological observations—review if condition deteriorates
Nursing—bed rest, elevate head of bed by 30°, protect pressure areas

Later priorities (first few days)
Maintain hydration—intravenous fluids if cannot drink safely
Consider nutrition—nasogastric (later via PEG tube) if cannot swallow safely

Other aspects
Hypertension—treat if blood pressure is extremely high (>200/ 120 mmHg), but with caution
Agitation—give the minimum sedation possible (often a difficult judgement)
Pain—use paracetamol or codeine
Bowels—use stool softeners, etc. to prevent straining

Clinical presentation

Subarachnoid haemorrhage can present with relatively minor symptoms, devastating neurological dysfunction, or be a cause of sudden death.

The typical presentation is with sudden onset of severe headache: 'the worst headache I've ever had'; 'like being hit on the back of the head with a hammer'. This usually occurs when the patient is active, rather than asleep, and often during exertion. There is frequently transient loss of consciousness, also vomiting.

Between 20 and 50% of patients with documented SAH report a distinct, unusually severe, 'warning headache' in the days or weeks prior to the episode of bleeding.

Physical signs

Many patients will have some or all of the following features:

- Impaired conscious level: GCS can vary from 3 (minimum) to 15 (maximum).
- Focal neurological signs, in particular: third nerve palsy (posterior communicating artery aneurysm); sixth nerve palsy (posterior fossa aneurysm, but also a false localizing sign with raised intracranial pressure); bilateral leg weakness (anterior communicating aneurysm); nystagmus or ataxia (posterior fossa aneurysm); aphasia, hemiparesis, hemianopia (middle cerebral artery aneurysm).
- Neck rigidity.
- Retinal haemorrhages, which are thought to result from an acute increase in intracranial pressure that causes obstruction to the venous outflow from the eye.

Patients may be hypertensive, have cardiac dysrhythmias, also ECG patterns mimicking myocardial infarction—all of which can lead to diagnostic confusion. Those whose SAH has led to syncope may have sustained a head injury, which can also make diagnosis difficult.

Investigation

Immediate

The investigation of choice in suspected SAH is immediate CT scan without contrast, taking very thin cuts through the base of the brain to optimize the chances of seeing small collections of blood (Fig. 43). The sensitivity of modern scanners for detecting SAH is very high: 98–100% if scanning is performed within 12 h of onset of symptoms, 93% within the first 24 h.

Lumbar puncture should be performed in suspected SAH if the CT scan is negative, equivocal or technically unsatisfactory. 'Traumatic taps' occur in up to 20% of procedures and need to be distinguished from true haemorrhage: the 'three tube' method, which looks for

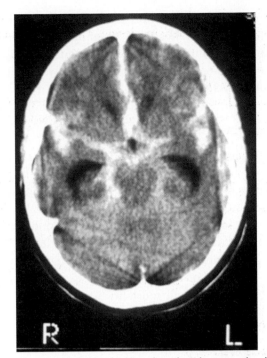

Fig. 43 CT scan showing blood in the subarachnoid space and early ventricular dilatation.

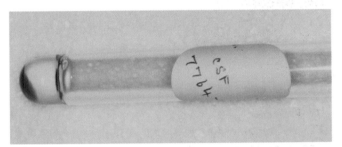

Fig. 44 Test tube of blood-stained CSF after being spun down in a centrifuge to reveal xanthochromic supernatant in a case of subarachnoid haemorrhage.

decreasing numbers of erythrocytes in successively collected specimens, is not entirely reliable. The diagnosis of SAH is established by centrifuging the CSF specimen without delay and demonstrating the presence of xanthochromia (due to the presence of oxyhaemoglobin and bilirubin) by spectrophotometry (Fig. 44). Note, however, that xanthochromia may not be present if the CSF is examined within 12 h of haemorrhage occurring, hence in the face of a normal CT scan lumbar puncture should be delayed until 24 h after the ictus.

Subsequent

In cases of proven SAH where intervention (radiological or surgical) is contemplated (see Treatment), imaging of the cerebral vessels by four-vessel angiography is required.

Differential diagnosis

Many studies have shown that about 30% of patients with

SAH are misdiagnosed at presentation. Differential is from infective causes of headache (meningitis, encephalitis, viral infection ('flu)), other causes of headache (migraine, cluster or tension headache; sinus-related headache), neck pain, and psychiatric disorder.

Complications

The patient may present with neurological deficit, recover, but then develop hemiplegia or other focal signs 4–10 days after rupture: this is due to delayed cerebral ischaemia.

Re-bleeding is the most feared complication. Series of patients admitted to hospital with SAH in the 1960s showed that about 10% died of the original haemorrhage, but 50% re-bled, with an 80% mortality in this group, i.e. the overall mortality was about 50%, with many survivors remaining neurologically disabled.

Treatment

General measures

Bed rest and treatment of hypertension, aiming to keep BP <160/100.

Specific measures

Nimodipine is used for prevention and treatment of ischaemic neurological deficit due to vascular spasm after SAH, for prevention at a dose of 60 mg p.o. every 4 h, for treatment by intravenous infusion at a rate of 0.5–2 mg/h. Once volume resuscitation (when necessary) has been completed, preventative treatment should be given to all patients with SAH who are not hypotensive. Intravenous nimodipine should only be administered in the setting of a neurological ICU because hypotension is a common and serious problem.

In appropriately selected patients, surgery prevents rebleeding and improves outcome. Indications for surgery are proven intracranial aneurysms in:
• patients with GCS greater than or equal to 12
• patients with GCS less than 12 who have space occupying intracranial haemorrhage associated with an aneurysm, or with hydrocephalus
• Age alone is not a contraindication to surgery.

After surgery, patients typically remain in hospital for 2 weeks. They should be treated for general vascular risk factors (hypertension, cholesterol, diabetes, stop smoking) and must inform the DVLA regarding driving (if they make a full recovery their licence is usually returned after 3 months). There are no long-term lifestyle restrictions (except smoking).

Prognosis

With modern medical and surgical management poor outcome (death or severe disability) occurs in 20% of all those with SAH admitted to hospital. A good clinical outcome is expected in 90–95% of those admitted in good clinical condition (GCS 14 or 15).

Prevention

Incidental aneurysms occur in up to 1% of the population. Any such patient should be referred for specialist advice, but the majority (aneurysms <10 mm in diameter) do not require surgery.

> Unruptured intracranial aneurysms—risk of rupture and risks of surgical intervention. International study of unruptured intracranial aneurysm investigators. *N Engl J Med* 1998; 339: 1725–1733.
> Edlow JA, Caplan LR. Avoiding pitfalls in the diagnosis of subarachnoid haemorrhage. *N Engl J Med* 2000; 342: 29–36.

2.9 Brain tumours

Pathology

Tumours can arise within the brain or adjoining structures, or invade by direct or haematological metastatic spread. Brain tumours can be benign or malignant,

Table 50 Classification of brain tumours.

Primary	Intraparenchymal	Gliomas
		Astrocytoma, many types
		Glioblastoma multiforme
		Oligodendroglioma
		Mixed glioma, e.g. oligoastrocytoma
		Ependymal tumours
		Neuronal tumours, e.g. gangliocytomas
		Primitive neuroectodermal tumours, e.g. medulloblastoma
	Extraparenchymal (extrinsic/extra axial)	Meninges: meningioma
		Cranial nerve sheath: schwannomas/neuromas
		Pituitary gland: micro- and macro-adenomas
		Bone: osteomas
		Blood vessel: haemangioblastomas
Secondary	Direct extension	Nasopharyngeal
		Chordoma
		Glomus jugulare tumours
	Metastasis	
	Haematological	Primary CNS lymphoma

Table 51 Age distribution of brain tumours by site.

Adult	Childhood
Supratentorial	
(70% of adult brain tumours)	Craniopharyngioma
Glioma	Pinealoma
Meningioma	Gliomas (mainly astrocytomas
Pituitary	of optic nerve and thalamus)
Metastasis (commonest)	
Infratentorial	
(Mainly cerebellar, brain stem rare)	Medulloblastoma (infancy)
Metastasis	Cerebellar astrocytoma
Acoustic neuroma	Ependymoma of IVth ventricle
Cerebellar haemangioblastoma	

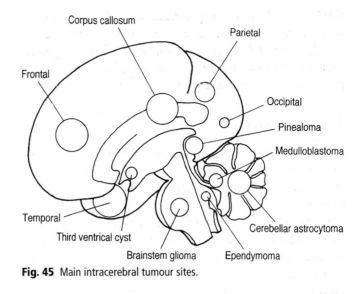

Fig. 45 Main intracerebral tumour sites.

malignancy implying rapid growth, poor differentiation, mitosis, necrosis and vascular proliferation, but metastasis to extracranial sites is infrequent. A benign tumour may be equally devastating by virtue of its position [1]. The classification of brain tumours is shown in Table 50, and their age distribution in Table 51.

Epidemiology

Primary brain tumours occur in 6 per 100 000 persons annually, 1 in 12 being in children under 15 years old.

Clinical presentation

The nature of the clinical presentation will reflect the site of the tumour (Figs 45 and 46) and its rate of expansion. Rapidly expanding tumours or those blocking CSF flow and causing obstructive hydrocephalus will present with symptoms (postural headache, nausea and vomiting, diplopia) and signs (papilloedema, and VIth nerve palsy)

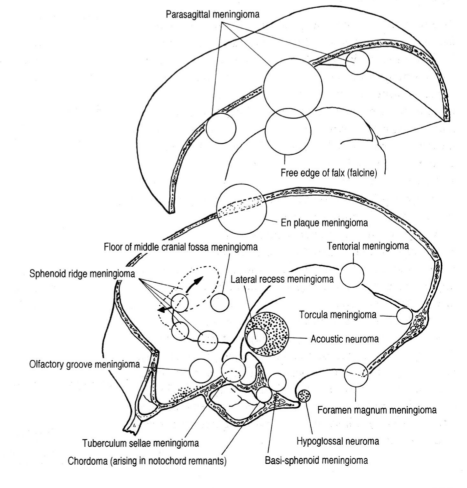

Fig. 46 Main locations of extracerebral intracranial tumours.

Table 52 Brain tumours: common presentations.

Site	Common symptoms and signs
Frontal	Personality change Contralateral motor signs Dysphasia (dominant hemisphere) (Note: Foster Kennedy syndrome: ipsilateral optic atrophy and contralateral papilloedema)
Parietal	Contralateral sensory change/cortical sensory loss Visual field defect (optic radiation) Neglect Apraxias (Note: Gerstmann's syndrome: agraphia, left/right disorientation, acalculia and finger agnosia)
Occipital	Homonymous hemianopia ± macular sparing
Temporal	Memory and behavioural disturbance
Parasagittal	Gait abnormality (small steps) Spastic paraparesis (consider in the differential diagnosis of spinal cord compression)
Posterior fossa	Raised intracranial pressure Ataxia and nystagmus Cranial nerve lesions
Pituitary	Bitemporal hemianopia (pressure on optic chiasm) Endocrine disturbance (see *Endocrinology*, Section 2.1) Cranial nerve III, IV, Va and b and VI (lateral extension to cavernous sinus) (Note: pituitary apoplexy: sudden blindness and subarachnoid haemorrhage)

of raised intracranial pressure. A VIth nerve palsy may be a 'false localizing' sign. Lesions involving the cortex may present with epilepsy. Stroke-like presentations usually reflect bleeding into a tumour. Common presentations are shown in Table 52. Rarely, patients may present with paraneoplastic syndromes (see Section 2.11.1, p. 104).

Investigation

The most important investigation is the CT or MRI scan. An MRI is preferable for:
• posterior fossa tumours
• detecting multiple lesions, more suggestive of metastases.

The high incidence of metastases compared to primary brain tumours makes a chest radiograph and blood tests (FBC, ESR, U+Es, LFTs, Ca, Phos) essential.

Lumbar puncture is unlikely to be safe and has a low positive yield.

Cerebral biopsy should be performed in most patients to exclude potentially treatable causes and also to help staging.

Differential diagnosis

The important conditions to consider in the differential diagnosis are as follows:

• Vascular causes such as haematoma with mass effect, giant aneurysm, arteriovenous malformation, cerebral infarct with oedema and venous thrombosis.
• Trauma resulting in haematoma/contusion.
• Infection of the CNS including abscess, tuberculosis, herpes simplex encephalitis and hydatid cysts.
• Many inflammatory conditions which may cause focal signs, particularly MS and neurosarcoidosis.

Treatment

There are several options to consider in the treatment of malignant primary brain tumours.

Symptomatic treatment

Consider steroids in the acute setting for the symptomatic treatment of oedema. Dexamethasone 12 mg intravenously, followed by 4 mg q.d.s. orally or intravenously for no more than a week (loses efficacy after this).

Surgery

Aggressive surgical resection for malignant lesions is impossible since the lesions are widely invasive beyond the macroscopic margins, and large-volume resections are associated with unacceptable morbidity. Surgery may be attempted if the lesion is situated in the frontal lobe or occipital pole.

Radiotherapy

Radiotherapy is not curative, but some tumours are sensitive. In the treatment of malignant cerebral glioma, radiotherapy offers a survival benefit of approximately 6 months [2].

Chemotherapy

The role of chemotherapy is not yet clear, but some patients may benefit [3].

Prognosis

This depends entirely on type, but a patient with a grade 1–2 glioma may survive for years, whereas the patient with a grade 4 tumour will survive for a maximum of months if treated with surgery alone.

Disease associations

Neurocutaneous syndromes

Brain tumours are cardinal features of the neurocutaneous

Table 53 Brain tumours as part of neurocutaneous disorders.

Syndrome	Genetics	Features
Von Hippel–Lindau disease	AD, 3p26–25	Brain: haemangioblastoma (cerebellar, less common in cerebral hemispheres and brain stem) Eyes: retinal angioma Skin: hamartomas Visceral organs: tumours and cysts Phaeochromocytoma
Neurofibromatosis 1	AD, 17q11.2	Brain: optic and chiasmatic nerve glioma, neurofibroma and plexiform neurofibroma Eyes: Lisch nodules Skin: café-au-lait spots (numerous), axillary ± inguinal freckles
Neurofibromatosis 2	AD, 22q11–13.1	Brain: bilateral acoustic neuromas. Less commonly, meningioma, glioma and other neuromas. Schwanomas compress in cranial or spinal roots in their foramina Eye: presenile cataracts Skin: cutaneous neurofibroma, café-au-lait spots (less numerous)
Tuberous sclerosis	AD, 9q34.1–34.2 (some families)	Brain: cortical tubers, subependymal nodules, astrocytoma Eye: hamartomas Skin: shagreen plaques, ungual fibroma, facial angiofibromata (adenoma sebaceum) Other: widespread hamartomatosis

AD, autosomal dominant.

syndromes. The prevalence of these is higher in the medical exam setting than in real life. Beware the patient with skin lesions and neurological signs! Table 53 summarizes these syndromes.

1 Allcut DA, Mendelow AD. Presentation and diagnosis of brain tumours. *Br J Hosp Med* 1992; 47(10): 745–752.
2 Delattre JY, Uchuya M. Radiotherapy and chemotherapy for gliomas. *Curr Opin Neurol* 1996; 8(3): 196–203.
3 DeAngelis LM, Burger PC, Green SB, Cairncross JG. Malignant glioma: who benefits from adjuvant chemotherapy? *Ann Neurol* 1998; 44(4): 691–695.

2.10 Neurological complications of infection

2.10.1 NEW VARIANT CREUTZFELDT–JAKOB DISEASE

Aetiology

There is increasing evidence supporting a causal association between bovine spongiform encephalopathy (BSE) and new variant creutzfeldt–Jakob disease (nvCJD).

Recent studies reveal that:
• Glycosylation patterns of the disease-associated prion protein (PrP) in nvCJD resembles that in BSE-infected cattle, but is not seen in sporadic CJD.
• In mice, the characteristics of the agents responsible for nvCJD and BSE were identical, but different from those in sporadic CJD [1].

Epidemiology

The only environmental risk factor identified is UK residence, but this may change. The size of the potential problem in the UK is difficult to predict as the time and source of exposure to BSE in the current cases of nvCJD is unknown. Genetic analysis indicates that BSE is transmitted only to humans who have the prion protein gene (PRNP) codon 129 methionine homozygous genotype.

Clinical presentation

In nvCJD, the mean age of onset is 29 years and mean disease duration is 14 months compared to the 60 years and 5 months, respectively, in sporadic CJD.

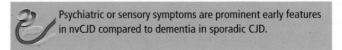

Psychiatric or sensory symptoms are prominent early features in nvCJD compared to dementia in sporadic CJD.

Physical signs

Cerebellar signs are prominent early on. Upgaze paresis, which is uncommon in sporadic CJD, often occurs in nvCJD. Pyramidal signs, primitive reflexes (such as grasp and pout reflexes) and myoclonus may also be seen [2].

Investigation

The following may be helpful:
- EEG may show slow waves, but not the periodic spike-and-wave complexes typical of sporadic CJD.
- Elevated levels of the neuronal protein 14.3.3 in CSF may be found.
- Post-mortem neuropathological examination is the only way of confirming the diagnosis, although there is one report of ante-mortem diagnosis using tonsillar biopsy [3].

Complications

The risks of transmission of nvCJD through blood are unknown but may be higher than the low risk associated with sporadic CJD [4]. There is concern that levels of PrP in lymphoreticular tissue of patients with nvCJD may be higher than in those with sporadic CJD. Therefore, blood and blood products from nvCJD cases are now withdrawn in the UK.

1 Stewart GE, Ironside JW. New variant Creutzfeldt–Jakob disease. *Curr Opin Neurol* 1998; 11: 259–262.
2 Zeidler M, Stewart GE, Barraclough CR *et al.* New variant Creutzfeldt–Jakob disease: neurological features and diagnostic tests. *Lancet* 1997; 350: 903–907.
3 Hill AF, Butterworth RJ, Joiner S *et al.* Investigation of variant Creutzfeldt–Jakob disease and other human prion diseases with tonsic biopsy samples. *Lancet* 1999; 353: 183–189.
4 Will RG, Kimberlin RH. Creutzfeldt–Jakob disease and the risk from blood or blood products. *Vox Sang* 1998; 75: 178–180.

2.11 Neurological complications of systemic disease

2.11.1 PARANEOPLASTIC CONDITIONS

Introduction

Non-neurological malignancies can affect the nervous system in many ways. This can be by infiltration or compression, either by direct spread of the primary tumour or by haematogenous metastatic spread. However, a wide range of non-metastatic remote complications are described. Many of these can be attributed to cachexia, competition between tumour and body tissues for substances such as glucose and tryptophan, or to adverse affects of chemotherapy such as vincristine and cisplatin. Others appear to have an immunological basis. It is this latter group that will be discussed as paraneoplastic conditions.

- Paraneoplastic syndromes can occur up to several years prior to detection of the underlying tumour. In some cases, the tumour is not identified until autopsy.
- The tumour is usually small, suggesting that it is being held at bay by the immune response.
- An immune response is directed against a tumour antigen also expressed on neural tissue (onconeural antigen). Paraneoplastic disorders are therefore autoimmune in nature.
- The pathogenesis of certain paraneoplastic conditions is antibody mediated (Lambert–Eaton myasthenic syndrome, LEMS) whereas in others it may be cytokine- or T-cell-mediated [1].
- Identification of a particular associated antineuronal antibody will direct the hunt for the underlying tumour.
- None of the paraneoplastic syndromes is invariably associated with malignancy.

Clinical presentation

Numerous neurological paraneoplastic syndromes are described. Given the broad range of symptoms, what is it that makes the clinician consider a diagnosis of paraneoplastic syndrome?
- Conditions that progress rapidly over weeks to months before reaching a plateau.
- Patients are usually significantly disabled at the time of presentation, and mild waxing and waning symptoms are unlikely to be paraneoplastic in origin.
- Presentations are usually stereotyped as described below.

Paraneoplastic conditions involving the central nervous system

Paraneoplastic encephalomyelitis (PEM)

LIMBIC ENCEPHALITIS

Symptoms are anxiety, depression, impairment of recent memory and fluctuating confusion. More than 70% are associated with small-cell lung carcinoma (SCLC). This is also described in Hodgkin's disease (HD).

BRAIN-STEM ENCEPHALITIS

There are variable brain-stem signs and there may be corticospinal tract involvement. Mainly associated with SCLC.

MYELITIS/ANTERIOR HORN CELL DISEASE

This can mimic MND. Any sensory signs are due to associated subacute sensory neuroneopathy (SSN). Often associated with brain-stem encephalitis.

Paraneoplastic cerebellar degeneration

Ataxia, dysarthria and nystagmus. May be associated PEM. Described with SCLC, gyaenecological tumours and HD.

Paraneoplastic opsoclonus/myoclonus syndrome

In children 50% have neuroblastoma. In adults, associated with cerebellar and brain-stem signs and encephalopathy. Clonazepam may offer relief.

Necrotizing myelopathy

Mimics transverse myelitis or cord compression.

Paraneoplastic conditions involving the eye

Cancer-associated retinopathy

Triad of photosensitivity, ring scotomatous visual field loss and attenuated calibre of retinal arterioles.

Paraneoplastic conditions involving the neuromuscular junction

Stiff man syndrome

Stiffness of proximal limbs and trunk. Described with breast cancer and HD. In association with breast cancer, antibodies to amphiphysin have been described.

> Stiff man syndrome is also associated with organ-specific autoimmune diseases and insulin dependent diabetes mellitus. Sixty per cent have antibodies to glutamic acid decarboxylase.

Lambert–Eaton myasthenic syndrome

Weakness of proximal muscles, mainly in the legs, and autonomic dysfunction. Post-tetanic stimulation of deep tendon reflexes. Antibodies to the presynaptic voltage gated calcium channel. Usually in association with SCLC.

Myasthenia gravis

Muscle fatigability, ptosis and ophthalmoplegia. Antibodies to the acetylcholine receptor. Associated with thymoma.

Paraneoplastic conditions involving the nerve

Subacute sensory neuroneopathy

Rapid progressive loss of all sensory modalities, especially proprioception, may result in pseudoathetosis. May be associated with myelitis. Usually in association with SCLC. The differential diagnosis of this striking neuropathy includes Sjögren's syndrome.

Motor neuroneopathy

Affects legs more than arms, often in a patchy distribution. Spares bulbar musculature. Associated with HD and other lymphomas.

Paraneoplastic vasculitic neuropathy

A mononeuritis multiplex associated with SCLC, endometrial cancer and others.

Brachial neuritis

Asymmetric pain, weakness and wasting in the muscles of the shoulder girdle is usually idiopathic, but can occasionally be associated with malignancy.

Autonomic neuropathy

May rarely be paraneoplastic.

Paraneoplastic conditions involving muscle

Dermatomyositis

Associated with cancer in 10% of cases. See *Rheumatology and clinical immunology*, Section 2.3.5.

Necrotizing myopathy

Necrosis without inflammation; rare.

Investigations

CSF analysis may show protein and a mild pleocytosis. Associated anti-neuronal antibodies may be identified in both serum and CSF. This is an emerging field [2]. Table 54 summarizes our knowledge of onconeural antigens to date.

Treatment

This is a difficult issue. There is limited evidence that complete cure of the malignancy driving the immune

Table 54 Onconeural antigens.

Antibody	Antigen	Associated cancer	Syndrome
Anti-Hu	All neuronal nuclei	SCLD and neuroblastoma	PEM, SSN
Anti-Yo	Purkinje cell cytoplasm	Gynaecological and breast	PCD
Anti-Ri	Neuronal nuclei	Breast, gynaeclogical, SCLC	PCD, opsoclonus
Antiamphiphysin	Synaptic vesicles	Breast	PEM, stiff man syndrome
Anti-VGCC	Presynaptic VGCC	SCLC	LEMS
Anti-AchR	AchR	Thymoma	Myasthenia gravis
Anti-Tr	Neuronal cytoplasm, Purkinje cells, spiny dendrites	HD	PCD

For abbreviations, see text.

response leads to partial or complete resolution of the paraneoplastic condition [3]. There is growing evidence, however, that immunosupressive therapies administered in an attempt to control the neurological symptoms may remove immunological control of the tumour, leading to more rapid growth and increased chance of metastasis.

1 Newsom-Davis J. Paraneoplastic neurological disorders. *J R Coll Physicians Lond* 1999; 33: 225–227.
2 Dalmau JO, Posner JB. Paraneoplastic syndromes. *Arch Neurol* 1999; 56: 405–408. [An up-to-date account of the onconeural antigens.]
3 Cher LM, Henson JW, Das A, Hochberg FH. Paraneoplastic syndromes. In: Vinken PJ, Bruyn GW, eds. *Handbook of Clinical Neurology*, Vol. 27 (71): Systemic Diseases, Part III. Amsterdam: Elsevier Science, 1998: 673–704. [Thorough, with historical perspective and in depth review of therapies.]

2.12 Neuropharmacology

Principles

This section will focus on the fundamental processes of chemical neurotransmission modulated by centrally acting drugs.

Chemical signalling in the CNS is responsible for normal neural function and is an important target for drug action. Only a handful of neurotransmitters are important in signalling at specific interneuronal connections.

Important CNS neurotransmitters are:
• dopamine
• 5HT (serotonin)
• γ-amino butyric acid (GABA)
• opioid peptides
• noradrenaline
• acetylcholine.
Failure of the neuronal signalling process is responsible for a wide variety of symptoms in disorders which include Parkinson's disease, depression, dementia, schizophrenia,

mania and epilepsy. Drugs used in the treatment of these disorders modulate neuronal signalling in the defective pathway to restore, as far as possible, normal neurotransmission.

There are several stages in the signalling process that are susceptible to modulation by drugs (Fig. 47). For a centrally acting drug to have clinical utility, it must target selectively a specific neurotransmitter at a specific set of interneuronal connections. Because a relatively small number of major neurotransmitters mediate chemical signalling in diverse central neuronal pathways, absolute selectivity of drug action is rarely achieved, with the result that side effects are particularly common with these agents.

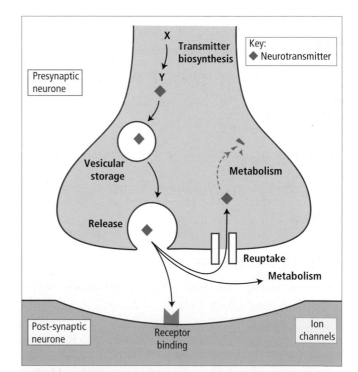

Fig. 47 Processes in neurotransmission susceptible to modulation by centrally acting drugs.

Dopamine

Dopamine (DA) neurones are found in the following.
• Nigrostriatal pathways where deficient dopaminergic neurotransmission is responsible for Parkinson's disease.

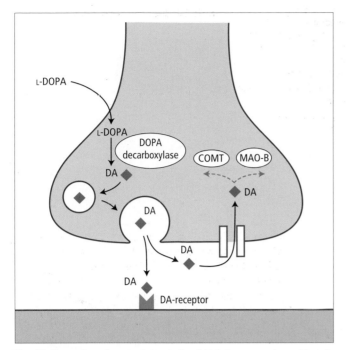

Fig. 48 Dopaminergic neurotransmission. MAO-B, monoamine oxidase B; COMT, catechol-O-methyl transferase; DA, dopamine.

- Mesolimbic and mesocortical pathways where excess dopaminergic neurotransmission has been implicated in schizophrenia.
- Tuberoinfundibular neurones, from where dopaminergic activity results in a tonic inhibition of prolactin secretion.
- The chemoreceptor trigger zone (outside the blood–brain barrier), where dopaminegic function is involved in emesis.

See Fig. 48.

DA receptors

There are two main families, D_1 and D_2, but a number of receptor subtypes. Most known functions are mediated by D_1- and D_2-like receptors.

DA-receptor agonists

These include bromocriptine, lysuride, pergolide, ropinirole (used in the treatment of Parkinson's disease) and cabergoline and quinagolide (used to treat hyperprolactinaemia). Dyskinesias are less common with DA-R agonists than L-DOPA in the treatment of Parkinson's disease, but hallucinations and confusion are common in the elderly.

DA-receptor antagonists

These are used in the treatment of schizophrenia (e.g. chlorpromazine, thioridazine, flupenthixol, haloperidol) and to treat nausea and vomiting (prochlorperazine, metoclopramide and domperidone). Side effects of long-term DA-R blockade in schizophrenia include depression, akathisia, Parkinsonism, tardive dyskinesia and neuroleptic malignant syndrome. Shorter-term treatment can result in hyperprolactinaemia and galactorrhoea. Acute dystonia and oculogyric cases are recognized side effects of DA-R blockade.

L-DOPA

L-DOPA is the precursor for dopamine synthesis used in the treatment of Parkinson's disease. It is given in combination with a peripheral DOPA decarboxylase inhibitor to prevent its metabolism in the gut wall and to enhance oral bioavailability. The long-term use of L-DOPA is associated with the development of dyskinesia.

Inhibitors of metabolism

DA is metabolized by monoamine oxidase B (MAO-B) and catechol-O-methyl transferase (COMT). Selegeline, an inhibitor of MAO-B, is used in the treatment of Parkinson's disease, as is entacapone, an inhibitor of COMT.

5-HT (serotonin)

5-HT-containing neurones are found in the midline raphe nuclei, with widespread projections to the cortex, limbic system, hypothalamus and cord. 5-HT is involved in the control of sleep, mood and emotion, appetite, sexual arousal and vomiting. The drugs that modulate the system are used in the treatment of migraine, depression, schizophrenia, to suppress appetite and to treat vomiting. Certain drugs of abuse including amphetamine, LSD and MDMA (ecstasy) promote 5-HT neurotransmission.

5-HT receptors

Many 5-HT receptor subtypes exist, the main targets for existing drug therapy being 5-HT_{1A}, 5-HT_{1B}, 5-HT_{1D}, 5-HT_2, 5-HT_3 and 5-HT_4. See Fig. 47.

Drugs affecting 5-HT release

Fenfluramine and dexfenfluramine promote 5-HT release and have been used as appetite suppressants. These drugs have been associated with the development of cardiac valve fibrosis and pulmonary hypertension. MDMA also promotes 5-HT release.

5-HT receptor agonists

The major 5-HT agonists used clinically are the triptans (sumatriptan, zolmitriptan and naratriptan), which are 5-HT receptor agonists used in the acute treatment of

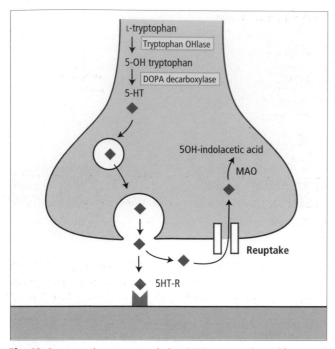

Fig. 49 Serotonergic neurotransmission. MAO, monoamine oxidase.

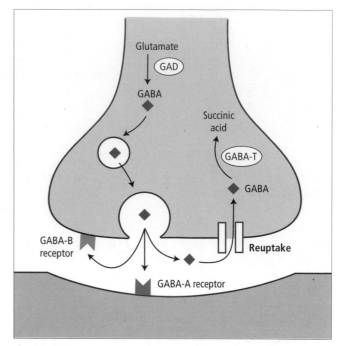

Fig. 50 GABA-ergic neurotransmission. GAD, glutamic acid decarboxylase; GABA-T, GABA transaminase.

migraine. Side effects include nausea and vomiting and, rarely, cardiac ischaemia caused by 5-HT receptor-induced coronary vasospasm. LSD is a partial agonist at the 5-HT$_2$ receptor and is a hallucinogen.

5-HT receptor antagonists

The 5-HT receptor antagonist pizotifen is used in the long-term prophylaxis of migraine. The 5-HT$_3$ receptor antagonists ondansetron and granisetron block the 5-HT$_3$ receptor in the chemoreceptor trigger zone and vagus nerve and are particularly effective in the nausea and vomiting associated with cancer chemotherapy.

Drugs blocking 5-HT reuptake

Selective serotonin reuptake inhibitors (SSRIs) such as fluoxetine, paroxetine and sertraline potentiate 5-HT neurotransmission by blocking reuptake (see Fig. 49). They have equivalent efficacy in the treatment of depression to tricyclics but are associated with a lower incidence of side effects and a better safety profile in overdose. Nefazodone and venlafaxine are newer antidepressants classified as serotonin noradrenergic reuptake inhibitors (SNaRIs) whose clinical efficacy and side-effect profile appears similar to SSRIs.

MAO inhibitors

MAO inhibitors reduce 5-HT metabolism and are used in the management of depression. Non-selective MAO inhibitors such as phenelzine and tranylcypromine are associated with significant dietary and drug interactions. Selective and reversible MAO inhibitors such as moclobemide are somewhat safer.

5-HT$_4$

5-HT$_4$ receptors in the enteric nervous system are involved in modulation of gut motility, and a variety of agonists and antagonists are under development for motility disorders.

GABA

γ-Aminobutyric acid (GABA) is a widely distributed inhibitory neurotransmitter in the CNS. Drugs which potentiate GABAergic neurotransmission in the CNS include benzodiazepenes, vigabatrin, valproate and probably gabapentin, all of which are used to treat epilepsy. See Fig. 50.

GABA release

Gabapentin, a newer anticonvulsant, increases the release of GABA by an unknown mechanism.

GABA metabolism

Vigabatrin is an inhibitor of GABA-transaminase (GABA-T) that enhances GABAergic neurotransmission by preventing GABA metabolism. It is used as add-on therapy in seizures resistant to monotherapy with first-line drugs.

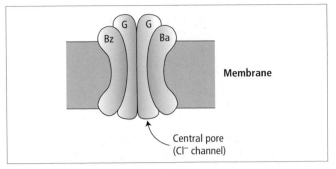

Fig. 51 GABA-A receptor. G, GABA binding site; Bz, benzodiazepine binding site; Ba, barbiturate binding site.

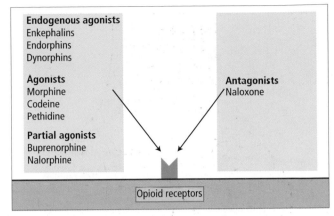

Fig. 52 Opioid peptides.

The action of sodium valproate may be mediated in part by the inhibition of GABA-T.

GABA-A receptor

The GABA-A receptor is a multisubunit, ligand-gated, Cl⁻ ion channel which, when activated, hyperpolarizes the postsynaptic membrane. GABA effects at this membrane are potentiated by benzodiazepines (Bz) and barbiturates (Ba), which have distinct binding sites (Fig. 51).

GABA receptor modulators

Benzodiazepines potentiate the action of GABA at the GABA-A receptor as do the barbiturates which are much less selective. Benzodiazepines are useful as sedatives, anxiolytics and anticonvulsants.

Opioid peptides

The endogenous opioid peptides, the enkephalins, endorphins and dynorphins, are derived from three distinct gene products, preproopiomelanocortin, preproenkephalin and preprodynorphin by sequential peptide cleavages. Neurones containing these peptides are distributed widely in the CNS where they modulate the perception of pain.

Opioid receptors

Three main classes of opioid receptor are recognized: μ, δ and κ. μ receptors are thought to be responsible for most of the analgesic effects of opioid receptor activation and also for respiratory depression, sedation and dependence. All three receptors are coupled to G proteins and the inhibition of adenylate cyclase. See Fig. 52, also *Cell biology*, Section 2.

Opioid receptor agonists

These include morphine and pethidine which are pure agonists, and pentazocine, nalorphine and buprenorphine which are partial agonists. All are used as analgesics. Heroin (diamorphine) has therapeutic use but like all opioid agonists, it is also a drug of abuse. See Fig. 52.

Opioid receptor antagonists

Nalaxone is a competitive antagonist at μ, δ and κ opioid receptors. Naloxone reverses opioid-induced analgesia, sedation and respiratory depression and is used in the treatment of opioid overdose. See Fig. 52.

Noradrenaline

In the CNS noradrenergic neurotransmission is involved in the control of mood, wakefulness and BP regulation. A functional deficiency in noradrenergic neurotransmission is thought to underlie some forms of depression and many drugs used to treat depression potentiate noradrenergic neurotransmission.

Interference with synthesis

Alpha-methyldopa is an antihypertensive that is metabolized by DOPA decarboxylase and dopamine β-hydroxylase to yield α methyl noradrenaline—a 'false transmitter' (Fig. 53). Depression is a recognized side effect of this agent.

Inhibitors of metabolism

Classical MAO-Is (pargyline and isocarboxazid) are irreversible, non-competitive inhibitors of MAO-A and MAO-B (Fig. 53). Moclobemide, a newer antidepressant, is a reversible competitive inhibitor of MAO-A.

Inhibitors of reuptake

Amphetamines and cocaine are stimulant drugs of abuse

109

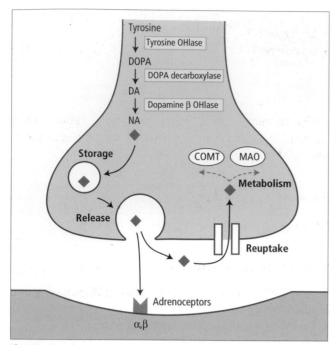

Fig. 53 Noradrenergic neurotransmission.

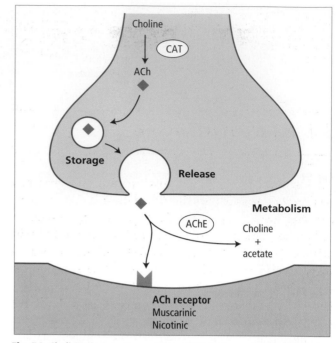

Fig. 54 Cholinergic neurotransmission. CAT, choline acetyltransferase; AChE, acetylcholinesterase.

that inhibit NA uptake (Fig. 53). Inhibition of NA reuptake underlies the antidepressant effect of reboxetine, a new class of antidepressant noradrenaline reuptake inhibitor (NARI).

> Dietary tyramine, found in some cheeses, red wine and Marmite, is normally metabolized in the bowel wall and liver by MAO-A. Patients taking classical MAO-Is are at risk of severe hypertensive reactions if they consume such foods, as the tyramine is absorbed systemically where it provokes NA release from sympathetic nerve terminals. Hypertensive crisis can be treated with alpha-adrenoreceptor antagonists (e.g. phentolamine) or Ca²⁺ channel blockers. Moclobemide is also an inhibitor of MAO-A, but because it is a competitive inhibitor it can be displaced by tyramine which is then metabolized.

Acetylcholine

Cholinergic neurones are widely distributed in the CNS. Major cholinergic pathways are found in the basal forebrain, striatum and nucleus accumbens. A functional over-activity of cholinergic neurotransmission is seen in Parkinson's disease and a loss of cholinergic neurones in Alzheimer's dementia.

Acetylcholinesterase inhibitors

Centrally acting acetylcholinesterose inhibitors (donepezil, rivastigmine and galantamine) have been used to treat Alzheimer's disease. Short-term improvement in objective measures of cognition has been shown, but the long-term value of these agents is unclear. See Fig. 54.

Muscarinic ACh receptor antagonists

Blockade of the mACh receptor with benzhexol, benztropine or orphenadrine is of limited therapeutic use in patients with Parkinson's disease, in particular where tremor is the prominent symptom. Side effects of these agents include confusion, blurred vision, urinary retention and dry mouth. mACh receptor antagonists are also used in the treatment and prevention of drug-induced extrapyramidal disorders. See Fig. 54.

3 Investigations and practical procedures

3.1 Neuropsychometry

An organized, thorough cognitive examination performed by the clinician is important both in the initial assessment and diagnosis of a patient's condition and in subsequent follow up. The most routinely used test is the Folstein 'Mini-Mental State Exam' (MMSE) which records a score out of 30 [1]. Use of this test, however, has its limitations: being heavily weighted toward verbal tasks, false 'normals' occur. A wider battery of tests allows for more sensitivity and specificity [2].

Orientation and attention

Is the patient orientated in place, person and time? Disorientation in person is seldom organic. Poor orientation should prompt examination of attention. This can be done by testing immediate recall of a string of digits. Normal forward digit span is 5–6 and backwards, 1–2 or less. Patients who perform poorly usually perform poorly on subsequent tests that require concentration. These areas are particularly impaired in acute confusional states.

Language

Listen carefully to the patient's general conversation. See Section 1.22, p. 49 for assessment of language.

> 💡 **Alzheimer's disease**
>
> Fluent speech with semantic or anomic errors. Errors on naming objects, the more severe the dementia, the less obscure the objects (high frequency words). Preservation of repetition.

Memory

Memory is divided into episodic memory (recollection of events) and semantic memory (our working knowledge of the world). Episodic memory is further divided into antegrade or retrograde, depending on the relation to the disease onset.

Episodic memory

Ask the patient to relate their life history from early childhood to the current day and have this verified by a relative. Antegrade episodic memory can be tested by the ability to remember a name and address after 5 min. Impairment of antegrade, episodic memory is characteristic of Alzheimer's disease.

Semantic memory

Naming and describing objects.

Frontal lobe dysfunction

This includes executive function, our ability to plan and reason.

Letter fluency

Ask the patient to give as many words (not proper nouns) beginning with a certain letter within one minute. Then ask them to name as many animals as possible within a further minute (beginning with any letter!). Normal individuals will name approximately 20 words and slightly more animals. In frontal lobe dysfunction, there is a decrease in letter frequency more than category (animal) frequency. This pattern of impairment is reversed in Alzheimer's disease.

Concrete thinking

Cognitive estimates

Ask the patient to estimate/guess the answers to the following questions:
- How high is the Post Office tower?
- How far is it to New York?
- How tall is the average man?
- How long is the average woman's spine?
- How many camels are there in Holland?
  Patients' answers may be both fixed and wildly out!

Proverbs

'Why should people in glass houses not throw stones?' The patient may translate proverbs literally.

Visuospatial

Test the following:
- Ask a patient to draw a clock face and to set the hand to ten-to-two. Look for signs of neglect.

- Copying of geometric figures.
- Line bisection.

Impairment in the ability to perform the above usually reflects non-dominant parietal lobe dysfunction.

Cortical and subcortical dementias

Dementias can be divided into those in which the pathology is predominantly subcortical or cortical [3]. Good examples of subcortical dementia are progressive supranuclear palsy and Huntington's disease. Typically, the patients are lethargic and withdrawn with slow thought processing. Memory impairment reflects frontal dysfunction with recollection aided by cues. Cortical dementia, as seen in Alzheimer's disease, is more rapid and the amnesia more severe. Dysphasia, dyspraxia and agnosia may be present. The lack of motivation and attention that characterize subcortical dementias are not usually seen, but as neurodegenerative diseases progress there is overlap of symptoms.

1 Folstein MF, Folstein SE, McHugh PR. 'Mini-mental state': a practical method for grading the cognitive state of patients for the clinician. *J Psychiatr Res* 1975; 12: 189–198.
2 Pasquier F. Early diagnosis of dementia: neuropsychology *J Neurol* 1999; 246(1): 6–15.
3 Savage CR. Neuropsychology of subcortical dementias. *Psychiatr Clin North Am* 1997 20(4): 911–931.

3.2 Lumbar puncture

Principle

Analysis of the CSF can yield valuable diagnostic information in a wide range of clinical circumstances.

Normal findings

- Pressure 80–200 mm of water (CSF)
- No more than 5 lymphocytes or mononuclear cells per μL
- No red blood cells
- Total protein 0.15–0.5 g/L
- Glucose 60–80% of blood glucose concentration
- No xanthochromia (see Section 2.8.4, p. 98).

A 'bloody tap' is not uncommon: if the patient has a normal blood count, then the ratio of white cells to red cells is approximately 1 to 1000. Hence, if the CSF contains 10 000 red cells per μL, the expected white cell count in the sample will be 10 per μL.

Indications

Inflammatory conditions

Central nervous system

Multiple sclerosis, acute demyelinating encephalomyelitis (ADEM), neurosarcoid.

Peripheral nervous system

Guillain–Barré syndrome, chronic inflammatory demyelinating neuropathy.

Neoplastic

Particularly malignant meningitis (diffuse meningeal infiltration). At least 5–10 mL of fresh CSF should be sent for cytological evaluation. Repeat sampling may be necessary.

Infective

Bacterial, viral and fungal. See *Emergency medicine*, Section 1.27.

Other indications

- Subarachnoid haemorrhage
- Benign intracranial hypertension
- Rapidly progressive dementia.

Contraindications

- Symptoms or signs of raised intracranial pressure without imaging.
- Focal neurological signs without imaging.
- Local infection (skin, bone, pustular acne).
- Thrombocytopenia, clotting disorder.

Practical details

Performed properly this should not be the painful terrifying experience that patients expect. As in all invasive procedures, allow adequate time for the local anaesthetic to work. Positioning of the patient is absolutely crucial to success, and without it failure is inevitable. While routinely performed with the patient lying on their left side (for a right-handed operator), knees drawn up to chest and the uppermost shoulder vertically over the other (Fig. 55), it is equally acceptable for the patient to be sat on the bed and leaning forward onto a chair or table. The latter position is often easier if the subject is obese.

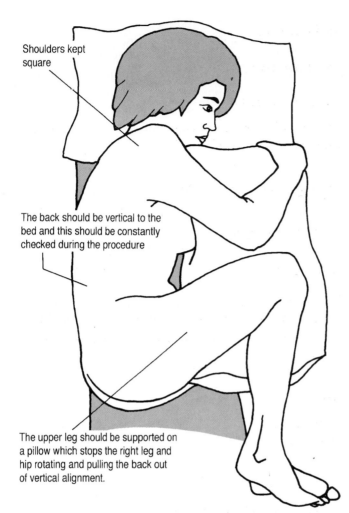

Shoulders kept square

The back should be vertical to the bed and this should be constantly checked during the procedure

The upper leg should be supported on a pillow which stops the right leg and hip rotating and pulling the back out of vertical alignment.

Fig. 55 The correct position for lumbar puncture.

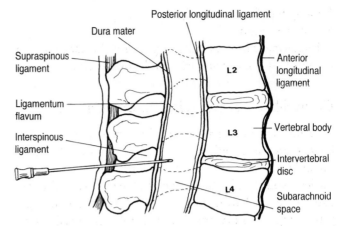

Posterior longitudinal ligament

Dura mater

Supraspinous ligament

Ligamentum flavum

Interspinous ligament

L2

L3

L4

Anterior longitudinal ligament

Vertebral body

Intervertebral disc

Subarachnoid space

Fig. 56 Lumbar puncture needle shown *in situ* at L3/4 level (often the easiest level). The needle is angled slightly headwards. If inserted at 90°, it tends to hit the upper surface of the arch of L4, producing a very characteristic grating sensation and an appropriate response from the patient.

> ❗ A common mistake is to insert the needle too low. Remember that the L3/4 space is located between the iliac crests (Fig. 56). Remember also that the spinal cord ends at approximately L1, so it is quite difficult to go too high.
>
> After injection of a small amount of local anaesthetic into the skin, massage it with finger or thumb in order to disperse the 'bleb'. This enables you to remain confident about the 'feel' of your anatomical landmarks, which is crucial to success [1].
>
> If anatomical landmarks cannot be discerned (scoliosis, etc.), lumbar puncture (LP) should be performed under radiological guidance. A pressure reading should be obtained with the patient relaxed, the legs uncurled and breathing normally. If the patient starts in a sitting position it is possible, after insertion of the needle into the subarachnoid space, to carefully move the patient into a lying position to allow pressure recording.
>
> After the procedure the patient need rest for no more than 30 min. Enforced bed rest has not been shown to reduce the incidence of post-LP headache (see below).
>
> For further information see *Emergency medicine*, Section 3.5.

Complications

Post-LP headache

This occurs in some degree in about 10% of LPs. It is not related to the amount of CSF taken but is likely to be due to continuous leak of CSF from the hole made in the dura. Incidence of post-LP headache (PLPH) is therefore related to the size of the hole, hence predictors of PLPH include:

• the gauge of the needle
• the angle the bevel is inserted (horizontally inserted the dural fibres will be parted, but with the bevel vertical the fibres will be sliced through)
• the number of attempts.

The headache is a typical low-pressure headache, worse on standing and ameliorated by lying down. Patients should be reassured. Symptoms normally resolve in a matter of days and, with the exception of bed rest, adequate fluid intake (occasionally intravenous) and simple analgesia, no further treatment is required.

Cerebral herniation

This is catastrophic and can be avoided by imaging prior to LP.

> 📕 1 Patten J. *Neurological Differential Diagnosis*, 2nd edn. London: Springer-Verlag, 1996: 273–281.

3.3 Neurophysiology

Neurophysiological investigation uses a variety of techniques to aid the diagnosis of disease processes affecting both the central and peripheral nervous systems.

3.3.1 ELECTROENCEPHALOGRAPHY

Principle

It is thought that the electroencephalography (EEG) signals reflect extracellular current flow from the summation of excitatory and inhibitory postsynaptic potentials.

Normal findings

The waking EEG pattern consists of mainly α (8–12 Hz) and β (>12 Hz) activity, with minimal θ (4–7 Hz) activity.

In sleep, there is increasing δ (1–3 Hz) activity with increasing depth of sleep. In drowsiness, there is disappearance of α activity, with increased θ and β activities.

Indications

To evaluate suspected epilepsy, altered consciousness (e.g. brain death), detect structural lesions (e.g. tumour) and detect certain diseases (e.g. herpes simplex encephalitis, CJD).

In epilepsy, the EEG is used to distinguish partial from generalized seizures, localize the epileptic focus in partial seizures and characterize epilepsy syndromes, e.g. 3-Hz spike-and-wave activity in absence attacks. Prolonged EEG monitoring or videotelemetry improves diagnostic accuracy in epilepsy. The EEG is not useful in aiding the diagnosis of a patient presenting with 'funny turns'. Minor asymmetries should not be considered pathological.

The typical sign of a focal cerebral lesion is polymorphic focal activity. In herpes simplex encephalitis, the EEG shows slowing with periodic sharp-wave complexes over the temporal lobe. EEG changes in CJD are discussed in Section 2.10.1, p. 103.

3.3.2 EVOKED POTENTIALS

Principle

Evoked potentials (EPs) measure electrical conduction through the nervous system in response to sensory stimulation.

Visual evoked potentials (VEPs) are elicited by monocular visual stimulation with a chequerboard pattern. Normally, a response is recorded from the visual cortex approximately 100 ms after eye stimulation, the P100 latency.

Brain-stem auditory evoked potentials (BAEPs) are elicited by monoaural stimulation with repetitive clicks, generating waves in the VIIIth cranial nerve and the brain stem. Normally, within 10 ms of the stimulus, five waveforms occur (I–V), representing sequential activation of structures of the auditory pathway.

Somatosensory evoked potentials (SSEPs) are generated by electrical stimulation of a peripheral nerve with recordings over the spine and scalp to assess central sensory processing. Responses depend on which nerves are stimulated.

Indications

VEPs

Abnormal (delayed P100 latency) in optic neuritis in MS, tumours compressing the optic nerve, ischaemic optic neuropathy, toxic amblyopias, glaucoma and Leber's hereditary optic atrophy.

BAEPs

Abnormal (as indicated by the presence, latency and interpeak intervals of waveforms I–V) in VIIIth nerve and brain-stem lesions, e.g. MS, acoustic neuromas and brain-stem gliomas.

SSEPs

Conduction delay or block arises in any disease affecting the CNS sensory pathways, e.g. MS. Abnormally large SSEPs may be seen in myoclonus of cortical origin.

3.3.3 ELECTROMYOGRAPHY

Principle

An electromyogram (EMG) records electrical activity of motor units from resting and voluntary muscle activity. Relaxed muscle normally shows no spontaneous electrical activity, except in the end-plate area where neuromuscular junctions are found. All voluntary muscle activity is recorded as motor unit potentials. A motor unit potential is the sum of muscle fibre potentials innervated by a single anterior horn cell.

Indications

• EMG is commonly used to evaluate anterior horn cell diseases, inflammatory muscle diseases, muscular dystrophies, myotonic disorders, neuromuscular junction disorders, axonal peripheral neuropathies and chronic radiculopathies.
• Single-fibre EMG is mainly used to diagnose myasthenia gravis and other neuromuscular junction transmission disorders, by the detection of jitter (see Section 2.2.5, p. 70).

3.3.4 NERVE CONDUCTION STUDIES

Principle

Motor nerve conduction studies (NCS) are done by recording the compound muscle action potential (CMAP) of a muscle to stimulation of its motor nerve.

Sensory NCS are done by recording sensory action potentials in sensory fibres when these fibres are stimulated. Supramaximal stimulation is used. Conduction velocity and amplitude of responses are measured.

F-waves can also be recorded in the muscle after the CMAP. Its latency represents conduction retrogradly up the motor nerve to the anterior horn cell and back to the muscle. Increased latency with normal motor conduction may be seen in radiculopathies (i.e. proximal disease).

See Fig. 57.

Indications

NCS are used to determine the presence and extent of peripheral nerve damage in entrapment neuropathies; whether the pathological process is axonal or demyelinating; or whether conduction block is present.

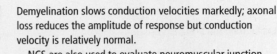

> **!** Demyelination slows conduction velocities markedly; axonal loss reduces the amplitude of response but conduction velocity is relatively normal.
>
> NCS are also used to evaluate neuromuscular junction disorders, e.g. myasthenia gravis where there is a decremental response to repetitive nerve stimulation.

> Daube JR. *Clinical Neurophysiology.* Philadelphia: F. A. Davis Company, 1996.

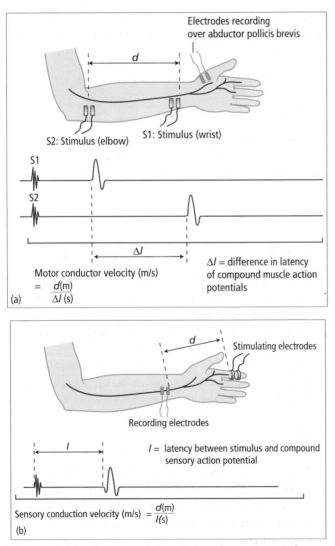

Electrodes recording over abductor pollicis brevis

d

S2: Stimulus (elbow)   S1: Stimulus (wrist)

S1

S2

Δ*l*

Motor conductor velocity (m/s)

$$= \frac{d(m)}{\Delta l (s)}$$

Δ*l* = difference in latency of compound muscle action potentials

(a)

d

Stimulating electrodes

Recording electrodes

l

l = latency between stimulus and compound sensory action potential

Sensory conduction velocity (m/s) $= \dfrac{d(m)}{l(s)}$

(b)

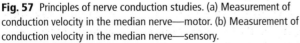

Fig. 57 Principles of nerve conduction studies. (a) Measurement of conduction velocity in the median nerve—motor. (b) Measurement of conduction velocity in the median nerve—sensory.

3.4 Neuroimaging

3.4.1 COMPUTED TOMOGRAPHY AND COMPUTED TOMOGRAPHIC ANGIOGRAPHY

Principle

Computed tomography (CT) images are produced by detecting X-rays that have been directed through tissue. The images depend on how much of the original beam has managed to passed through the tissue, known as X-ray attenuation. Contrast agents improve the sensitivity and specificity of CT. Enhancement occurs when the blood–brain barrier (BBB) is compromised, e.g. in inflammatory lesions or tumours.

Computed tomographic angiography (CTA) is based on detecting enhancement of arterial vessels after injection of contrast using fast helical CT scanners [1,2].

Indications

CT is best used to detect acute bleeding and calcium (bone). It is the initial investigation of choice in stroke, subarachnoid haemorrhage (SAH) and head trauma. It is also used to assess bony pathology, e.g. bony erosion from tumours and when MRI is contraindicated. In stroke, CT may not reveal an infarct within the first 48 h. MRI will detect an infarct within a few hours of a stroke. However, CT is preferred because it detects intracranial haemorrhage better than MRI in the first 48 h. In head trauma, CT is indicated because it detects bony injuries and traumatic intracerebral or subarachnoid haemorrhage.

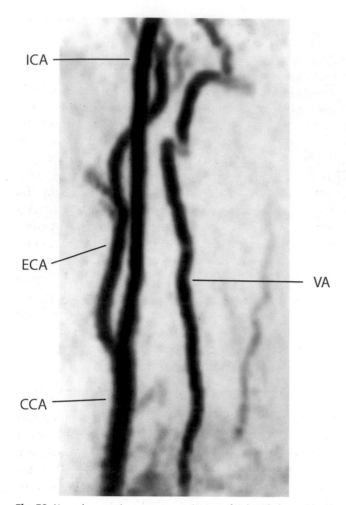

ICA

ECA

VA

CCA

Fig. 58 Normal magnetic resonance angiogram of right sided carotid and vertebral artery systems. CCA, common carotid artery; ICA, internal carotid artery; ECA, external carotid artery; VA, vertebral artery.

If SAH is strongly suspected, a lumbar puncture must be performed, even if CT is normal.

CTA may be used in patients who decline catheter angiography and have contraindications for MRA to detect carotid artery stenosis, carotid dissection, arteriovenous malformations and cerebral aneurysms. However, CTA is inferior to angiography or MRA.

Contraindications

Contrast agents are contraindicated in patients with asthma or who are allergic to the contrast itself. Renal failure is a relative contraindication. In pregnancy, the fetus must be shielded from the harmful radiation.

3.4.2 MRI AND MRA

Principle

An MR image is obtained when a radiofrequency pulse excites the protons in the tissue, producing radio wave

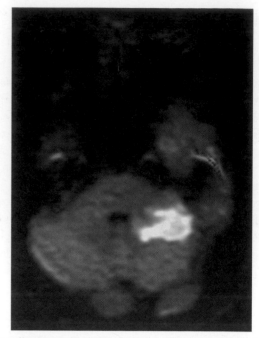

Fig. 59 Diffusion weighted MRI scan demonstrating acute infarction in the right cerebellar hemisphere. Courtesy of Professor M. Brown, Institute of Neurology, University of London.

emissions [3,4]. The signal intensity depends on the mobile hydrogen nuclei concentration of tissues. T1 (spin-lattice) and T2 (spin-spin) relaxation time constants depend on physical properties of the tissue. As in CT, contrast enhancement is due to disruption of the BBB.

MRA is performed using the time-of-flight (TOF) or phase-contrast (PC) techniques. In TOF MRA, vessels are detected because of inflow of unsaturated spins into the imaging plane. In PC MRA, vessels are detected because moving protons within vessels accumulate phase shifts proportional to their velocity as they cross a magnetic gradient (Fig. 58).

Indications

MRI is best for soft tissue and vascular abnormalities, and is superior to CT in detecting posterior fossa or spinal cord (e.g. syrinx and epidural abscess) lesions. Indications for MRI include stroke, tumour, degenerative diseases, MS, vascular lesions, e.g. aneurysm and vascular malformation, epilepsy, myelopathy and cerebral infections, e.g. abscess, herpes simplex encephalitis and meningitis.

In stroke, after taking into the account the advantages of CT, note that haematomas of more than 2–3 days old are better seen with MRI.

Diffusion-weighted MRI (DWI) is exquisitely sensitive to acutely infarcted tissue (Fig. 59) and perfusion-weighted MRI (PWI) detects cerebral tissue which is underperfused in the setting of acute stroke. If the defect in PWI is greater than that seen on DWI, it may be that this tissue is under threat from ischaemia, but is not infarcted, and would survive if perfusion could be reinstated, for example using thrombolytic therapy (see Section 2.8.1, p. 90).

Indications for MRA are similar to CTA but the former provides better quality images. In the investigation of carotid artery stenosis, if MRA and carotid dopplers are concurrent, then arterial angiography (and its risk of stroke) should not be required.

Contraindications

Metallic objects, e.g. shrapnel in eyes, intracranial clips and pacemakers are contraindications for an MRI.

3.4.3 ANGIOGRAPHY

Principle

Angiography is performed by introducing a catheter via the femoral or brachial artery, up the aorta, into the carotid or vertebral arteries and injecting radio-opaque contrast to allow detailed visualization of vessels.

Indications

Angiography is used to diagnose aneurysms, arterial stenosis (e.g. thromboembolism, dissection, vasculitis, atherosclerosis), arteriovenous malformations and cerebral venous sinus thrombosis. Therapeutic interventional procedures can also be carried out, e.g. embolization of aneurysms, arteriovenous malformations or blood supply to tumours, arterial thrombolysis and angioplasty.

Complications

These include local haematoma or bleeding, infection, pseudoaneurysm formation, vessel damage, renal failure, contrast reaction, stroke or transient ischaemic attack and death. In experienced hands, diagnostic angiography carries a risk of stroke of less than 1%. However, interventional procedures carry a risk of major complications of up to 10%, including vessel perforation.

1 Gilman S. Imaging the brain. First of two parts. *N Engl J Med* 1998; 338: 812–820.
2 Gilman S. Imaging the brain. Second of two parts. *N Engl J Med* 1998; 338: 889–896.
3 Edelman RR, Warach S. Magnetic resonance imaging (1). *N Engl J Med* 1993; 328: 708–716.
4 Edelman RR, Warach S. Magnetic resonance imaging (2). *N Engl J Med* 1993; 328: 785–791.

3.5 SPECT and PET

Single-photon emission computed tomography (SPECT) and positron emission tomography (PET) are two methods by which functional, rather than conventional structural, neuroimaging can be performed. Functional neuroimaging can be divided into techniques that demonstrate synaptic activity or regional activation (called functional mapping) based on the close association between blood flow and neuronal activation/synaptic activity, and techniques that allow detection of particular neurotransmitter or neuro-chemical substances. Tracer design is therefore based on physiological molecules involved in metabolic turn over (such as oxygen, glucose and amino acids) and enzyme activation or on neurotransmitters and their receptors. The specific tracers are labelled with gamma-emitting radioisotopes for SPECT and positron-emitting radio-nucleotides for PET.

3.5.1 SPECT

Gamma-emitting radionucleotides are commercially available and images are taken with a routine nuclear medicine camera. This makes SPECT less expensive and more widely available compared with PET. The disadvantages are inferior spatial resolution and less quantification than are possible with PET.

3.5.2 PET

PET depends on positron (positively charged electrons)-labelled radionucleotides, which have a short half-life and are generated by a cyclotron. PET can only be performed, therefore, in a centre with a cyclotron. Commonly used positrons are oxygen (^{15}O), carbon (^{11}C) and nitrogen (^{13}N). Fluorine (^{18}F) is used to replace hydrogen. The image gathered represents the distribution of emitted positrons. The increased sensitivity of PET over SPECT allows for less radioactive exposure.

Functional imaging

Functional imaging techniques are concerned with describing activity of neurones in the brain associated with some physiological, cognitive or pathological state, i.e. function of the brain as opposed to structure. Studies using PET may be steady-state or activation studies, in which a physical or cognitive task is associated with changes in cerebral blood flow in discrete brain regions.

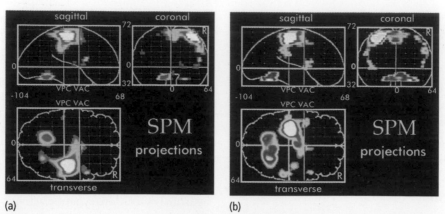

(a)   (b)

Fig. 60 Statistical parametric maps (SPM) of brain areas activated (in comparison with rest) by a paced, sequential, finger-to thumb opposition task in patients with lesions of left internal capsule (a) using left hand, and (b) recovered right hand. The SPMs are presented as projections through the brain seen from side (sagittal), back (coronal), and top (transverse) views. The frontal pole is on the right side of the transverse section. Highly significant changes of activity between active and resting states are shown in colour, coded to represent levels of significance (white, greatest significance). In comparing (b) with (a) it can be seen that the same task has led to activations that are not only bilateral but are more extensive, reflecting recruitment of other motor areas not normally activated by simple motor tasks. Reprinted from Chollet *et al. Ann Neurol* 1991; 29: 63–71 with permission of Lippincott, Williams and Wilkins Inc.

Steady-state studies

• Characteristic pattern of impaired metabolism in parietal and posterior temporal regions seen in early Alzheimer's disease.
• Patchy abnormalities, particularly in the distribution of the middle cerebral artery in vascular dementia.
• Reduced uptake of ^{18}F-DOPA in the basal ganglia in Parkinson's disease.
• Hypometabolism in the striatum in Huntington's disease.

Activation studies

• Localization of cerebral function in normal volunteers, e.g. language, memory, attention, motor control.
• Studies of the reorganization of the brain in the recovery of function following brain injury, e.g. after stroke (Fig. 60).

3.6 Carotid Dopplers

Principle

The technique utilizes the fact that sound waves reflected off red blood cells give an indication of the flow velocity within the vessel (Fig. 61). A stenosed vessel gives a high-flow velocity. The accuracy of the test compared to angiography (gold standard) is operator-dependent, but should approach at least 90% in good centres.

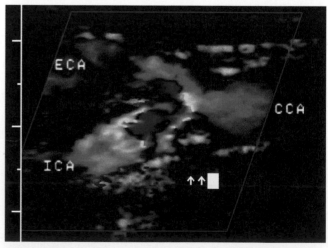

(a)

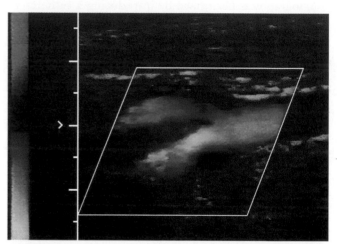

(b)

Fig. 61 Colour flow Doppler ultrasound scans. (a) Normal carotid bifurcation; (b) internal carotid artery stenosis causing turbulent blood flow (seen in blue). CCA, common carotid artery; ICA, internal carotid artery; ECA, external carotid artery. Courtesy of Professor M. Brown, Institute of Neurology, University of London.

Carotid Dopplers cannot distinguish between absence of flow (complete occlusion) and very low flow (tight stenosis with a patent vessel).

Indications

To screen for carotid artery stenosis when clinically suspected. If this technique is used in conjunction with MRA and the results are in agreement, then arterial angiography (and its risk of stroke) should not be required.

Acknowledgement

We are grateful to Springer Verlag for allowing reproduction and re-drawing of illustrations from Patten J. *Neurological Differential Diagnosis*, 2nd edn. London: Springer, 1996.

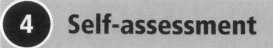

Self-assessment

Answers on pp. 210–215.

Question 1

A 44-year-old male presents with a partial right foot drop. Which of one of the following would be most suggestive of a L5 radiculopathy?

A Absent right ankle jerk

B Abnormal sensation over the lateral border of the right calf

C Associated weakness of ankle plantar flexion

D Associated weakness of ankle eversion only

E Associated weakness of ankle eversion and inversion.

Question 2

A 62-year-old male smoker presents with a 6-week history of a rapidly progressive gait disturbance. On examination there is a profound loss of all sensory modalities distally. Power is maintained.

1 What is the most likely diagnosis?

2 What investigations should be carried out?

3 How should this man be managed?

Question 3

A 15-year-old boy presents with gradually progressive muscle weakness and wasting. CK is raised. Muscle biopsy has revealed reduced, though present, dystrophin when compared to controls. There is no family history, his three sisters being well. His mother asks if this is Duchenne's muscular dystrophy (DMD).

1 How would you respond to the mother's question?

2 What is the most likely diagnosis?

3 How would you confirm your suspected diagnosis?

Question 4

Neurocutaneous disorders

A Lisch nodules

B Inguinal freckles

C Shagreen patch

D Cerebellar haemangioblastoma

E Plexiform neurofibroma

F Hamartomas

G Cortical tubers

H Bilateral acoustic neuromas

I Phaeochromocytoma

For each of the following neurocutaneous disorders, which of the above is associated? Each option may be used once, more than once, or not at all.

1 Neurofibromatosis type 1 (select 3 options)

2 Neurofibromatosis type 2 (select 1 option)

3 Von Hippel–Lindau disease (select 3 options)

4 Tuberous sclerosis (select 3 options).

Question 5

Presentation of brain tumours

A Homonymous hemianopia

B Marked personality change

C Bitemporal hemianopia

D Ataxia

E Spastic paraparesis

F Apraxia

G Weight loss

H Nystagmus.

For each site of primary intracranial tumour below, which of the above is a common mode of presentation? Each option may be used once, more than once or not at all.

1 Posterior fossa

2 Occipital lobe

3 Parietal lobe

4 Frontal lobe.

Question 6

The following would lead one to suspect a parkinsonian syndrome rather than idiopathic Parkinson's disease? (T/F):

A Unilateral presentation

B Associated tardive dyskinesia

C Lack of tremor

D Failure to respond to L-DOPA

E L-DOPA-induced dyskinesias.

Question 7

A 33-year-old woman presents with a 48-h history of pain behind the right ear followed by drooping of the right side of her face. She also describes having an 'odd taste' in her mouth. She had previously been fit and well. On examination, there is right-sided facial weakness affecting both the upper and lower parts of the face and impaired taste sensation over the right anterior part of the tongue. There is no sensory loss over the face or any rash in the external auditory meatus and soft palate.

1 What is the diagnosis in this case?

2 Which other three symptoms may this patient have?

3 If a vesicular rash is present on the pinna, what diagnosis must you consider?

Question 8

A Mutation in the PMP22 gene
B Mutation in the connexin 32 gene
C Diabetes mellitus
D B_{12} deficiency
E Amyloid
F Vasculitis.

For each type of neuropathy, select possible causative factors from the list above. Each option may be used once, more than once or not at all.

1 Subacute painful neuropathy (select 1 option)
2 Chronic demyelinating neuropathy (select 2 options)
3 Autonomic neuropathy (select 2 options)
4 Chronic axonal neuropathy (select 4 options).

Question 9

You are asked to see a 27-year-old woman with multiple symptoms. Six years ago she developed mild numbness and weakness of her right upper limb which resolved after about a week. Since then she has had intermittent episodes of facial numbness, dizziness, unsteadiness, slurring of speech, poor coordination, limb weakness and paraesthesiae. After each episode of weakness and incoordination she is left with more disability, although there is little progression between attacks. She frequently has urinary urgency. Recently she complained that her eyes 'have gone all funny'. On examination she has impaired adduction of the eyes bilaterally with nystagmus in the abducting eye on both directions of lateral gaze. Jaw jerk is brisk. Tone is generally increased in the limbs. Muscle power is 3–4/5 in the lower limbs and 4–5/5 in the upper limbs. Deep tendon reflexes are generally brisk with bilateral extensor plantar responses. She has a coarse intention tremor, dysmetria and dysdiadochokinesia. Sensation is mildly impaired to all modalities distally. Her gait is ataxic.

1 What name is given to the eye abnormalities?
2 Where is the lesion causing the eye abnormalities?
3 What is the underlying neurological disease?
4 Name two investigations to aid diagnosing the neurological condition.

Question 10

A 26-year-old female with known epilepsy presents with increasing seizure frequency.

A Headache, nausea and vomiting
B Recently commenced the oral contraceptive pill (OCP)
C Pregnancy
D Non-synchronous limb movements
E Recently started night shift.

For each explanation below select the clues available in the history from the list above. Each option may be used once, more than once or not at all.

1 Expanding lesion (select 1 clue)

2 Non-organic seizures (select 1 clue)
3 Fall in plasma drug concentration (select 2 clues).

Question 11

How may typical absences and complex partial seizures (CPS) be distinguished?

Question 12

Based on a knowledge of the functions of nerve fibre of different diameters, what are the clinical features of a small-fibre neuropathy?

Question 13

Which disc protrusions affect L4 and L5, respectively?

Question 14

What features in the history suggest that stroke is the likely diagnosis?

Question 15

Poor prognostic indicators in multiple sclerosis include (T/F):

A Sensory symptoms at the onset of the disease
B Visual symptoms dominating the disease
C Male gender
D Progressive form of the disease from the onset
E Age of onset before age 40.

Question 16

The Holmes–Adie syndrome (T/F):

A Affects women more commonly than men
B Commonly affects both pupils
C Is associated with a dilated pupil that reacts sluggishly to light and accommodation
D Is associated with brisk deep tendon reflexes
E Is usually caused by neurosyphilis.

Question 17

A New variant Creutzfeldt–Jakob disease
B Herpes simplex encephalitis
C Normal awake adult
D Normal asleep adult
E Absence seizures
F Hepatic encephalopathy.

For each of the EEG changes, select the most likely condition from the list of options above. Each option may be used once, more than once or not at all.

1 Triphasic waves
2 Prominent δ wave activity
3 3-Hz spike-and-wave pattern
4 Periodic lateralizing sharp-wave complexes.

Question 18

A Amyloid precursor protein

B Superoxide dismutase
C α-synuclein
D Prion protein
E Ataxin-3.

For each of the neurodegenerative diseases, select the most likely abnormal protein conformation it is associated with from the list of options above. Each option may be used once, more than once or not at all.

1 Amyotrophic lateral sclerosis
2 Parkinson's disease
3 Creutzfeldt–Jakob disease
4 Alzheimer's disease.

Question 19

A 53-year-old woman is referred to you, complaining of a burning sensation on the anterolateral aspect of her right thigh, extending from her groin to almost her knee. The patient is diabetic and is taking warfarin for atrial fibrillation. She has had a recent chest infection for which she was prescribed an antibiotic. Examination reveals normal muscle power and reflexes, but reduced pin prick sensation over the affected area. What is the most likely diagnosis?

A Diabetic femoral amyotrophy
B Ruptured intervertebral disc
C Iliopsoas haematoma from warfarin causing a femoral neuropathy
D Compression of the lateral cutaneous nerve
E Femoral hernia.

Question 20

A 64-year-old man presents with a week's history of lower back pain, weakness of and paraesthesias in the legs and difficulty in initiating micturition. He is an insulin-dependent diabetic and has pressure sore ulcers on both his feet which the district nurse cleans and dresses for him regularly. His diabetic control is not tight and his most recent HbA_{1c} is 9%. On examination, he is mildly febrile. He has mild increase in tone and weakness in his lower limbs. Reflexes are brisk in the lower limbs with extensor plantars. Sensory examination is variable. Straight leg raising produces pain.

1 What is the most likely diagnosis in this man?
2 What two investigations will you carry out?
3 What is the management?

Question 21

With regard to the treatment of Parkinson's disease, which of the following are true statements?

A Peripheral dopa decarboxylase (DDC) increases the bio-availability of dopamine in the central nervous system
B Pergolide, a dopamine agonist, is well tolerated in the elderly
C Levodopa preparations usually contain an inhibitor of catechol o-methyl transferase (COMT).

D Selegiline is an irreversible monoamine oxidase B inhibitor
E Dyskinesias may limit levodopa dosage.

Question 22

The following are classical in Alzheimer's disease patients (T/F):

A Fluent speech
B Impaired repetition
C Impairment of retrograde episodic memory
D Concrete thinking
E Impaired category fluency.

Question 23

The following are complications of Guillain–Barré syndrome (T/F):

A Cardiac dysrhythmias
B Livedo reticularis
C Profound postural hypotension
D Pulmonary emboli
E Frequent relapses.

Question 24

A 17-year-old woman is referred because of loss of sensation of the left hand. A month earlier she had burned the tip of her left little finger on a hot stove and had not realized it until she smelled burning skin. She also describes weakness of her left hand with difficulty gripping things and a constant pain in the neck. On examination she has atrophy of the small muscles of the left hand, and weakness in the small muscles of the hands bilaterally, with the left side more severely affected than the right. There is impaired pain and temperature sensation over the medial two fingers and palm of both hands and the medial part of the left forearm. Light touch, vibration and joint position sense are all normal. Reflexes are brisk in the legs with extensor plantar responses bilaterally.

1 Which dermatomes of the left upper limb are affected on sensory examination?
2 What type of sensory deficit does the patient have?
3 What is the diagnosis in this case?
4 Give one investigation you would carry out.
5 What eye abnormality may occur in this condition?

Question 25

The following are recognized features of metabolic muscle disease (T/F):

A Muscle pain at rest
B Myoglobinuria
C Gower's manoeuvre
D Maternal inheritance
E 'Second wind' phenomenon.

Question 26

A 30-year-old man is referred with a 5-year history of an

increasing problem with tripping over things, with his left leg more severely affected than his right. With the onset of the problem, he also noticed a dull aching pain over his lower back. More recently, he describes having numbness extending from his buttocks down the back of his legs into the soles and dorsum of both feet. He has been impotent with no early-morning erections for the last year. Over the last 6 months he has had problems with urinary incontinence and one episode of faecal incontinence. On examination, he has wasting of muscles of his buttocks and calves. There is asymmetrical weakness of dorsiflexion and plantar flexion of the ankles, and eversion of the feet, with the left side being more severely affected. Ankle jerks are absent and plantar responses downgoing bilaterally. There is generalized impairment of sensation extending from the anal margin down the buttocks, back of the legs, over the soles and dorsum of the feet, and on the lateral aspect of the left shin. The anus is patulous.

1 Which nerve roots are responsible for the parasympathetic reflex arc required for penile erection?
2 Where is the lesion causing this man's symptoms and signs?

Question 27

The following considered important to take into account when advising a patient with epilepsy whether they can come off medication (T/F):

A Age over 75
B Taking more than one antiepileptic drug
C A history of seizures after starting antiepileptic drugs
D Previous history of non-compliance
E A history of myoclonic seizures
F An abnormal EEG in the previous year
G Whether the patient drives or not.

Question 28

A 58-year-old man is referred to you with weakness. His symptoms started 2 months ago with his lower limbs being mainly affected. He describes increasing difficulty climbing up stairs and getting up from a chair. On direct questioning, there is no suggestion of fatigability with exercise. He also complains of dry mouth and impotence. There are no speech, swallowing or visual problems. On systemic questioning, he has a long history of mild breathlessness on exertion and a chronic cough which he attributes to his heavy smoking. However, over the last 2 weeks he has noticed blood streaks in his sputum. On examination, muscle power is 3/5 proximally and 4/5 distally in the lower limbs and 4/5 proximally and 5/5 distally in the upper limbs, muscle power improving on repeated testing. Deep tendon reflexes are depressed but improve with repeated muscle contraction. There are no sensory changes or extraocular muscle abnormalities.

General examination reveals no evidence of a rash but dullness to percussion over the left upper zone and reduced breath sounds bilaterally, especially in the left lung.

1 What two investigations would you do?
2 What is the neurological diagnosis?
3 What is the most likely underlying cause of the neurological condition in this case?
4 Explain the pathophysiology of the neurological condition.

Question 29

Myoclonus is a common feature of the following conditions (T/F):

A Lewy body dementia
B Huntington's disease
C Cortical-basal degeneration
D Juvenile myoclonic epilepsy
E Vascular encephalopathy
F Creutzfeldt–Jakob disease.

Question 30

A 40-year-old ex-miner is seen by you in the outpatient's clinic with progressive lower limb weakness over the last 2 years. He describes heaviness of his lower limbs and frequent tripping which is preventing him from walking long distances. He also suffers from frequent night cramps. Over the last 6 months he has noticed increasing difficulty with swallowing, especially of liquids. He denies any sphincter or visual disturbances. His father suffered from the same condition. Examination reveals occasional muscle twitching in the upper and lower limbs, and muscle thinning in the lower limbs. There is bilateral foot drop and lower limb weakness, the left leg being more affected than the right. Deep tendon reflexes are depressed with bilateral extensor plantar responses. There are no sensory abnormalities. Apart from a brisk jaw jerk and spastic tongue, cranial nerve examination is unremarkable.

1 What is the diagnosis?
2 What investigation would you do to confirm the diagnosis in this patient?

Question 31

The following are associated with insomnia (T/F):

A Parkinson's disease
B Hypothyroidism
C Phenytoin
D Pain
E Alcohol.

Question 32

A 55-year-old woman with known myasthenia gravis is admitted in acute respiratory failure. She has severe generalized weakness and is too weak to give a history. Her present medications include pyridostigmine bromide and azathioprine.

1 What two possible diagnoses would you consider in this case?

2 What test may distinguish between the two possible diagnoses?

3 Apart from ventilatory support, what initial treatment would you specifically institute to treat each of the two possible diagnoses?

Question 33

The neuropathy associated with the following is typically painful (T/F):

A Guillain–Barré syndrome

B Vasculitis

C Paraneoplastic neuroneopathy

D Hereditary motor and sensory neuropathies

E Leprosy.

Question 34

A 25-year-old man presents with a week's history of bilateral shoulder and arm pain. The pain on occasion has been so severe as to awaken him from sleep several times over the last few days. He has also noticed increasing weakness of his arms and describes difficulty lifting things at work where he is a shop assistant. On examination there is weakness of abduction and adduction of the arms, elbow flexion, and wrist extension and flexion bilaterally, the right side being more severely affected than the left. The biceps and supinator reflexes are depressed. There is mild impairment of sensation over the lateral aspect of the arms extending down to the thumbs and index fingers bilaterally.

1 What is the diagnosis?

2 Which nerve segments are affected?

Question 35

A unilateral spinal cord lesion at T1 produces (T/F):

A Ipsilateral loss of proprioception and vibration sense below T1

B Ipsilateral loss of temperature sense below T1

C Contralateral brisk knee reflex and upgoing plantar reflex

D Ipsilateral lower motor neurone paralysis at the level of the lesion

E Normal superficial abdominal reflexes.

Question 36

A 46-year-old woman with a marked change in personality over the last 2 years is referred to you. She has become increasingly sexually flirtatious with inappropriate behaviour in social situations. Impairment of abstract thinking, memory and planning has become increasingly obvious.

However, the ability to perform arithmetic tasks is relatively preserved. Speech output is diminished. There is no motor impairment. Physical examination is unremarkable except for the presence of grasp reflexes.

1 What is the most likely diagnosis?

2 What do grasp reflexes indicate?

Question 37

Features suggestive of new variant Creutzfeldt–Jakob disease rather than sporadic Creutzfeldt–Jakob disease include (T/F):

A Mean age of onset is younger

B Depression at presentation

C Upgaze paresis

D Changes in mentation at presentation

E Time between onset of symptoms and death is longer in the former.

Question 38

Which of the following statements on the EEG in normal adults are true?

A The waking pattern consists mainly of δ activity

B The α rhythm is attenuated by eye opening

C δ activity is normally present when asleep but not when awake

D β activity is faster than 12 Hz

E In drowsiness there is disappearance of α activity.

Question 39

A Superior orbital fissure

B Foramen rotundum

C Foramen ovale

D Foramen spinosum

E Internal acoustic meatus

F Jugular foramen

G Foramen magnum.

For each structure below, select the opening in the cranial floor above which it passes through. Each option may be used once, more than once or not at all.

1 Middle meningeal artery

2 Facial nerve

3 Ophthalmic division of trigeminal nerve

4 Oculomotor nerve

5 Maxillary division of trigeminal nerve.

Question 40

A Expressive aphasia

B Receptive aphasia

C Global aphasia

D Conduction aphasia

E Motor transcortical aphasia

F Sensory transcortical aphasia

G Mixed transcortical aphasia

For each of the locations of the lesion below, select the

type of aphasia it is associated with above. Each option may be used once, more than once or not at all.

1 Arcuate fasciculus
2 Superior temporal gyrus
3 Surrounding inferior frontal gyrus
4 Surrounding superior temporal gyrus and inferior frontal gyrus
5 Inferior frontal gyrus.

Question 41

Regarding visual hallucinations, which of the following statements are true?

A Visual hallucinations secondary to eye disease often disappear with eye closure.

B Visual hallucinations secondary to occipital lobe lesions may disappear with saccadic eye movements

C Peduncular hallucinosis is a syndrome of complex visual hallucinations secondary to lesions in the occipital cortex

D Epileptic visual hallucinations are more likely to be complex

E Complex hallucinations are more likely to result from lesions in the visual association areas or connections with the temporal lobe than from lesions in the occipital lobe.

Question 42

1 Pins and needles and heaviness spreading down the right arm and then the right leg over minutes followed by generalized headache in a 62-year-old hypertensive man

2 Dysarthria and weakness in the right hand of sudden onset in a 54-year-old diabetic woman

3 Left facial pain, blurred vision, and a heavy sensation in the right-sided limbs, of sudden onset in a 29-year-old woman.

For each of these clinical scenarios, pick the most likely diagnosis based on the history given, from the list below.

A Migraine with aura

B Subarachnoid haemorrhage with middle cerebral artery vasospasm

C Acute episode of central nervous system demyelination

D Internal carotid artery dissection followed by middle cerebral artery territory ischaemia

E Lacunar infarct.

Question 43

Which of the following are true?

A Vertigo worsened by movement is the cardinal feature of benign positional vertigo (BPV)

B Hallpike's manoeuvre is positive when a patients symptoms are reproduced

C Short-duration vertigo is more characteristic of BPV than Menières disease

D Vertical nystagmus always indicates a central nervous system lesion

E Downbeat nystagmus localizes the lesion to the cranio-cervical junction.

Question 44

A 74-year-old man attends outpatients with his wife. She gives a history of an episode of transient loss of memory and confusion in her husband. After showering, he came downstairs and appeared not to know where he was, or who his wife was, although he seemed to remember who he was. His memory for past events was also impaired. He was able to carry on normal conversations concerning his surroundings. His symptoms lasted for much of the rest of the day, but when he awoke the next morning, his retrograde amnesia was limited to a short period of time before the shower. His past history includes mild hypertension and migraine.

Which of the following diagnoses best suit this clinical picture?

A Transient ischaemic attack affecting the left temporal lobe

B Transient global amnesia

C Subdural haematoma affecting predominantly right frontal lobe

D Complex partial seizure

E Migraine equivalent

F Frontal lobe dementia.

Question 45

You are referred by the casualty officer a 60-year-old woman with a 2-week history of pain in the right eye and double vision. The patient has type 2 diabetes mellitus and hypertension. On examination, there is ptosis of the right eye and diplopia on looking up with the right eye abducted. The right pupil is dilated with no direct or consensual pupillary light reflexes. The left eye is normal. Visual fields are full to confrontation and visual acuity is 6/6 corrected bilaterally. Blood pressure is 175/100 mmHg. The rest of the examination is unremarkable.

1 What is the cranial nerve abnormality?

2 What is the value of pupillary involvement in diagnosing the cranial nerve abnormality and why does it occur?

3 What is the most likely underlying cause of the cranial nerve abnormality?

4 What is the investigation of choice in this patient?

Question 46

In patients with Parkinson's disease (T/F):

A metoclopramide is useful in reducing nausea

B chorea is a recognised side-effect of L-DOPA treatment

C L-DOPA should be given with an inhibitor of DOPA decarboxylase

D ropinirole acts as a dopamine receptor agonist

E anticholinergic drugs can be used to treat tremor.

Question 47

A Edrophonium

B Pyridostigmine

C Pralidoxime mesylate

D Atropine

E Pilocarpine

F Donepezil

For each clinical situation listed, select the most appropriate drug from the list of options above.

1 Treatment of Alzheimer's disease

2 Diagnosis of myasthenia gravis

3 Antidote for organophosphate poisoning

4 Treatment for acute angle closure glaucoma.

Question 48

A lithium

B ondansetron

C methylenedioxymethylamphetamine (MDMA; ecstasy)

D sumatriptan

E olanzapine.

Select the from the list above the drug whose mechanism of action most closely fits the descriptions below

1 $5HT_3$ receptor antagonist

2 $5HT_1$ receptor agonist

3 selective serotonin reuptake inhibitor

4 $5HT_2$ receptor blocker.

Ophthalmology

AUTHORS:
P. Frith and H. Towler

EDITOR:
P. Frith

EDITOR-IN-CHIEF:
J.D. Firth

1 Clinical presentations

1.1 An acutely painful red eye

Case history

A 25-year-old man presents with a red eye that has become increasingly painful over the past 3 days. The eye aches badly, bright light makes the pain worse and his vision has become slightly blurred.

Clinical approach

There are many causes of a red eye (Table 1): most can be immediately discounted in this case as the association of redness with pain suggests that this is not merely an episode of conjunctivitis. The following are most likely:
• Iritis—inflammation of the front chamber of the eye, also known as anterior uveitis
• A corneal lesion such as an ulcer.
These are difficult to distinguish, except by slit-lamp examination. Both may give rise to photophobia and blurring of vision.

Iritis is a prime cause of a painful red eye, especially if photophobia is also present.
   Danger signals in the patient with a red eye are pain and visual blurring—these are **not** features of a benign condition: the patient requires urgent ophthalmological assessment, including slit-lamp examination.

Relevant history

Change in vision—Distinct impairment of vision, as in this case, suggests a serious problem and must never be ignored (see Table 1).
Discharge—a purulent discharge suggests bacterial conjunctivitis.
Characteristics of pain—patients with conjunctivitis may complain of grittiness but they do not have pain. Photophobia is common in corneal diseases and intraocular inflammation. Pain made worse by reading, which requires accommodation, suggests iritis. Severe pain suggests scleritis (see Section 1.2).

Table 1 Differential diagnosis of a red eye.

	Disease	Discriminating clinical features
Common	Bacterial conjunctivitis	Sticky eye; normal vision
	Viral conjunctivitis	Less sticky eye; pre-auricular lymphadenopathy; URTI; discomfort
	Chlamydial conjunctivitis	Conjunctival follicles; recurrent stickiness
	Allergic conjunctivitis	Itchy; sometimes atopic history
	Episcleritis	Discomfort; sectoral; self-limiting
	Iritis	Pain; photophobia; visual blurring; irregular pupil; keratitic precipitates
Unusual	Scleritis	Pain; may be worse at night; systemic associations. See Section 1.2
	Corneal abscess	Soft contact lens wear or trauma; white corneal infiltrate; pain; blurred vision
Rare	Endophthalmitis	Trauma or eye surgery; i.v. drug use; poor vision
	Acute glaucoma	Hazy cornea; mid-dilated unreactive pupil; hard eye

Relevant history

Ask specifically about:
• Previous similar episode
• Features to suggest a systemic disease. Note particularly the presence of erythema nodosum, dysuria or urethral discharge, oral or genital ulceration, joint or back pain, shortness of breath or diarrhoea, immune status (AIDS) and intravenous drug use. See Sections 2.1 and 2.2 for further discussion of causes of iritis and scleritis
• Soft contact lens wear—risk of acute bacterial infections of the cornea, particularly if lenses are worn overnight.

Examination

Check the eye for the following:
• Where is it red?—in conjunctivitis or diffuse scleritis the redness may involve the whole of the visible portion of the eye. Redness that is localized around the corneal limbus is suggestive of intraocular inflammation, and sectoral redness is commonly seen in conjunctival haemorrhage, nodular scleritis and episcleritis (see Section 1.2). The conjunctiva may show prominent follicles in chlamydial and viral conjunctivitis.

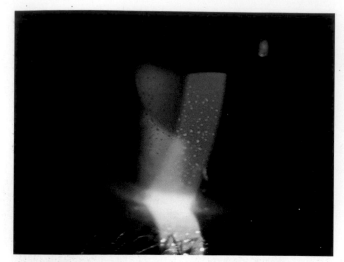

Fig. 1 Slit-lamp view shows multiple white keratitic precipitates characteristic of iritis. These are deposited in the front chamber from the aqueous as a sediment on to the inner surface of the cornea.

- Is it sticky?—this would suggest conjunctivitis.
- Visual acuity—measure with the glasses normally worn and through a pinhole. Acuity worse than 6/9 may indicate serious ocular pathology.
- The pupil—in iritis this may be irregular due to the formation of adhesions. In acute glaucoma it is characteristically mid-dilated and unreactive. A relative afferent pupillary defect (see Section 3.1.3) always indicates serious retinal or optic nerve disease.
- The cornea—fluorescein staining will reveal a corneal ulcer.
- Slit-lamp examination is required (see Section 2.1 and Fig. 1), although larger precipitates on the corneal surface can sometimes be seen with a direct ophthalmoscope.

Measurement of intraocular pressure is mandatory to exclude secondary glaucoma in those with inflammatory disorders of the eye. Always check the contralateral eye carefully: a systemic cause is more likely if there is simultaneous bilateral inflammation. In the absence of systemic symptoms, examining the rest of the patient is unlikely to give valuable clues.

Approach to investigations and management

Investigations

In most patients with a unilateral red eye the diagnosis can be made on clinical grounds and confirmed by targetted investigation (Table 1). Conjunctival infection can be confirmed by culture if chlamydial or viral cause is suspected. A first uncomplicated attack of unilateral acute iritis does not require investigation. For iritis associated with systemic symptoms, initial investigation should be as follows:

- Chest radiograph, biochemistry (particularly serum calcium and angiotensin-converting enzyme (ACE) level, or biopsy of involved tissue may suggest sarcoidosis
- C-reactive protein (CRP) may be raised in any active systemic inflammatory process
- Look for HLA-B27 positivity if ankylosing spondylitis is possible.

Management

Viral conjunctivitis is most commonly due to RNA viruses and is self-limiting. Herpes simplex corneal disease is treated with topical aciclovir. Acute iritis is treated with topical steroids and mydriatics. The patient should be told that iritis can recur, which is much more likely if they are HLA-B27 positive, when there is a 50% chance of a further attack.

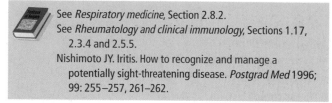

See *Respiratory medicine*, Section 2.8.2.
See *Rheumatology and clinical immunology*, Sections 1.17, 2.3.4 and 2.5.5.
Nishimoto JY. Iritis. How to recognize and manage a potentially sight-threatening disease. *Postgrad Med* 1996; 99: 255–257, 261–262.

1.2 Two painful red eyes and a systemic disorder

Case history

A woman of 60 has felt unwell for several weeks, with malaise, anorexia and joint swelling. For the first time in her life, she has had sinus congestion with some bleeding when blowing her nose and a feeling of her ears being blocked up. In the past week, both eyes have become very bloodshot and last night the pain around her eyes became severe enough to stop her from sleeping properly. She now feels very unwell and is sure the red eyes are something to do with her illness.

Clinical approach

The adult who presents simultaneously with red eyes and severe pain has scleritis until proved otherwise. This is much less common than iritis but should prompt a search for an active underlying systemic vasculitis, especially rheumatoid arthritis or Wegener's granulomatosis.

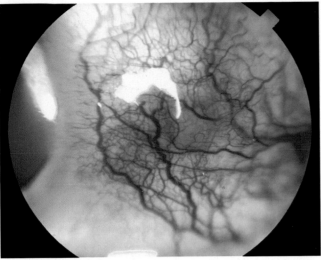

Fig. 2 Anterior nodular scleritis, pretreatment. The episcleral vessels are markedly dilated and the underlying sclera swollen. There is scleral translucency with the underlying darker choroid visible in the centre of the nodule.

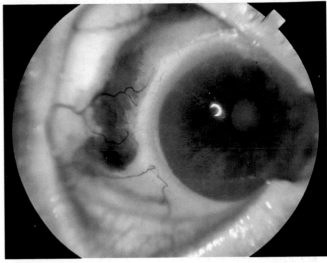

Fig. 4 Necrotizing scleritis in rheumatoid arthritis (scleromalacia perforans) with full-thickness scleral loss. Only thin conjunctiva and episclera cover the choroid.

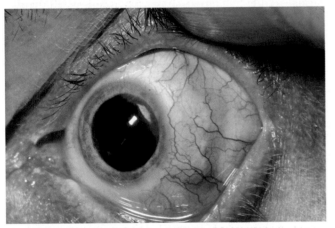

Fig. 3 Healed anterior scleritis. After treatment with prednisolone and cyclosporin, the sclera has returned to normal thickness but is more translucent, allowing the darker choroid to show through.

The degree of pain associated with scleritis is variable, but some characteristics are particular pointers to this diagnosis:
• Pain interrupting sleep, which may even lead to pacing about or banging the head against a wall
• Pain worse on eye movement (but see also Section 2.5, p. 146)
• Pain that is so unbearable that the patient asks for the eye to be removed.

Relevant history

This woman has upper respiratory symptoms, but ask anyone who may have scleritis about systemic symptoms such as:
• arthritis
• shortness of breath
• upper respiratory problems—especially sinusitis, epistaxis and deafness.

Examination

The eye is red, although the pattern varies and often redness of the sclera is patchy (Fig. 2); there may also be swelling or thinning (Fig. 3). Loss of full-thickness sclera, called scleromalacia perforans and usually associated with rheumatoid arthritis, is uncommon but sight threatening (Fig. 4).

Approach to investigations and management

Investigations

Investigations for scleritis are important, because it is an uncommon, capricious and sight-threatening condition, especially compared with the related but milder condition of episcleritis, which causes a similar pattern of redness, but much lesser intensity of symptoms, signs and significance.
• Ultrasonography of the eye coat should be done by an expert, because both getting a reliable image and interpreting the results need care and experience; in scleritis, the affected sclera is thickened.
• For the systemic element, check the mid-stream urine (MSU) for red cells or casts, and do a full blood count (FBC), renal and liver function tests, inflammatory markers (CRP), and serological tests for rheumatological or vasculitic conditions (rheumatoid factor, antineutrophil cytoplasmic antibody [ANCA]), and chest radiograph.

> History and investigation of the patient with scleritis may show a systemic vasculitis such as rheumatoid arthritis or Wegener's granulomatosis.

131

Management

If scleritis is confirmed, treatment for the eye—as for systemic features—should be with systemic immunosuppression, usually initially using corticosteroids in an oral dose of 1 mg/kg per day. Threatened perforation may require a pulsed intravenous regimen and other cytotoxics.

 See *Nephrology*, Sections 1.9 and 1.12.
See *Rheumatology and clinical immunology*, Sections 1.20, 1.21, 2.4 and 2.5.

1.3 Acute painless loss of vision in one eye

Case history

A bricklayer aged 60 reports that earlier this evening, as he was watching TV, he suddenly noticed 'something wrong with his vision'. He says that he 'found he could see nothing'.

Clinical approach

 Abrupt painless loss of vision in one eye may be caused by a retinal arterial or venous occlusive event.

Patients with acute loss of vision need to be talked through the event to unearth those exact details that will provide a diagnosis, and which can easily become garbled in the telling. Ask about the following points if the information does not emerge spontaneously:
• Has vision recovered completely, back to normal?
• Was the loss in one eye (as transpired in this case) or both; did he check each eye separately at the time or is there some doubt about this?
• Was the blindness complete—total loss of vision—or was it partial?
• If partial, which area was affected most?
• How long did the episode last—was it for seconds, minutes or hours?

Differential diagnosis

Look for features to make the following diagnoses listed below.

Arterial occlusion

If loss was complete, even if only in part of the field of vision, in one eye only and with vision in the other eye

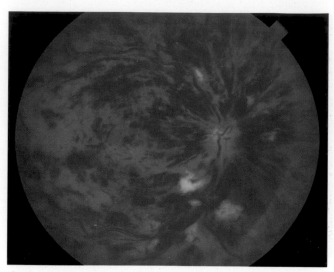

Fig. 5 Central retinal vein occlusion with characteristic 'bloodstorm' appearance and cotton-wool spots.

entirely normal, this is likely to be an arterial event in the retina—either amaurosis fugax or a completed stroke. Retinal transient ischaemic attacks (TIAs), like others, are usually brief—less than 30 min—and are by definition strictly uniocular. They almost always imply an embolic event, most commonly from the ipsilateral carotid bifurcation. By contrast, the patient with a post-chiasmal TIA affecting vision will rarely report the episode. Transient disturbance of vision with vague characteristics cannot allow a definite diagnosis, although they may be regarded as possible TIAs.

Retinal vein occlusion

Patients who occlude the retinal vein will present with an acute onset, often coming on overnight, although the onset is not as abrupt as with an arterial event, nor is the loss transient. Loss of vision, although pronounced, is less complete than with an arterial occlusion; the retinal appearance is of flame and blot haemorrhages in a global pattern if the central vein is blocked (Fig. 5) or wedge-shaped if a branch vein is occluded (Fig. 6).

Other

Other causes of acute painless loss of vision include the following:
• Retinal detachment, in which a uniocular visual field defect may be present corresponding to the site of the lesion
• Vitreous haemorrhage, in which the patient may describe acute onset of floaters and the red reflex may be obscured (Fig. 7).
• Acute optic neuropathy: see Section 1.5 (p. 135).
• Migraine equivalent: a possible homonymous loss, a geometric pattern, persistence with the eyes closed and

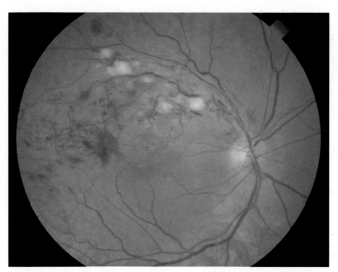

Fig. 6 Branch retinal vein occlusion in a sector above the fovea. Vision may be affected, depending on changes at the fovea itself, such as haemorrhage or oedema.

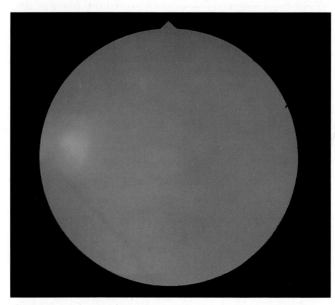

Fig. 7 Vitreous haemorrhage: the optic disc can just be seen through a diffuse vitreous haze caused by red cells. With a dense haemorrhage the red reflex may be entirely obscured.

scintillation all suggest a migraine equivalent even if headache was not a feature.

• Giant cell arteritis: the visual loss may not be painful, but headaches and/or other systemic features are associated (see Section 1.5, p. 135).

Relevant past history

Cerebral TIAs, vascular events elsewhere and vascular risk factors should be explored (see *Cardiology*, Section 1.5). Has the patient got multiple sclerosis, or had any previous neurological episodes that might support this diagnosis? (See *Neurology*, Section 2.5.)

Examination

The eye

With a retinal TIA there may be no eye signs, although emboli should be sought after dilating the pupil with 1% tropicamide.

With a completed retinal stroke, in the acute event the fundus looks pale with narrowed arterioles and a 'cherry red spot' usually appears at the fovea, as the underlying choroidal circulation shows through (Fig. 8). Emboli may be visible at the disc within the main retinal artery or at retinal arteriolar bifurcations (Fig. 9). Later, within days, the fundus may look normal; optic atrophy supervenes within weeks as the nerve fibres die back. At all stages there will be a relative afferent pupillary defect.

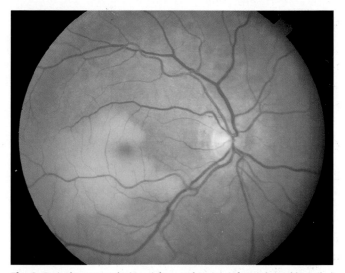

Fig. 8 Retinal artery occlusion: right eye showing inferotemporal branch retinal artery occlusion with a cherry red spot and surrounding retinal oedema and pallor. Visual loss is profound and may be total.

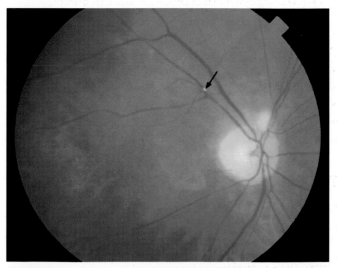

Fig. 9 Branch retinal artery embolus (Hollenhorst's plaque): a well-defined refractile opacity is seen in the superotemporal branch artery at the first bifurcation (arrow). There is also a cotton-wool spot at the edge of the optic disk at 1 o'clock.

Examination for a relative afferent pupillary defect is crucial in cases of acute visual loss.

Move a bright light from one eye to the other, watching each direct pupil response—asymmetry suggests a defect on the side of the pupil that tends to dilate.

See Section 3.1.3 for further information.

General

Has the patient got atheromatous vascular disease? Check for a bruit at the ipsilateral carotid bifurcation, listening with the diaphragm below the angle of the jaw, and asking the patient to hold his breath; check also for vascular bruits elsewhere and for absent peripheral pulses.

Are there any abnormal cardiovascular findings? Is the patient in atrial fibrillation? What is the blood pressure? Are there any murmurs? Are the temporal arteries thickened, tender or pulseless? (See Section 1.5, p. 135.)

Approach to investigations and management

Investigations

In all cases check FBC, renal and liver function, inflammatory markers (erythrocyte sedimentation rate/C-reactive protein [ESR/CRP]), blood sugar and lipids. Check ECG for myocardial ischaemia or even an occult myocardial infarct.

Carotid imaging is warranted if surgery is to be considered. Patients with bilateral episodes require particularly careful assessment, including an echocardiogram to look for a cardiac source of embolism.

Management

All patients need attention to cardiovascular risk factors such as smoking, diabetes, hyperlipidaemia and hypertension.

Carotid endarterectomy should be considered for stenosis of 70% or more; otherwise daily aspirin is beneficial, if tolerated. If this patient has a completed retinal arterial occlusion with permanent loss of vision in one eye, he may have difficulty laying bricks accurately for a week or so until he adjusts to judging depth monocularly. He is entitled to drive, once adjusted to monocularity, because the good eye provides the acuity and visual field that are legally necessary.

Internal carotid stenosis of greater than 70% may warrant endarterectomy as well as control of other vascular risk factors. Otherwise, consider aspirin.

1.4 Acute painful loss of vision in a young woman

Case history

A 25-year-old woman reports that the vision in one eye has become blurred over the past 3 days, so that now she can see very little. The eye has been aching. She is otherwise well but consulted a neurologist a few years ago for 'peculiar sensations', although no precise diagnosis was given.

Clinical approach

In a patient of this age, with this particular pattern of visual loss and the vague neurological history, this is very likely to be an attack of demyelinating optic neuritis. There are certain key features that might pin this diagnosis down. Ask about the following:
• How much of the visual field is affected? In optic neuritis, the loss of vision particularly affects the central field, blurring the whole face at a conversational distance, and is larger than that found with retinal (foveal) oedema.
• The pain in optic neuritis may be worse on eye movement, with an unpleasant 'pulling' feeling.
• One hallmark of optic neuritis is a tendency for visual acuity to improve spontaneously over the following weeks.

Other optic nerve lesions are less common and usually painless. If other features of an optic nerve lesion are not found, and even if the retina appears normal, there is still a possibility of foveal oedema as a cause of central scotoma, in which case a fluorescein angiogram may be helpful (see Section 3.3, p. 156).

Relevant history

The neurological history is important and full details should be sought: what can the patient remember, what tests were performed, and what do the neurologist's notes and letters reveal? It may be that a diagnosis of multiple sclerosis (MS) was considered likely but the patient was not informed at the time of a suspected first event.

Examination

The eye

The signs of an optic nerve lesion should be checked, expecting to find some or all of the following:
• Reduced visual acuity to a variable degree, although total loss of vision is rare

• Central scotoma, partial to colour or total, best mapped with a small coloured target, perhaps the conventional red hatpin, although any small coloured object will do
• Impaired colour appreciation so that, compared with the normal eye, colours look 'washed out'
• Imbalance of the symmetry of pupil response to an alternating bright light, so a 'relative afferent pupil defect' is present
• Swollen optic nerve head in the acute stage (Fig. 10), unless the inflammation is 'retrobulbar', when its appearance is normal. Optic atrophy follows months later (Fig. 11).

General

Is there any evidence of neurological deficit, e.g. cerebellar signs, or those of a spinal cord lesion? These would support the diagnosis of MS in this context.

Fig. 10 Optic disc swelling: if vision is normal, this may be papilloedema secondary to raised intracranial pressure. If vision is reduced, an acute optic neuropathy is likely.

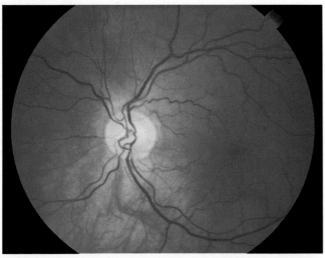

Fig. 11 Optic disc atrophy: there are many causes of this important sign, including past neuritis or ischaemia, or compression. Visual acuity will depend on the cause.

Approach to investigations and management

The eventual level of recovery of visual acuity is difficult to predict and hence a guarded prognosis must be given.

Has the patient got MS? Referral back to the neurologist may be appropriate, as may tests such as brain MRI, electrophysiological testing (e.g. visual evoked potentials) and lumbar puncture. The implications of this episode will need to be discussed (see *Neurology*, Section 1.25) and whether treatment for MS is warranted.

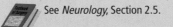
See *Neurology,* Section 2.5.

1.5 Acute loss of vision in an elderly man

Case history

A 75-year-old man reports that he suddenly noticed loss of vision in one eye. Recently, he has felt unwell, has lost weight, finds it difficult to get out of bed in the morning and has begun to have headaches.

Clinical approach

> Consider giant cell arteritis in any elderly patient with acute loss of vision that may be caused by acute optic nerve ischaemia. This condition is a medical emergency: visual loss in the affected eye is irreversible, and the second eye is at immediate risk.

An elderly patient with acute and painful visual loss has giant cell arteritis (synonymous with 'temporal' or 'cranial' arteritis) until proved otherwise. Although there may be diagnostic clinical features, many cases hinge on a high index of suspicion in the face of conflicting clinical evidence. In general, the older the patient, the less likely a non-arteritic event. Diagnosis can be confirmed by temporal artery biopsy. Loss of vision, when it occurs in giant cell arteritis, is pronounced and irretrievable—the second eye is at immediate risk.

Relevant history

This man has many obvious clues to the diagnosis of giant cell arteritis, but ask any patient of middle age

135

or older presenting with acute loss of vision about the following:

- Headaches—which tend to be lateralized
- Scalp tenderness—usually noted when brushing the hair
- Jaw pain, which may be the result of claudication
- Symptoms of polymyalgia rheumatica, including muscular pain (particularly of shoulder girdle), stiffness, general malaise, weight loss, fever.

Examination

The eye

If there is established ischaemia of the optic nerve head, there will be signs of an optic nerve lesion (see Section 1.4, p. 134) with the following:

- A pale swollen optic disc visible on ophthalmoscopy (Fig. 12)
- Vision may be totally lost, without even perception of light
- The visual field may show a partial pattern of loss, often altitudinal, i.e. affecting the upper or lower part (Fig. 13)
- A relative afferent pupil defect.

General

Examine specifically for tenderness of cranial arteries —not only temporal, but also occasionally facial or occipital—with swelling and/or loss of pulsation. These findings are characteristic of, but not necessary for, the diagnosis.

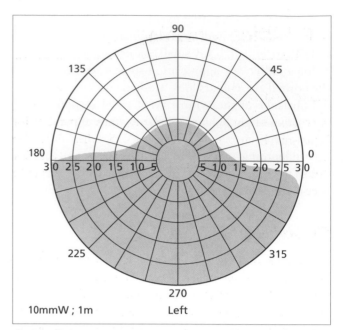

Fig. 13 Inferior altitudinal field defect in giant cell arteritis with ischaemic optic neuropathy. The field of the right eye was normal. Uniocular altitudinal defects are secondary to an anterior lesion, in either the retina or the optic nerve.

Approach to investigations and management

Investigations

Check the ESR and CRP urgently. The pre-steroid CRP is especially important; if normal, this virtually excludes the diagnosis of giant cell arteritis. Although temporal artery biopsy may be negative, finding a positive result is so important for future strategy that biopsy should be performed whenever feasible.

Management

If giant cell arteritis is possible, give corticosteroids immediately rather than withhold them: visual loss can progress rapidly and once present is irretrievable, and the second eye could become affected. Arterial biopsy can be done within the next 24 h and then a further decision made about strategy. If both eyes are affected there is even greater urgency in beginning treatment.

Corticosteroid dose should be tailored to the circumstances:

- If vision is little affected, an initials oral dose of prednisolone 1 mg/kg per day is adequate
- If both eyes are affected, some clinicians advocate intravenous administration of methylprednisolone, although there is no conclusive evidence of superiority over oral prednisolone.

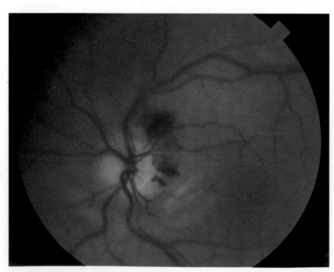

Fig. 12 Optic disc in the acute stage of giant cell arteritis. The infarcted optic nerve head is pale and swollen with blurred and haemorrhagic margins. Visual loss is usually irreversible in this situation, and the second eye is at immediate risk.

See *Medicine for the elderly*, Section 1.5.
See *Rheumatology and clinical immunology*, Section 2.5.1.

1.6 Difficulty reading

Case history

A 50-year-old author with diabetes finds that the vision in one eye is blurred when she reads. She last visited her optometrist 3 years ago to get new reading spectacles, but has not gone back for the annual check that he recommended.

Clinical approach

Visual impairment more marked for reading than distance is very suggestive of macular disease. The likely cause of her symptom is diabetic maculopathy, when the central fovea becomes affected by retinal oedema or frank hard exudate, which extends from areas of leakage within the surrounding macula. A retinal vein occlusion may also cause blurring of central vision as a result of macular oedema (see Section 1.3, p. 132). Age-related macular degeneration, which may cause similar symptoms, is unlikely in a woman of this age. A vitreous haemorrhage, associated with proliferative retinopathy, will give rise to acute onset of floaters or of generally blurred vision in one eye, rather than the specific central pattern, noted only on reading, that she describes.

Differential diagnosis of difficulty reading includes:
- Incorrect focus, correctable by an optometrist
- Something wrong with the clarity of the eye interior, often a cataract
- Something wrong with the central retina at the fovea, especially age-related macular degeneration in elderly people
- Something wrong with the brain, especially a homonymous visual field defect, usually caused by a stroke.

Exactly what is the visual defect? Take a careful history, thinking of the following diagnostic possibilities as you do so.

Macular oedema

The vision is often blurred in a patchy way. Patients can often draw this fairly accurately in relation to the fixation point corresponding to the fovea itself, perhaps using the squared chart devised by Amsler (Fig. 14). They may also admit that straight lines—on a page or the bathroom tiles—look bent, or that the image seems smaller or larger in the affected eye, all of which are symptoms of macular oedema.

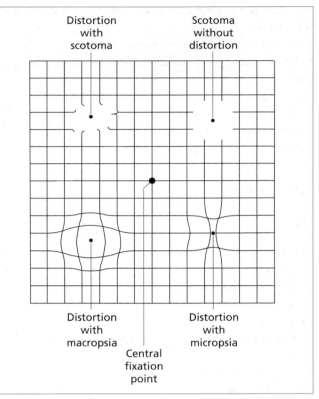

Fig. 14 Amsler chart patterns: the patient is able to draw the defect in central vision produced by a lesion near the fovea.

Floaters

If the patient with diabetes describes a sudden onset of floaters, the diagnosis may be of an acute vitreous haemorrhage, indicating posterior vitreous separation and usually proliferative retinopathy in this context. A small haemorrhage is like 'a cloud of midges', a moderate one like 'a net curtain waving about' and a dense bleed interferes alarmingly with vision.

Cataract

Another cause of difficulty reading is cataract. Lens changes producing cataract occur at a younger age in diabetes (Fig. 15), a tendency also increased by systemic corticosteroid treatment.

The presentation is usually with gradual change in vision, but in the first affected eye the patient may not notice this until quite advanced, thus presenting as if the loss is acute. Characteristic associated symptoms are of difficulty in bright light or from sunlight due to glare, such as in car headlights when driving at night.

Glaucoma

Glaucoma can present in many ways, although difficulty reading would be unusual because central vision is usually preserved until late.

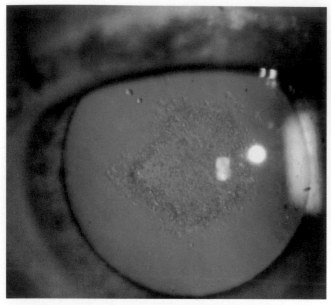

Fig. 15 Early cataract seen against the red reflex. The granular appearance in the centre of the pupil is typical of posterior subcapsular cataract, secondary to the use of systemic corticosteroids.

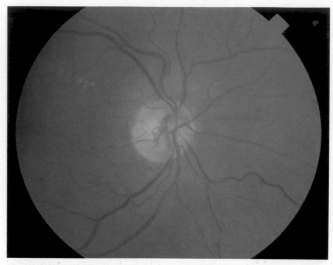

Fig. 16 New vessels on the optic disc, centrally.

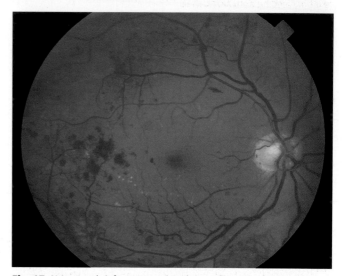

Fig. 17 New vessels inferotemporal to the macula. Large blot haemorrhages temporal to the fovea are indicative of retinal ischaemia in this watershed area.

Stroke

Stroke may cause sudden onset of reading difficulty and can be surprisingly hard to pin down when not associated with another neurological deficit. Characteristically the patient has difficulty finding his or her way on the page, even if the letters seem clear and central acuity is normal. If the homonymous visual loss is to the right side, there is difficulty completing the line whereas, to the left, the difficulty is finding the beginning of the next line—this may become clear if the patient is asked to read aloud.

Relevant past history

The optometrist should be consulted; they will almost certainly have an accurate record of the previous visual acuity and the retinal appearance—background retinopathy, with a few dots, blot haemorrhages and sparse hard exudate, although not involving the fovea itself. Quite rightly, he had recommended an annual check to see whether these changes were progressing, even if vision was normal and the patient was happy with her reading spectacles.

Examination

The eye

Visual acuity for both distance and near should be tested; they will be appreciably reduced—to perhaps 6/9 or 6/12, or font size 6–8—and improve little with a pinhole or new spectacles.

The eye should be examined carefully for any of the changes described above, which can be seen only after dilating the pupil with 1% tropicamide for 20 min.

• Is there a cataract? This may be visible against the red reflex using the ophthalmoscope, and is certainly seen with the slit lamp, these appearances being more obvious if the pupil is dilated.

• Is there an acute vitreous haemorrhage? A small bleed can best be detected with the slit lamp when red cells appear in the vitreous, behind the lens; a large bleed will obscure the ophthalmoscopic red reflex (see Fig. 7).

• Is there macular oedema or hard exudates near the fovea? If the patient looks directly into the beam the fovea is seen, but the subtle textural change of oedema is not easy to detect without stereoscopic viewing techniques. The second eye should also be examined for sight-threatening features close to the fovea.

• Are there other retinal changes? Both eyes should be examined carefully for diabetic changes, taking particular

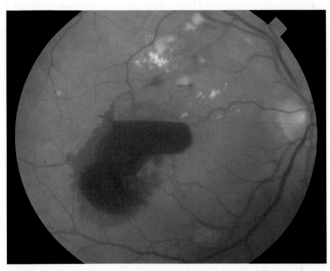

Fig. 18 Preretinal haemorrhage, which shows a horizontal fluid level, as a result of bleeding from new vessels.

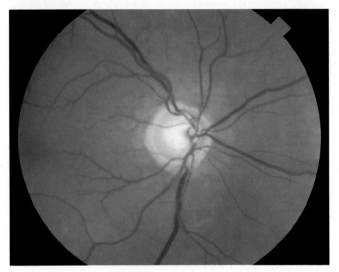

Fig. 19 Optic disc cupping in chronic glaucoma. The peripheral rim is narrow and pale, the central cup wide.

concern to exclude signs of proliferation of new vessels, which can coexist with macular changes (Figs 16 and 17) and may cause acute central visual loss if blood collects in front of the fovea (Fig. 18). In central retinal vein occlusion, the distribution of haemorrhage has a different pattern from that of diabetes, especially in being focal and uniocular rather than widespread and bilateral (see Fig. 6). In advanced glaucoma, cupping of the optic disc should be apparent (Fig. 19).

General

If examination of the eye does not reveal a cause for the difficulty in reading, then the woman may have had a stroke. Is there any evidence, perhaps subtle, to suggest this? Ask her to extend her arms in front of her and close her eyes—has she got a slight drift of one arm? Keeping her eyes closed, ask her to touch the tip of her nose with her right index finger and then her left—can she do this accurately on both sides? Ask her to 'play the piano' as fast as she can with both hands simultaneously—are movements clumsier on one side than the other? Does she have a homonymous visual field defect, or visual or sensory inattention on one side?

> In the patient with difficulty reading that is not due to incorrect focus, examine the following carefully and logically:
> • Retinoscopy will distinguish diabetic maculopathy from age-related macular degeneration, retinal vein occlusion and cataract
> • If none of these is present, check for a homonymous visual field defect that would probably indicate a stroke, and look hard for evidence of other neurological deficit
> • If still puzzled, refer to an ophthalmologist who is able to assess visual fields, measure ocular pressure, examine the macula and offer appropriate treatment.

Approach to investigations and management

Investigations

More precise assessment of macular function may require fluorescein angiography. Macular oedema can be difficult to see otherwise, and this test may both establish the diagnosis and help target focal laser treatment to leaking areas.

Management

Clinically significant diabetic macular oedema may require laser treatment, delivered either as focal burns to leaking microaneurysms or more scattered applications (grid laser) for difficult oedema.

Annual screening of all patients with diabetes should be performed with the aim of detecting treatable areas early, preferably before vision is affected, because the earlier treatment is given the better the chance of maintaining normal vision for a longer time. Hard exudate at the fovea itself soon becomes irreversible and unfortunately some patients with diabetes present in this way.

Overall control of blood sugar and blood pressure is also important in the longer-term strategy to preserve vision.

> See *Endocrinology*, Section 2.6.

1.7 Double vision

Case history

A financial management consultant aged 35 has come to hospital accident and emergency in a taxi, leaving a party

139

at which he became unwell. He is not able to give a clear history because he is distressed by headache. His wife says that, after several drinks, but before the meal, he complained of not feeling well, developed a headache and said that his vision was double. He has vomited once in the taxi on the way to hospital and is still nauseated, clutching a vomit bowl.

Clinical approach

The difficulty here is to distinguish alcohol intoxication from migraine or a more serious problem such as enlargement of an intracranial aneurysm, specifically an acute third nerve compression caused by an aneurysm arising from the posterior communicating artery of the circle of Willis. Analysis of the double vision and a search for other neurological signs are therefore crucial. If the third nerve is compressed from outside—an extrinsic lesion—it is more likely that the passenger parasympathetic fibres supplying the pupil will be involved and the ipsilateral pupil dilated. If the aneurysm has leaked, signs of subarachnoid haemorrhage may be found.

History of the presenting problem

It is likely that a clear history will be difficult to obtain from the patient, so obtaining details from the wife is particularly important. He has never had an episode like this before, he does not get migraine and he does not get drunk. Although he has suffered from headaches occasionally in the past, he has never before become distressed in this way. He cannot describe his double vision clearly, but he says that at present if he opens both eyes his vision is still double 'most of the time'. He is still nauseated but not photophobic.

Other relevant history

There is no history of hypertension, diabetes or other cardiovascular disease. He has been under considerable stress at work recently.

Examination

The examination is crucial and should be thorough, despite the patient's distress.

Vision and the eye

Answer the following questions:
- What is the general appearance? Although the patient has not noticed drooping of the left upper eyelid, his wife agrees that this is not the way it usually looks.
- What are the pupils like? Examining carefully, the left pupil is also slightly dilated compared with the right and is less brisk to light reaction, both direct and consensual.
- What about the double vision? In which direction is this worst, and which best? The patient's vision is double when looking in most directions, with both horizontal and vertical separation, but becomes single if either eye is covered, which confirms that this is truly binocular and so caused by an ocular muscle imbalance. Vision is least double on looking to the left, indicating that the left lateral rectus is functioning, but movements of the left eye are restricted in other directions with doubling of the images, looking up, down and to the right.
- What does the ocular fundus look like? This is normal: the optic disc margins are clearly defined on both sides, meaning that intracranial pressure has not been raised for any length of time.

General

There are no signs of meningeal irritation such as neck stiffness, and there are no other neurological signs. Blood pressure is 160/95 mmHg.

Approach to investigations and management

The clinical diagnosis is of a left third nerve palsy. Urgent cranial imaging is warranted, looking for a compressive cause, specifically a posterior communicating aneurysm on the left side. Immediate surgical clipping of the aneurysm will need to be considered by neurosurgical colleagues. Despite lack of other clinical signs, headache and nausea suggest that subarachnoid haemorrhage may be present: this could be detected by magnetic resonance imaging (MRI) and/or confirmed by lumbar puncture.

See *Emergency medicine*, Section 1.22.
See *Neurology*, Sections 1.14, 1.15, 1.16, 1.19, 2.6 and 2.8.4.

2 Diseases and treatments

2.1 Iritis

Aetiology

Most cases of iritis are of unknown aetiology: some recognized causes are shown in Table 2.

Clinical presentation

Symptoms are of a red, aching eye with photophobia, which tends to worsen over hours to a few days. Vision may be blurred, but acuity is not severely affected. The pupil tends to be small and may be irregular because the iris has adhered to the anterior lens, in which case it festoons on dilatation. There may be symptoms or signs to suggest an underlying cause (Table 2), but this would be unusual. Diagnosis is made by slit-lamp examination, which is essential whenever iritis is suspected.

> **Slit-lamp examination**
>
> The features of iritis include:
> - 'Flare'—leak of protein from inflamed vessels into the anterior chamber makes the fluid in the aqueous look hazy.
> - Keratitic precipitates—inflammatory cells in the anterior chamber sometimes deposit on the inner surface of the cornea, forming keratitic precipitates (see Fig. 1). Large precipitates are characteristic of granulomatous iritis such as that caused by sarcoid.
> - Hypopyon—if iritis is severe, inflammatory cells may sediment at the bottom of the anterior chamber characteristic of Behçet's disease or endophthalmitis.

Investigation

A first uncomplicated attack of unilateral acute iritis does not require investigation. However, investigation should obviously be guided by any clues to an underlying cause (Table 2) in the history. Appropriate investigations include:
- Chest radiograph—looking in particular for evidence of sarcoidosis
- Serum C-reactive protein—suggests systemic inflammatory process if raised
- Full blood count; MSU and renal function (for TINU), liver and bone chemistries—serum calcium may be raised in sarcoidosis
- Serum angiotensin converting enzyme—may be raised in sarcoidosis

Table 2 Causes of iritis.

Autoimmune	Drug induced
Ankylosing spondylitis	Rifabutin
Sarcoidosis	Cidofovir
Behçet's syndrome	
Inflammatory bowel disease	
Juvenile chronic arthritis	
Psoriasis	
Reiter's syndrome	
TINU (tubulointerstitial nephritis)	
Infectious	
Herpes zoster	
Herpes simplex	
Leptospirosis (uncommon)	
Lyme disease	
Syphilis	
Tuberculosis	
Leprosy	

Note. There is a clear association of iritis with HLA-B27 positivity. The most likely causes of acute iritis with systemic associations are HLA-B27/spondylitis/sacroiliitis and sarcoidosis.

- Serology for syphilis is selected cases
- Test for HLA-B27 positivity—this does not influence immediate management, but those with HLA-B27 are much more liable to recurrent attacks. 'Birdshot choroidopathy' is a very rare disease in which there is reduced vision as a result of inflammation within the vitreous rather than the aqueous: this is uniquely correlated with HLA-A29.

Treatment

Iritis responds promptly to topical treatment with steroids and pupil dilators in the vast majority of cases: drops are preferrable by day and ointment by night. A typical regimen would include dexamethasone 0.1% every 2 h for the first 48 h, then four times daily until review in a week, together with cyclopentolate 1% three times daily. The latter prevents the formation of adhesions between iris and lens whilst inflammation is active, but will also blur vision, especially for reading.

Prognosis

Iritis settles without sequel provided that treatment is not delayed. Vision is expected to return to normal.

Repeated attacks are more likely if iritis is associated with a persistent systemic disease or if the patient is

HLA-B27 positive, when the risk of recurrent iritis is 50%, some fifteen times greater than if they are HLA-B27 negative.

See *Respiratory medicine*, Section 2.2.8 and *Rheumatology and clinical immunology*, Sections 2.3.4, 2.5.2 and 2.5.5. Nishimoto JY. Iritis. How to recognize and manage a potentially sight-threatening disease. *Postgrad Med* 1996; 99: 255–257, 261–262.

2.2 Scleritis

Aetiology

Scleritis is an inflammatory disease of the vessels supplying the sclera which may be associated with rheumatoid arthritis and systemic vasculitis, especially Wegener's granulomatosis (see *Rheumatology and clinical immunology*, Sections 1.19, 2.3.3 and 2.5.2), or other autoimmune rheumatic tissue diseases in about 50% of cases.

Clinical presentation

Scleritis may be anterior or posterior, and anterior scleritis may be nodular, diffuse or necrotizing. Posterior scleritis may be associated with anterior disease, but can also occur in isolation unassociated with systemic disease.

Pain is the most common symptom of scleritis, and is typically severe, worse at night and on eye movement, and wakes the patient from sleep. Redness, photophobia and lacrimation are other common symptoms of anterior scleritis. However, severe necrotizing scleritis in patients with vasculitis associated with polyarticular rheumatoid arthritis may occur without preceding pain or redness. Uncommonly, posterior scleritis may present with ocular pain, reduced visual acuity, proptosis and limitation of extraocular movements, but with a white eye.

When a patient presents with pain in the eye, remember that:
- severe eye pain worse at night is highly suggestive of scleritis, but also that
- severe necrotizing scleritis associated with rheumatoid arthritis is usually painless.

Physical signs

The sclera is usually red and thickened with dilatation of episcleral vessels (Fig. 2). The redness may be localized as in nodular scleritis, or diffuse. The brick-red colour is best seen in daylight.

In very severe scleritis, the sclera may appear white and is necrotic as a result of vascular occlusion. This is an important sign that can easily be overlooked; it is an indication for urgent treatment with systemic steroids. Scleral thinning and increased scleral transparency show through the underlying bluish choroid, either after scleritis has healed (Fig. 3) or in acutely necrotizing scleritis (Fig. 4).

Investigation

Any associated systemic disease should be identified by FBC, ESR, CRP, rheumatoid factor, anti-neutrophil cytoplasmic antibody (ANCA), antinuclear antibody (ANA) and anti-DNA antibodies. Ocular ultrasonography is essential to diagnose posterior scleritis, showing thickening of the posterior eye coat which may also be evident on computed tomography (CT) or MRI of the eye and orbit. Scleral biopsy may rarely be required, specifically only if lymphoma or infection is suspected.

Differential diagnosis

Episcleritis is a mild, non-sight-threatening disease that resolves spontaneously over 6–8 weeks. By contrast to scleritis, pain is not a feature, and the redness will usually blanch with phenylephrine drops. Iritis (anterior uveitis) is less painful and the redness is more marked around the cornea. Slit-lamp examination will distinguish these conditions. Rarely, lymphoma may present with scleral inflammation.

Treatment

Non-steroidal anti-inflammatory drugs, especially flurbiprofen, may be effective for milder cases, but systemic steroids are frequently required to control disease, and immunosuppressive therapy is essential immediately for severe or necrotizing disease. In the short term, flurbiprofen 100 mg three times daily will produce symptomatic improvement within 48 h if effective. Necrotizing or severe disease requires systemic steroid therapy as oral prednisolone 1 mg/kg per day initially or intravenous pulse methylprednisolone 500–1000 mg. Unresponsive disease may require additional immunosuppressive therapy with cyclophosphamide.

Longer-term, steroid-sparing treatment may be required if therapy is necessary and the steroid dose cannot be reduced to acceptable maintenance levels. Agents used include azathioprine, cyclosporin and methotrexate.

Complications

Frequent complications include keratitis, uveitis, cataract, glaucoma and exudative retinal detachment in posterior scleritis. Rarely, the globe actually perforates.

Prognosis

Twenty-five per cent of scleritis patients lose two or more lines of vision over 3 years, usually as a result of cataract or corneal involvement. Less than 5% of eyes lose useful vision in the longer term.

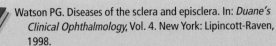
Watson PG. Diseases of the sclera and episclera. In: *Duane's Clinical Ophthalmology*, Vol. 4. New York: Lipincott-Raven, 1998.

McCluskey PJ, Watson PG, Lightman S, Haybittle J, Restori M, Branley M. Posterior scleritis: clinical features, systemic associations, and outcome in a large series of patients. *Ophthalmology* 1999; 106: 2380–2386.

2.3 Retinal artery occlusion

Aetiology

Retinal arterial occlusion is caused by acute obstruction of the central retinal artery or its branches as a result of embolism, or less commonly of thrombosis; it occurs most commonly in the fifth or sixth decade. Associated conditions include carotid vascular disease, diabetes, hypertension, valvular heart disease, dysrhythmias—especially atrial fibrillation with left atrial thrombus—and, less commonly and especially in younger patients, atrial myxoma, coagulopathies and haemoglobinopathies, and with intravenous drug abuse.

Clinical presentation

Patients present with sudden, painless loss of vision. The visual loss may be transient (amaurosis fugax) or sustained, depending on whether or not arterial blood flow is re-established. Central artery occlusion results in total visual loss and branch occlusion in altitudinal (upper or lower) field loss.

Uncommonly, visual loss may primarily affect the peripheral field with preservation of central vision if the macula is supplied by a cilioretinal artery arising from the short posterior ciliary vessels. This pattern occurs in 25–30% of the population (Fig. 20). Rarely, the converse situation of cilioretinal artery occlusion with sparing of the central retinal artery may also occur (Fig. 21). Retinal artery occlusion may occasionally result from giant cell arteritis

Physical signs

Visual acuity is usually profoundly reduced (to hand move-

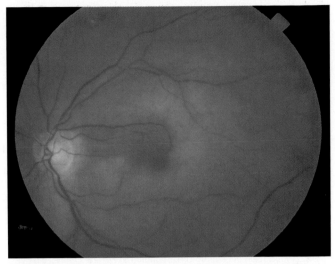

Fig. 20 Retinal artery occlusion with macular sparing as a result of a patent cilioretinal artery. The central macula/fovea is perfused, but there is surrounding retinal pallor with oedema which causes a 'cherry red patch' rather than a 'cherry red spot'. The visual acuity in that eye recovered to 6/9, but with a permanently restricted peripheral field.

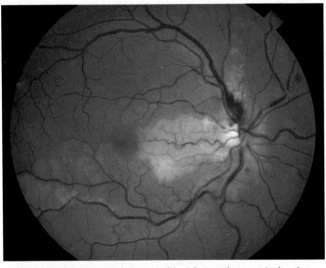

Fig. 21 Cilioretinal artery occlusion. This right eye shows retinal oedema between the optic disc and macula, the opposite of Fig. 20. Visual acuity is poor and there is a large central scotoma which will persist.

ments or even to no light perception), a relative afferent pupillary defect is present, retinal pallor may be sectoral or generalized, the retinal arteries are attenuated and a 'cherry red spot' may be seen at the macula as a result of the underlying choroidal circulation visible through the fovea (see Fig. 8). A bruit may be audible over the ipsilateral carotid, but absence of a bruit does not exclude significant stenosis; look for clinical evidence of dysrhythmias (especially atrial fibrillation) and hypertension.

Sometimes an embolus may be visible within the arterial lumen—a Hollenhorst plaque (see Fig. 9) and/or 'cattle-trucking' of the blood column in the arteries may be seen.

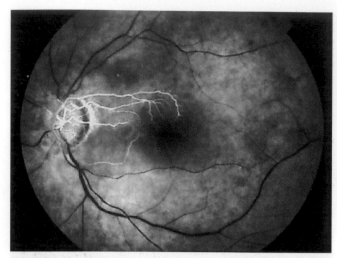

Fig. 22 Fluorescein angiogram corresponding to Fig. 20. Fluorescein dye (which appears white) fills the central cilioretinal circulation in contrast to the non-perfused retinal arteries and veins, which appear black.

Investigation

Look for hypertension and cardiac dysrhythmias, and assess ECG and chest radiograph, ESR, CRP, FBC, lipids, haemoglobin electrophoresis and coagulation studies —especially in younger patients with no other identifiable risk factors.

Carotid Doppler studies and an echocardiogram are important in identifying a remediable source of emboli that may also threaten the brain (see *Cardiology*, Section 3.11 and *Neurology*, Section 3.6).

Fluorescein angiography (Section 3.3, p. 156) may be of value in atypical situations (Fig. 22).

Differential diagnosis

The clinical features of retinal artery occlusion are difficult to confuse with other causes of acute unilateral visual loss such as retinal vein occlusion, retinal detachment or acute ischaemic optic neuropathy.

Treatment

No treatment has been shown to be effective in restoring vision and randomized controlled studies are lacking. Most treatments attempt to improve ocular perfusion either by lowering intraocular pressure or by vasodilatation. Any treatment undertaken more than an hour after the onset is unlikely to improve visual recovery and it should be emphasized to patients that any visual improvement is a bonus.

In the very early stages, emergency ocular massage is easy to perform and may assist in dislodging an embolus. Intraocular pressure can be dramatically reduced by removal of aqueous humour from the anterior chamber through paracentesis with an insulin syringe after instilling povidone–iodine solution.

Short term, treat any identifiable risk factors, such as hypertension, or anticoagulate for embolic thrombus from the heart or coagulopathy. Consider aspirin therapy for lesser degrees of carotid stenosis. Longer term, patients shown to have >70% carotid occlusion should be considered for carotid endarterectomy. Consider management of obesity, smoking and hyperlipidaemia.

Complications

Long-term ocular complications after retinal artery occlusion are uncommon, and much fewer than after retinal vein occlusions. Iris neovascularization may occur, leading to neovascular glaucoma, but retinal neovascularization is rare. The risk of a similar event in the second eye is very small, unless there is bilateral carotid disease or a cardiac source for emboli.

Prognosis

Thirty per cent of affected eyes recover visual acuity of 6/60 or better, although 5% have no light perception in the affected eye. Retinal artery occlusion is associated with serious life-threatening conditions which determine the overall mortality.

> Retinal artery occlusion:
> • usually causes permanent visual damage in spite of therapeutic intervention
> • is frequently associated with serious, potentially life-threatening conditions such as carotid vascular or cardiac disease, the treatment of which will reduce morbidity and mortality.

Prevention

Identification of treatable risk factors should reduce the risk to the contralateral eye and prolong life.

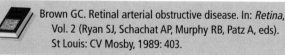

> Brown GC. Retinal arterial obstructive disease. In: *Retina*, Vol. 2 (Ryan SJ, Schachat AP, Murphy RB, Patz A, eds). St Louis: CV Mosby, 1989: 403.

2.4 Retinal vein occlusion

Aetiology

Retinal vein occlusion occurs when the central retinal vein (central retinal vein occlusion [CRVO]) or its branches (branch retinal vein occlusion [BRVO]) become obstructed as a result of thrombosis within the lumen, often preceded by changes within the vessel wall. Hypertension, diabetes, hyperlipidaemia, hyperviscosity syndromes, hypercoagulability and raised intraocular pressure all predispose to this condition. Occlusion usually occurs at the optic disc itself within the central vein, or at an arteriovenous crossing of a branch vein.

Epidemiology

Retinal vein occlusion is the second most common retinal vascular disease after diabetic retinopathy.

Clinical presentation

Presenting symptoms result either from the onset of the occlusion or from the development of complications. Vein occlusions are usually unilateral and, if bilateral, rarely simultaneous.

Common

Sudden onset of painless loss of vision. Branch retinal vein occlusion causes visual loss when the macula is involved, but if the macula is spared the occlusion may be an incidental finding.

Uncommon

Painless loss of vision may arise from vitreous haemorrhage as a complication of ischaemic CRVO.

Rare

A red painful eye may result from neovascular (rubeotic) glaucoma—a late complication.

Physical signs

In CRVO, there are widespread flame and blot retinal haemorrhages (see Fig. 5), often with cotton-wool spots (microinfarcts) throughout the retina, in contrast to the sectoral distribution in BRVO (see Fig. 6). A relative afferent pupil defect (RAPD) is indicative of significant retinal ischaemia, as are numerous cotton-wool spots. BRVO will produce a corresponding visual field defect, but not a RAPD because much of the retina remains perfused and healthy.

Uncommonly, if vitreous haemorrhage is significant, the red reflex will be obscured (see Fig. 7). Rarely, in neovascular glaucoma, the cornea is hazy, the eye rock hard and the conjunctiva red.

Investigations

A fluorescein angiogram may be helpful in cases where

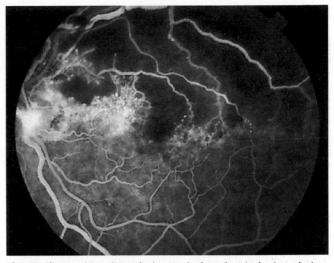

Fig. 23 Fluorescein angiography in superior branch retinal vein occlusion showing darker areas where there is loss of capillary circulation and profound retinal ischaemia.

there is diagnostic uncertainty, but is mainly used to demonstrate the site of occlusion, the degree of retinal ischaemia and determine the risk of complications (Fig. 23).

Directed at establishing the aetiology of the vein occlusion, investigations may include blood pressure, ECG, FBC, ESR, blood glucose, lipids, immunoglobulins and coagulation studies, in addition to ocular pressure estimation. The younger the patient, the greater the chance of finding a cause.

Differential diagnosis

Characteristic CRVO and BRVO are readily distinguished from most other causes of retinal haemorrhage. Bilateral CRVO is rare and may be mimicked by severe nonproliferative diabetic retinopathy. Waldenström's macroglobulinaemia may produce retinal changes similar to bilateral CRVO. Accelerated hypertensive retinopathy should not be forgotten (see *Cardiology*, Section 2.17.1).

Treatment

Emergency treatments such as haemodilution and anticoagulation are of no reliable benefit. Short term, identifiable risk factors should be treated to reduce the risk of systemic complications and retinal vein occlusion in the other eye. Long term, laser photocoagulation may be beneficial for macular oedema in some cases of BRVO but not in CRVO. Panretinal photocoagulation should be performed in ischaemic eyes at risk of neovascularization.

Complications

Permanent visual impairment from macular damage is more common in CRVO than in BRVO. Uncommonly, retinal and iris neovascularization may occur secondary to significant retinal ischaemia, leading to vitreous haemorrhage and/or rubeotic glaucoma.

Prognosis

Morbidity

A quarter of eyes with BRVO recover visual acuity of 6/9 or better without treatment—sufficient for driving. The risk of a similar event in the fellow eye is appreciable, although not high.

 Patz A. Argon laser photocoagulation for macular oedema in branch vein occlusion. *Am J Ophthalmol* 1984; 98: 271–282.
Branch Vein Occlusion Study Group. Argon laser scatter photocoagulation for prevention of neovascularization and vitreous haemorrhage in branch vein occlusion. A randomized clinical trial. *Arch Ophthalmol* 1986; 104: 34–41.
Laatikainen L, Kohner EM, Khoury D, Blach RK. Panretinal photocoagulation in central retinal vein occlusion: a randomised controlled clinical study. *Br J Ophthalmol* 1977, 61: 741–753.

2.5 Optic neuritis

Aetiology

Optic neuritis may present in isolation, but ultimately more than 50% of patients will develop clinical evidence of MS (see *Neurology*, Section 2.5).

Clinical presentation

There is moderate-to-severe loss of central vision of rapid onset, often associated with pain on eye movement. Visual loss may increase during the first week, then slowly recover, although improvement in acuity may be incomplete. Vision may be worse when body temperature is increased after a bath or exertion—Uhthoff's phenomenon.

Rarely, optic neuritis may be bilateral and associated with a transverse myelitis causing paraparesis or paraplegia (Devic's disease). Occasionally a more chronic onset is suggestive of local inflammatory disease, such as sinusitis or Wegener's granulomatosis associated with posterior scleritis.

Physical signs

Reduced visual acuity, reduced colour perception, central or centrocaecal scotoma, relative afferent pupil defect (RAPD) and swollen optic disc may be expected. Uncommonly, the peripheral retinal veins are sheathed.

Investigations

Investigation is usually not necessary at first presentation in a previously healthy patient (unless steroid treatment is planned) because the prognosis for visual recovery is good. MRI may show evidence of demyelination and visual evoked potentials (VEPs) may show delay and/or reduction in amplitude (see *Neurology*, Section 3.3.2).

Differential diagnosis

• Acute anterior ischaemic optic neuropathy in older patients, when the visual field defect is usually altitudinal.
• If bilateral, consider Leber's optic neuropathy found predominantly in young men, or nutritional or toxic optic neuropathy such as that caused by alcohol, tobacco, ethambutol, quinine or vitamin B_{12} deficiency. In children, consider a postviral phenomenon.

Treatment

If visual loss or pain is severe, intravenous methylprednisolone should be administered (1 g/day for 3 days) because visual function recovers more rapidly and pain is controlled. Oral steroids should not be used because they are associated with an increased risk of new episodes of optic neuritis, as found by the Optic Neuritis Study Group. Longer term, there is no proven visual benefit from the use of corticosteroids.

Prognosis

Visual recovery after a first episode is normally good or complete; recurrent episodes may be associated with progressive visual impairment that can be profound. Steroid treatment only hastens recovery during acute episodes and does not improve the ultimate visual outcome. The risk of a similar event in the second eye is appreciable but low. The development of MS is associated with increased mortality.

Lightman S, McDonald WI, Bird AC *et al*. Retinal venous sheathing in optic neuritis: its significance for pathogenesis of multiple sclerosis. *Brain* 1987; 100: 405.
Optic Neuritis Study Group. A randomised, controlled trial of corticosteroids in the treatment of acute optic neuritis. *N Engl J Med* 1992; 326: 581–588.
Optic Neuritis Study Group. The effect of corticosteroids for acute optic neuritis on the subsequent development of multiple sclerosis. *N Engl J Med* 1993; 329: 1764–1769.

2.6 Ischaemic optic neuropathy in giant cell arteritis

Aetiology

Giant cell arteritis (GCA) is an inflammatory disorder of unknown aetiology affecting small to medium-sized arteries of the head and neck. It is characterized by disruption of the internal elastic lamina, with an inflammatory cell infiltrate of giant cells, lymphocytes and plasma cells (see *Rheumatology and clinical immunology*, Section 2.5.1). Visual loss is most commonly caused by involvement of the posterior ciliary arteries, resulting in acute anterior ischaemic optic neuropathy (AION) and rarely central retinal artery occlusion.

It is extremely rare in people younger than 60 years, and is twice as common in women. It was first described by Sir Jonathan Hutchinson in 1890, some 2 years after the description of polymyalgia rheumatica by William Bruce—the two syndromes constituting the opposite extremes of a single clinical disorder.

Clinical presentation

In unselected series visual loss occurs in about 5–10% of all patients with GCA. It is usually unilateral and marked. Altitudinal field loss may occur (see Fig. 13). Systemic symptoms include scalp tenderness and headache, pain on chewing (jaw claudication), proximal muscle weakness or stiffness, and general malaise.

> Patients with polymyalgia rheumatica rarely complain of proximal muscle weakness, but may be aware of being unable to roll over in bed or get out of a chair or the bath.

Uncommonly, amaurosis fugax may precede more profound central visual loss and diplopia occurs in about 10% of patients before visual loss. Rarely, occipital blindness may occur as a result of involvement of the vertebrobasilar circulation.

Physical signs

The optic disc is pale and swollen, and there are often haemorrhages at the disc margin (see Fig. 12). There is a RAPD and visual acuity is severely reduced, often to hand movements or light perception. The temporal arteries may be tender and pulseless, although clinically normal arteries may be pathologically involved. Uncommonly, eye movements may be impaired as a result of involvement of cranial nerves III and VI.

Investigation

An ESR, CRP, temporal artery biopsy or biopsy of other clinically involved artery such as facial or occipital should be performed within 48 h of starting steroids, to avoid compromising the histology. A normal ESR does not reliably exclude GCA, although a normal CRP effectively does (there is only one documented case report with normal CRP precorticosteroid), but a positive biopsy is absolute confirmation of the diagnosis which may prove important in longer-term strategy. FBC may show a normochromic/normocytic anaemia.

> **Giant cell arteritis**
> - A pre-steroid normal ESR does not reliably exclude GCA, although a normal CRP effectively does—there is currently only one case report of confirmed GCA with normal CRP
> - A positive biopsy is absolute confirmation of the diagnosis.

Differential diagnosis

The major differential diagnosis is between non-arteritic AION and retinal artery occlusion. It is important to establish the diagnosis because steroid therapy is necessary for GCA, but inappropriate or even hazardous for non-arteritic AION associated with hypertension or diabetes. In cases of doubt, steroids should be given pending the outcome of investigations.

Treatment

The primary aim of treatment is to suppress the arteritis and minimize the risk of damage to the fellow eye or other organs. Recovery of vision in the presenting eye is unlikely. Urgent steroid treatment can be initiated almost immediately after blood has been taken for ESR and CRP. Prednisolone can be given by mouth in a dose of 1 mg/kg per day: there is no evidence that intravenous steroids are more effective than those given orally, providing that initial treatment is supervised.

In the short term, the steroid dose is tapered according to the response of clinical features such as headache and fall in ESR and CRP. This can usually be achieved by 10-mg decrements per week to 30 mg, then by 5-mg decrements to 10 mg, followed by a much more cautious reduction in 1-mg steps.

Longer term, the median duration of steroid therapy for GCA is 2 years, so it is important to begin prophylaxis against osteoporosis. It is unusual for GCA to recur after successful treatment, unless steroids have been withdrawn too quickly.

Complications

It is more appropriate for the follow-up of patients with GCA to be undertaken by a physician rather than an ophthalmologist, because the risk of long-term complications is greater from the treatment than from the disease. Steroid-induced cataract may occur in the fellow eye.

Prognosis

Visual recovery is uncommon in the presenting eye. A small number of patients lose vision in the second eye even when treatment has been initiated. Intravenous steroids such as methylprednisolone have been advocated, but evidence of their extra efficacy is lacking.

Hayreh SS. Steroid therapy for visual loss in patients with giant cell arteritis. *Lancet* 2000; 355: 1572–1573.

2.7 Diabetic retinopathy

Aetiology

Retinopathy takes time to develop and is extremely rare before puberty or at presentation in type 1 diabetes. After 10 years of diabetes, approximately 80% of patients with type 1 diabetes have detectable retinopathy. In type 2 diabetes, where the onset is uncertain, retinopathy may be established in up to 25% at the time of diagnosis of the diabetes. Retinopathy is a consequence of chronic hyperglycaemia, and poor diabetic control is now established as contributing to the risk of developing significant retinal changes.

Clinical presentation

Diabetic retinopathy is asymptomatic until sight-threatening complications occur, by which time the disease is in an advanced state. When symptoms do arise, gradual blurring of vision is more common than acute loss of vision, unless there is a vitreous haemorrhage or the patient suddenly becomes aware of the problem and panics.

Sight-threatening yet asymptomatic retinopathy must therefore be detected by screening, and maculopathy in type 2 diabetes is the most common cause.

 Diabetic retinopathy

• People with type 1 diabetes are more likely to develop proliferative disease than maculopathy, and the reverse applies to those with type 2 diabetes
• In type 2 diabetes, retinopathy may already be established when diabetes is diagnosed
• Prevention of retinopathy is far better for the patient than laser treatment when retinopathy is established.

Examination

It is essential to examine the fundus through dilated pupils using at least 1% tropicamide, best combined with 2.5% phenylephrine drops (see p. 154) to allow proper assessment of the macula—the central area between the major retinal vessels, temporal to the optic disc. Diabetic retinopathy is classified into four types.

Background

Mild-to-moderate non-proliferative retinopathy is characterized by microaneurysms and haemorrhages, sometimes referred to as 'dots and blots' (Fig. 24). Leakage from these can result in retinal oedema and hard exudates, but this is asymptomatic unless the fovea at the centre of the macula is involved (maculopathy).

Maculopathy (exudative or ischaemic)

Clinically significant oedema, hard exudates (Fig. 25) or ischaemia may affect the macula either alone or in combination. The critical area is within a disc diameter (1.5 mm) of the central fovea. Hard exudates are easily recognized, but retinal oedema and ischaemia are more readily identified by fluorescein angiography. Maculopathy may coexist with pre-proliferative and proliferative retinopathy.

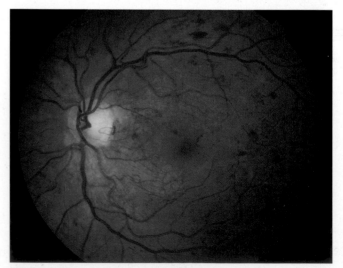

Fig. 24 Background diabetic retinopathy with dot and blot haemorrhages, although no hard exudate.

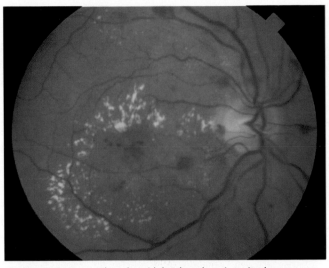

Fig. 25 Diabetic maculopathy with hard exudates in a circular or circinate pattern at the fovea. Vision will already be reduced as the fovea is involved.

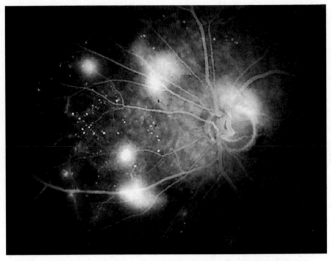

Fig. 27 Fluorescein angiography of proliferative retinopathy showing profuse focal leakage of fluorescein (white patches) from retinal new vessels.

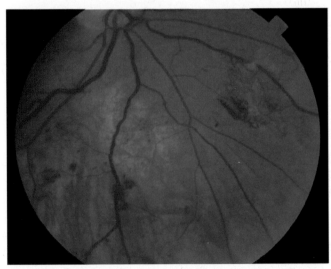

Fig. 26 Venous beading and proliferative diabetic retinopathy with a fan of new vessels at 2 o'clock.

Pre-proliferative (ischaemic)

The signs of this stage of severe retinopathy indicate retinal ischaemia. These include multiple cotton-wool spots, large haemorrhages (more than half a disc in diameter), venous dilatation and irregularity, venous beading (Fig. 26) or loops, and intraretinal microvascular abnormalities (IRMAs). This stage is also asymptomatic.

Proliferative

The hallmark of this stage of retinopathy is the growth of new vessels from the surface of the retina at the disc (NVD, see Fig. 16) and/or elsewhere along the vascular

arcades (NVE, Fig. 27 and see Fig. 17). Traction on new vessels may result in preretinal (see Fig. 18) and vitreous haemorrhage (see Fig. 7), and contraction may lead to retinal detachment.

Differential diagnosis

People with diabetes are at increased risk of retinal vein occlusion, which can usually be distinguished from diabetic retinopathy by the greater extent of haemorrhage and asymmetry of findings. Occasionally, diabetic retinopathy may be asymmetrical in the presence of significant carotid stenosis, which appears to 'protect' the ipsilateral eye.

Investigation

Fluorescein angiography (see Section 3.3, p. 156) can be useful if clinical findings are unclear, or if focal treatment is to be accurately targeted. Ocular ultrasonography can be helpful in detecting whether the retina is detached or if the retina cannot be visualized because of vitreous haemorrhage or cataract. Assessment of diabetic control and blood pressure are relevant.

Treatment

Maculopathy is treated by laser coagulation, either focally or as a 'grid'. The primary goal is maintenance of vision by sealing leaking areas close to the fovea. Proliferative retinopathy is treated by more extensive scatter, or panretinal, laser. Vitreous haemorrhage and advanced retinal fibrosis with detachment may require surgical treatment by vitrectomy and retinal microsurgery.

Complications

Common

Irreversible visual loss from untreatable or unresponsive maculopathy or proliferative disease.

Uncommon

Neovascular (rubeotic) glaucoma caused by neovascularization of the iris and obstruction to the drainage mechanism of the eye.

Prognosis

Risk of loss of vision depends on the stage of retinopathy. The approximate percentage of eyes that will lose useful vision irretrievably within 5 years if not treated rises from 3% for background retinopathy, through 20% for exudative and 30% for pre-proliferative, up to 50% for proliferative.

In addition to the visual morbidity of diabetic retinopathy, there is increased morbidity and mortality from other diabetic complications, including nephropathy, hypertension, ischaemic heart disease and peripheral vascular disease. In the UK and USA, diabetic retinopathy is still the most common reason for registration as partially sighted or blind in the working age group.

Prevention

Primary

In both types 1 and 2 diabetes, the most important means of preventing blindness from diabetic retinopathy is good diabetic control, proven by well-conducted clinical trials in the UK and USA. Other risk factors to be addressed include hypertension, hyperlipidaemia and smoking.

Secondary

The risk of visual loss from diabetic retinopathy can be reduced by regular eye examination by a trained observer such as an optometrist, physician or GP, or by retinal photography. If sight-threatening retinopathy is identified, treatment by laser photocoagulation will reduce the risk of blindness from maculopathy and proliferative disease by an estimated 60%. Patients with background or no retinopathy should be examined once a year, pre-proliferative eyes more frequently—every 3–6 months.

Photocoagulation treatment of proliferative diabetic retinopathy

Diabetic Retinopathy Study Research Group. Clinical application of Diabetic Retinopathy Study (DRS) findings, DRS Report Number 8. *Ophthalmology* 1981; 88: 583–600.

Photocoagulation for diabetic macular oedema

Early Treatment Diabetic Retinopathy Study Research Group. Early Treatment Diabetic Retinopathy Study report number 1. *Arch Ophthalmol* 1985; 103: 1796–1806.

Diabetes Control and Complications Trial Research Group. The effect of intensive treatment of diabetes on the development and progression of long-term complications in type 1 diabetes mellitus. *N Engl J Med* 1993; 329: 977–986.

UK Prospective Diabetes Study (UKPDS) Group. Intensive blood-glucose control with sulphonylureas or insulin compared with conventional treatment and risk of complications in patients with type 2 diabetes (UKPDS 33). *Lancet* 1998; 352: 837–853.

General

Towler HMA, Patterson JA, Lightman SL. *Diabetes and the Eye*. London: BMJ Publishing Group, 1996.

3 Investigations and practical procedures

3.1 Examination of the eye

Examination of the eye by the non-specialist requires the following assessments:
- Visual acuity
- Visual fields
- Pupil responses
- Ocular media and fundus using the ophthalmoscope
- Ocular movements.

Measurement of the intraocular pressure using specialized equipment is an important part of the ophthalmologist's and optometrist's routine examination.

3.1.1 VISUAL ACUITY

Each eye should be tested, where possible with a Snellen chart, usually at a distance of 6 m, and wearing spectacles or contact lenses if normally worn. Near vision can be tested with standard reading test types, although a magazine or newsprint is a good functional test. A pinhole to overcome moderate refractive errors can be created with a large safety pin and a piece of thin card.

3.1.2 VISUAL FIELDS

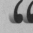 The visual field is 'an island of vision surrounded by a sea of blindness'. (H.M. Traquair, 1957)

The visual fields can be assessed by subjective clinical method or by objective perimetry. The choice is determined by the clinical circumstances, the necessity for long-term comparison and medicolegal requirements, such as for driving.

Confrontation fields

Clinical examination of visual fields can be very precise, and may be the only method of detecting an abnormality such as an inattention. The extent of the normal visual field is learned through experience.

How to assess the visual fields by confrontation

- Sit comfortably facing the patient and at the same level.
- Cover one of the patient's eyes.

- Ask the patient to look steadily at your own eye.
- Ask the patient to say YES each time they first see the target (hand, finger, hat pin, plug of biro) as it appears in the peripheral field, 'out of the corner of their eye'.
- Bring the target into the expected area of vision in each quadrant—superonasal, inferonasal, superotemporal and inferotemporal, corresponding to NW, SW, NE and SE compass points. Testing at the horizontal or vertical meridians requires particular care.
- Assess whether or not the extent of the field is normal, allowing for prominent eyebrows, a large nose or ptosis.
- If a defect is found, examine its extent, looking especially carefully for demarcation along the horizontal or vertical meridian.
- Look for any deficit within the observed field of vision—a scotoma—and map its extent by moving from the non-seeing into a seeing area. This element of testing can be refined by using a smaller target, such as a 2–5 mm red hat pin. Ask also if the quality of the colour changes. It should be possible to identify the normal blind spot using this technique.
- Repeat the process for the other eye.

How to detect visual inattention

This can be very disabling: patients are usually unaware of any visual problem but may have noticed that they bump into objects. This inattention is usually in the patient's left field of vision and is caused by a right parietal lesion. Test each eye separately by confrontation to check that a visual field defect is *not* present. Then:
- ask the patient to keep both eyes open
- hold your hands up in each temporal visual field
- ask the patient to point to whichever hand moves
- assess whether the patient can see your fingers move, first each side alone and then both simultaneously.

If the patient can see both stimuli in isolation, but not on one side when presented simultaneously, visual inattention is present on that side.

Interpretation of visual field defects

Common visual field defects are shown in Table 3. Two major principles apply to the assessment:
- Visual field defects that respect the vertical meridian involve the visual pathways at or behind the optic chiasm —occipital cortex to optic tract—usually homonymously

151

Field defect	Anatomical site	Aetiology
Central scotoma, unilateral	Retina or optic nerve	Macular disease, optic neuritis
Central scotoma, bilateral	Retina or optic nerve	Age related, toxic, hereditary
Altitudinal, unilateral	Retina or optic nerve	Vascular occlusion, glaucoma
Homonymous hemianopia (congruous)	Visual cortex or optic radiation	Stroke
Homonymous hemianopia (incongruous)	Optic tract (rare)	Stroke or compression
Homonymous quadrantanopia	Optic radiation	Stroke or compression
Bitemporal hemianopia	Optic chiasm	Pituitary or hypothalamic compression

Table 3 Common visual field defects.

• Visual field defects that respect the horizontal meridian involve the visual pathways anterior to the chiasm—optic nerve or retina—usually uniocularly.

If a hemianopic defect is identified, the degree of congruity or similarity in each eye should be assessed. The more congruous the field defect, the more posterior the lesion in the visual pathway (common); very incongruous homonymous field defects may indicate a lesion in the optic tract (rare).

Visual field testing by perimetry

Modern computerized visual field analysers have greatly enhanced the speed, reliability and reproducibility of visual field testing, particularly for conditions associated with progressive visual field change such as glaucoma. Specific field testing strategies can be used to look for particular patterns of field loss associated with differing diseases, and the present generation of field analysers can compare a current test with previous observations, as well as provide indices of reliability of the examination.

Visual fields for driving

Homonymous hemianopia, which precludes driving, can be assessed by confrontation testing but may need formal perimetry to convince the patient of its extent. The binocular Estermann field is most commonly used. Fig. 28 is a simplified cartoon showing the critical area. Subtle defects, such as field changes resulting from glaucoma or diabetes retinopathy or its treatment, always require objective testing. Visual inattention is normally a bar to driving.

Patten JP. *Neurological Differential Diagnosis* (2nd edn). Berlin: Springer-Verlag, 1999.
Kline LB, Bajandas FJ. *Neuro-Ophthalmology Review Manual* (4th edn). Slack, New Jersey, 1996.

3.1.3 PUPIL RESPONSES

The pupils should be examined for size and the pupil response to light should be assessed with a bright pen

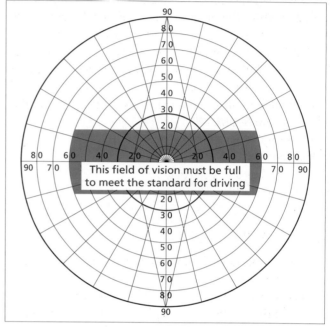

This field of vision must be full to meet the standard for driving

Fig. 28 Simplified version of the visual field required for driving, assessed with both eyes open (binocular), extending 120° horizontally and 20° vertically either side of the horizontal meridian.

torch, noting both the direct and consensual responses and their symmetry.

Relative afferent pupil defect

If light is shone into one eye, both pupils constrict to a similar degree, meaning that both the direct and consensual responses are equally active. The 'swinging light test' is a simple and rapid method of finding out whether this is so. After checking both direct and consensual responses for each eye, proceed as follows:
• Shine a bright light into the right eye for 5 s.
• Observe the pupil of the left eye.
• Move the light swiftly to shine in the left eye.
• Does the pupil of the left eye dilate?
• If so, there is a relative afferent pupillary defect on the left side.
• Now observe the pupil of the right eye.
• Move the light swiftly back to shine on the right eye.
• Does the pupil of the right eye dilate?

• If so, there is a relative afferent pupillary defect on the right side.

This test effectively compares the afferent pathway (within the retina or optic nerve, anterior to the chiasm) of the light reflex of the right eye with that of the left. If there is a relative afferent pupillary defect on one side, i.e. that pupil dilates when the light is shone directly into it, then there is a problem in the retina or optic nerve on that side.

The near response

The near response should be tested by asking the patient to refocus from the distance on to a close object, such as small print, to ensure that accommodation is stimulated. Normally, pupil responses to light and near are similar, but in a handful of uncommon diagnoses the response to light is sluggish and less complete than the near response —so called light–near dissociation—which is found in the following conditions:
• Adie's pupil (large at first but later smaller)
• Aberrant regeneration of the third nerve
• Argyll Robertson pupil (small)
• Parinaud's midbrain syndrome (large).

Unequal pupils (anisocoria)

A difference in pupil size may be physiological or pathological (Table 4).

Consider the following, if pupils are unequal:
• Is the light reaction normal? A large unreactive pupil with normal eye motility may be caused by blunt injury, pharmacological substances or an Adie's pupil.
• Is the eyelid position normal? A small ptosis with small pupil may be a Horner's syndrome; a large ptosis with large pupil may be a palsy of nerve III, especially a compressive palsy.
• Are eye movements full? If not, consider a palsy of nerve III if the pupil is large, especially if the eye is turned down and out. Remember to lift the eyelid when testing for diplopia!

3.1.4 OPHTHALMOSCOPY

The direct ophthalmoscope is an invaluable instrument for examining the eye. The image that it provides is magnified and upright but of a very limited area, so that the retina has to be 'scanned' to provide the observer with a composite view. It also lacks depth perception and examination of the peripheral retina is restricted. Its advantages are its ease of use, relatively simple construction and maintenance, and ability to examine the retina through an undilated pupil. It is salutary to remember that von Helmholtz invented the ophthalmoscope while still a medical student!

How to use the direct ophthalmoscope

1 First, check that the batteries and bulb are satisfactory: halogen bulbs produce a whiter, brighter light, especially when rechargeable batteries are used which have the advantage of not leaking and ruining the instrument.
2 It is always preferable to examine the eye through dilated pupils, although this may not always be possible (see below). Select the larger aperture if the pupil is dilated; the smaller if not.
3 Stand about 1 m from the patient and rotate the lens dial to provide the sharpest image. You should remove spectacles if normally worn by you or the patient, unless either of you has a high error of focus.
4 Shine the ophthalmoscope light at the patient's pupils and look for the normal red reflex from the retina (the same as the 'red eye' from flash photography). Any opacity within the eye's media such as a cataract (see Fig. 15) or vitreous haemorrhage (see Fig. 7) will darken the red reflex. A subluxed lens may be evident, especially if the pupil is dilated.
5 Examine each eye in turn, using your right hand and eye for the patient's right eye and vice versa. Try to remain as upright as possible because this allows the patient to look beyond you and maintain fixation on a distant object. It is also important to approach from a slightly temporal direction, which means that the optic disc is easily identified and sharp focus on it is possible. If you approach the eye straight on, the pupil will constrict and the rather featureless retina at the macula may be difficult to identify.
6 Once the optic disc is identified it should be systematically assessed for colour, swelling, cupping, haemorrhage,

Table 4 Common causes of unequal or irregular pupils.

Condition	Pupil features	Greatest anisocoria	Light reaction	Near reaction	Response to dilating drops
Simple anisocoria	Round and regular	Dark	Normal	Normal	Normal
Horner's syndrome	Small and regular	Dark	Normal	Normal	Moderate
Adie's pupil	Dilated and irregular	Light	Poor or absent	Sustained (tonic)	Normal
Argyll Robertson pupil	Small and irregular	(Bilateral)	Absent	Present	Poor
Palsy of nerve III	Dilated	Light	Absent	Absent	Normal
Pharmacological	Dilated or small	Light or dark	Absent	Absent	Poor
Traumatic	May be irregular/oval	Light	Reduced	Reduced	Variable
Iritis (synechiae)	Irregular	Dark	Normal	Normal	Poor and festoons

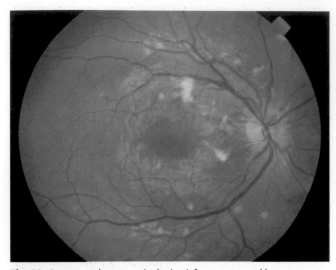

Fig. 29 Cotton-wool spots: retinal microinfarcts, scattered between branches of major retinal vessels.

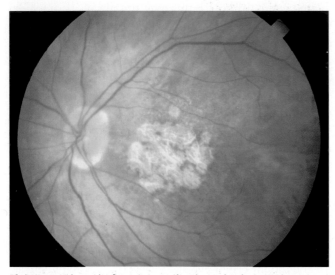

Fig. 30 Atrophy at the fovea in age-related macular degeneration. Pigmentation may also be found.

Use the green filter ('red-free') on the ophthalmoscope to give better contrast, especially when examining for diabetic retinopathy or vascular changes. Fine red structures are more clearly defined.

Indirect ophthalmoscopy

This method uses either a head-mounted binocular indirect ophthalmoscope or a slit lamp and hand-held lens. These techniques afford two major advantages: depth perception and a wider field of view, allowing the entire retina to be inspected. The image is, however, upside down and less magnified than with the direct ophthalmoscope, and dilatation of the pupil is mandatory. Indirect ophthalmoscopy is essential for examining the peripheral retina and vitreous.

Dilatation of pupils

Indications
Examination of the fundus of the eye is complete only if the pupil is dilated. It is possible to examine the optic disc through an undilated pupil, particularly if the room is dark, but the macula or more peripheral retina will not be seen adequately.

Contraindications
Contraindications to pupil dilatation for fundoscopy:
• Patients with acute head injury or in coma, in whom it is important to observe serial neurological signs including pupil size and reactivity
• Patients at risk of acute angle-closure glaucoma, if an inappropriate dilating agent is used (see below).

Practical details

Before dilatation
Before dilating the pupils, assess and record the pupil reactions, including the relative afferent responses. Patients should be warned of the following:
• Near vision especially will be blurred for about 2 h
• Bright lights may be uncomfortable
• Driving is not advisable
• If they develop eye pain or discomfort, they should phone back immediately or attend an eye A&E department.

Choose a dilating agent (Table 5). For diagnostic purposes, tropicamide drops are ideal—1% for adults and 0.5% for children—which block the parasympathetic terminals in the pupillary constrictor muscle. A brown iris dilates more slowly than a blue one, and dilatation is more prolonged; in very dark eyes cyclopentolate 1% drops can be used but the patient should be warned to expect a more sustained blurring of vision. Phenylephrine 2.5% drops stimulate the sympathetic system and act synergistically with tropicamide to allow maximum pupil dilatation. Phenylephrine should be used with caution both in children and in adults with ischaemic heart disease, because it may induce hypertension, exacerbate angina or cause dysrhythmias as a result of its sympathomimetic action when absorbed.

venous pulsation (often present, so try to count the pulse), neovascularization and pigmentation (see Figs 9–11).

7 Next follow the four main vascular arcades peripherally—temporal and nasal, above and below—assessing vessel calibre and regularity, arteriovenous (AV) crossing changes for AV nipping, while looking for neovascularization or vascular occlusion. Cotton-wool spots are most frequently seen between vascular branches along the major arcades or close to the optic disc (Fig. 29).

8 Next, examine the macula looking for the normal bright light reflex from the fovea, while assessing any pigmentary change (Fig. 30), haemorrhage or hard exudates. Subtle macular changes may not be readily seen with the direct ophthalmoscope.

9 Finally, examine the more peripheral retina in all quadrants by asking the patient to look up and down, right and left.

Table 5 Dilating drops.

Agent	Mode of action	Duration (h)	When to use
Tropicamide 1%	Parasympathetic block	2–4	Adult
Tropicamide 0.5%	Parasympathetic block	2–4	Child
Cyclopentolate 1%	Parasympathetic block	6–8	Very dark iris
Phenylephrine 2.5%	Sympathomimetic	2–4	Full examination of peripheral retina, or photography
Phenylephrine 10%	Sympathomimetic	2–4	Very dark iris

Practical details (*continued*)

The procedure

One or two drops are placed in the lower conjunctival fornix of each eye and 15–20 min allowed for the pupils to dilate. Tropicamide drops sting: if children are reluctant to allow drops, lie the child down, place a drop at the inner corner of each closed eye and wait—the child will always open the eye and so the drop rolls in with minimum fuss.

Complications

Dilatation of the pupil can precipitate acute glaucoma in susceptible eyes, but this is rare, occurring in less than one in 1000 patients and lower with tropicamide than cyclopentolate. The onset of acute glaucoma is during the recovery phase of pupil dilatation, usually several hours after the drops have been instilled. Eyes at risk are typically long sighted (hypermetropic), with spectacle lenses that are convex and magnifying. These eyes have shallow anterior chambers and are predisposed to obstruction of the drainage angle between the iris and cornea when the pupil is mid-dilated. Shallowing of the anterior chamber can also occur as a result of the progressive enlargement of the lens with age, particularly if there is coexisting cataract. Short-sighted (myopic) eyes are not predisposed to acute glaucoma. Patients with known common chronic glaucoma may be safely dilated.

3.1.5 EYE MOVEMENTS

Pursuit and saccadic movements

Eye movements to pursuit of a slowly moving target should be examined to the extreme of gaze right and left horizontally, then vertically looking to both right and left in upgaze and downgaze, and also to convergence. The pattern of diplopia should be carefully analysed (see below) because this gives important information about a likely cause. Nystagmus and broken pursuit may be seen.

To test rapid (saccadic) movements, ask the patient to switch gaze between dissimilar targets such as a pen and a thumb on command, from right to left or up to down.

Analysis of diplopia

Lesion of nerve VI

Doubling that is horizontal—'dead level'—and parallel, worse on looking to the affected side and improving as distant objects come closer is likely to be caused by a sixth-nerve palsy. Nerve VI is a single nerve supplying a single muscle with a single action, and it is very rare to have a single isolated lateral rectus lesion for any other reason. Doubling occurs to either side if the palsy is bilateral. These patterns are so characteristic that they constitute a reliable 'telephone' diagnosis, although it is still wise to confirm this by examining the patient!

Lesion of nerve IV

Doubling that is worst looking down and in, as in reading, eating or going downstairs, may be the result of a fourth-nerve lesion. The two images are separated horizontally and vertically and tilted, as a result of the complex action of the superior oblique muscle. Lesions of a single superior oblique muscle do occur, so the fourth nerve itself is not necessarily at fault. Fourth-nerve palsies may be bilateral as the two nerves cross at the level of the tentorial fold.

Lesion of nerve III

Doubling that is present in most directions and complex to analyse, but least on looking outwards, may be caused by a third nerve palsy. Inspect the ipsilateral eyelid position and pupil size carefully.

Other

Doubling that is in none of these patterns, especially if it is variable or diurnal, may be caused by an ocular muscle disorder, such as thyroid eye disease or myasthenia gravis.

3.2 Biopsy

3.2.1 TEMPORAL ARTERY BIOPSY

Indications

This is used to establish the diagnosis of GCA (cranial or temporal arteritis) in patients presenting with symptoms or signs suggestive of this condition.

Contraindications

There are no contraindications, except known extra-cranial–intracranial collateral circulation via the super-ficial temporal artery.

Practical details

1 Written informed consent should be obtained.

2 Performed under aseptic conditions in a designated clean area or operating room. Equipment: fine-toothed skin forceps, sharp and blunt scissors, skin retractors (cats' paws), D15 scalpel, suture forceps, absorbable and non-absorbable sutures, local anaesthetic (a dental syringe is ideal).

3 Identify the frontal branch of the temporal artery, where it runs across the forehead, and mark its course with an indelible pen for about 3 cm.

4 Infiltrate the skin with local anaesthetic in two parallel lines adjacent to, but not directly over, the artery.

5 Remove any overlying hair, cleanse the skin with 5% povidone–iodine solution (or equivalent), then drape with sterile towels or plastic adhesive drape.

6 Incise the skin with a scalpel (e.g. D15 blade) along the skin mark.

7 Dissect the subcutaneous tissues to expose the artery for the length of the skin incision. Avoid injury and path-ological artefact to the artery by minimizing any direct handling.

8 Ligate the ends of the artery and any branches with 5/0 chromic catgut (or similar suture), then excise the artery specimen.

9 Close the skin in two layers and dress the wound.

10 Place the arterial specimen in fixative and send for histopathology.

11 External, non-absorbable skin sutures can be removed at 5–6 days.

Complications

Haemorrhage can occur early or late, and is the result of either inadequate ligation or secondary infection. The latter risk is increased by concomitant steroid therapy. Collateral flow from the extracranial to the intracranial circulation can occur through the temporal artery. Temporary occlusion of the artery before permanent ligation will identify the unlikely problem of a stroke—remember that a stroke can also occur as a direct result of GCA. It has been known for a facial nerve to be biopsied in error.

 Kline LB, Bajandas FJ. *Neuro-Ophthalmology Review Manual* (4th edn). Slack, New Jersey, 1996.

3.2.2 CONJUNCTIVAL BIOPSY FOR DIAGNOSIS OF SARCOIDOSIS

Occasionally, the tarsal conjunctiva lining the lower lid may show visible granulomas. These are a very conveni-ent site for biopsy to demonstrate non-caseating granu-lomas diagnostic of sarcoidosis. The conjunctival surface is anaesthetized topically with drops, the affected site is gently grasped with forceps and a snip of tissue is taken. If the tissue sample is small, to prevent it being lost, place it gently at the centre of a small square of card and put this into formol saline, with a note for the technician to indic-ate where the tissue is located.

3.3 Fluorescein angiography

Principle

The retinal circulation is normally impervious to fluor-escein because of the blood–retinal barrier, similar to the blood–brain barrier. Transit through the retina and choroid can be recorded either on film, digitally, by video or by direct observation. Indocyanine green (ICG) angio-graphy, a very similar technique, gives better assessment of choroidal disease.

Indications

To allow assessment of the retinal circulation in a variety of diseases, in particular to determine the presence and degree of leakage (see Fig. 26) and ischaemia (see Fig. 23) within the retina.

Contraindications

Contraindications are previous allergy to fluorescein, recent myocardial infarction and pregnancy (relative).

Practical details

Before the procedure

Written informed consent should be obtained and the patient warned that the skin and urine will be discoloured for 24 h. Resuscitation facilities must be available. The pupils should be fully dilated.

The procedure

The dye (3 mL of 20% or 5 mL of 10% sodium fluor-escein) is rapidly injected into an antecubital vein with the patient seated at the camera. Venous access must be secure because extravasation is painful. A series of photographs or continuous video is recorded over the initial minute and periodically over the next 5–10 minutes as the dye enters the eye and is distributed throughout the circulation.

Complications

Complications are transient nausea or vomiting (occurs in 5% of patients), local extravasation and thrombophlebitis, anaphylaxis and circulatory shock. Mortality is less than 1 in 200 000.

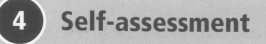

4 Self-assessment

Answers on pp. 214–216.

Question 1
Drug effects on the eye:
A Prednisolone
B Amiodarone
C Ethambutol
D Rifabutin
E Tamoxifen
F Thalidomide
G Sildenafil (Viagra)
H Cyclosporin
I Canthaxanthin (Orobronze)
K Hydroxychloroquine

For each ocular side effect below, select the most likely causative drug(s) from the options listed above. Each option may be used once, more than once or not at all.
1 Drug deposition in the cornea
2 Optic neuropathy
3 Cataract
4 Drug deposition in the retina
5 Uveitis.

Question 2
Which of the following statements about diabetic retinopathy are true?
A It is the most common cause of blindness in people of working age in the Western World
B Visual impairment is most commonly caused by proliferative retinopathy
C Maculopathy is best treated with lipid-lowering drugs
D Background diabetic retinopathy should be treated with laser because vision is likely to be threatened within a year
E Screening for diabetic retinopathy is not cost-effective.

Question 3
The relative afferent pupil defect (RAPD) (T/F):
A Is characteristic of a nerve palsy of cranial nerve III
B Is associated with a contralateral ptosis
C May be caused by ischaemic central retinal vein occlusion
D Is a characteristic finding in an eye affected by giant cell arteritis
E Is a cause of unequal pupil size (anisocoria).

Question 4
Figure 31: the most likely cause of this retinal appearance (with similar findings in the other eye) in a 25-year-old man is:
A Hypertensive retinopathy
B Proliferative diabetic retinopathy
C Subarachnoid haemorrhage
D Infective endocarditis
E Carotid atherosclerotic disease.

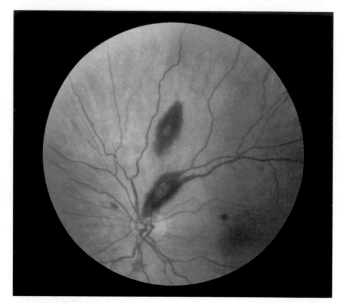

Fig. 31 Question 4.

Question 5
A 45-year-old woman with type 2 diabetes who is on long-term tamoxifen therapy complains of blurred vision in both eyes (Figs 32 and 33). Visual acuity is 6/12 in each eye. Which of the following statements are true?
A Tamoxifen retinopathy is present and the drug should be stopped
B Both retinas show hard exudates, indicating diabetic retinopathy that requires laser treatment
C Choroidal metastases are present in both fundi
D Ocular radiotherapy would be contraindicated because of the risk of secondary cataract and radiation retinopathy.

Question 6
This fundus photograph (Fig. 34) in a 16-year-old boy shows (T/F):
A Deep retinal haemorrhage
B Vitreous haemorrhage

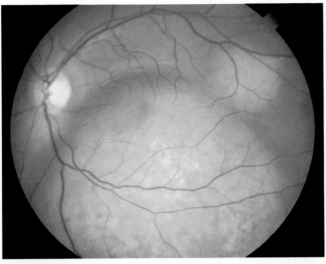

Fig. 32 Question 5.

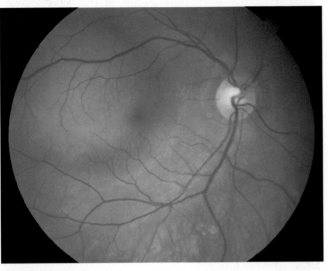

Fig. 33 Question 5.

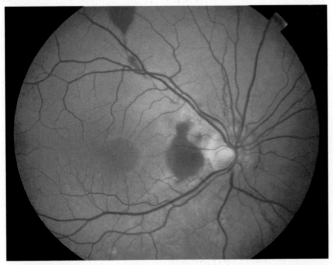

Fig. 34 Question 6.

C Ocular features consistent with blunt trauma

D Angioid streaks

E Ocular features consistent with pseudoxanthoma elasticum.

Question 7

Figure 35: the most likely cause of this optic disc appearance is (select the best answer):

A Papilloedema

B Giant cell arteritis

C Toxoplasma chorioretinitis

D Myelinated nerve fibres

E Accelerated (malignant) hypertension.

Question 8

Figure 36: this eye of a 21-year-old man has 6/6 acuity with contact lens correction. Which of the following statements are true?

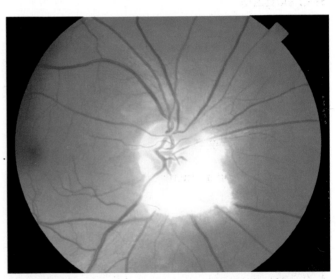

Fig. 35 Question 7.

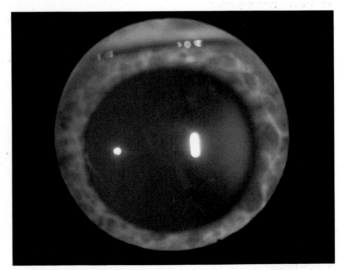

Fig. 36 Question 8.

A This appearance is consistent with Marfan's syndrome
B This appearance is consistent with homocystinuria
C This appearance is consistent with blunt trauma
D This patient has an increased risk of retinal detachment
E This patient could be a firefighter in the UK.

Question 9

Figure 37: this 25-year-old stevedore complained of disturbance of vision in his left eye after lifting a heavy box at work. Select the most appropriate description from the list below:

A The macula shows a cherry red spot
B There is a retinal haemorrhage adjacent to the fovea, most probably caused by a Valsalva type of manoeuvre
C The retinal appearance is consistent with diabetic retinopathy
D The optic disc shows pathological cupping
E The patient should be treated with strict bedrest and aspirin for one week.

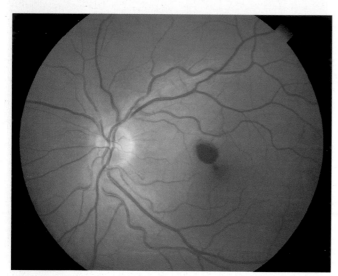

Fig. 37 Question 9.

Question 10

Figure 38: which of the following statements about this appearance in a 24-year-old woman with diabetes are true?

A The pigmentary disturbance is typical of retinitis pigmentosa
B Preretinal haemorrhage is present

C Laser photocoagulation is required
D Sight-threatening diabetic maculopathy is present
E This appearance is consistent with normal visual acuity.

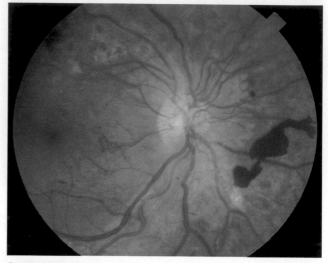

Fig. 38 Question 10.

Question 11

Figure 39: this photograph of a clinically and biochemically euthyroid woman shows (T/F):

A Lid retraction
B Lid lag
C Ptosis
D Optic nerve compression
E Thyroid eye disease.

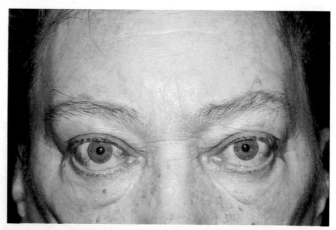

Fig. 39 Question 11.

Psychiatry

AUTHORS:
V. Kirchner, M. Lipsedge

EDITOR:
M. Lipsedge

EDITOR-IN-CHIEF:
J.D. Firth

1 Clinical presentations

1.1 Acute confusional state

Case history

A middle-aged man has an acute confusional state after cardiac surgery. His mental state had appeared normal on admission. Forty-eight hours after the operation he has removed his intravenous line, refuses to allow the nurses anywhere near him and is cowering in a corner of the ward. He is clearly terrified and suspicious, and accuses the staff of trying to kill him.

Clinical approach

The most likely cause of this disruptive behaviour is delirium (acute confusional state), but occasionally patients might develop a brief psychosis (see Section 2.3, p. 182) or a severe affective (mood) disorder (see Sections 2.11, p. 198, and 2.12, p. 201) after major surgery.

Does the patient show the cardinal features of delirium?
- Clouding of consciousness which may fluctuate
- Disorientation in time, place and person
- Impaired grasp of their situation and diminished attention
- Reversal of sleep–wakefulness cycle
- Confusion worsens at night with a morning lucid interval.

The common causes of delirium are shown in Table 1.

> After coronary artery surgery, delirium which follows a lucid interval is probably due to metabolic disturbance, medication or sleep deprivation [1].

History of the presenting problem

Try to establish the underlying cause of the delirium by asking relatives:
- to estimate the patient's usual daily alcohol intake
- whether there has been increasing absentmindedness and progressive impairment of memory over the preceding 6 to 12 months or so, indicating dementia with superimposed delirium.

Ask nursing staff:
- about early warning signs, e.g. daytime drowsiness
- if there was a lucid interval in the morning which might have given a misleading impression of normality during the morning ward round?

Table 1 Common causes of delirium.

Systemic
Infection (e.g. pneumonia, septicaemia, urinary tract infection)
Respiratory or cardiac failure
Electrolyte imbalance
Metabolic disorder, e.g. renal or hepatic failure
Severe hypotension due to reduced cardiac output secondary to myocardial infarction, pulmonary embolus or dysrhythmia
Severe anaemia

Intracranial
Cerebrovascular accident
Intracranial space-occupying lesions: subdural haematoma, brain abscess, brain tumour
Postictal states

Drug-induced
Steroids, theophylline, β-blockers
Drug intoxication (e.g. with analgesics)
Withdrawal of alcohol or benzodiazepines

Relevant past history

Ask about the following:
- Has there been a recent head injury (possibility of subdural haematoma)?
- Is there a history of previous psychiatric disorder which might point towards a relapse of schizophrenia or manic–depressive disorder precipitated by psychological stress of operation?
- Is there a history of seizures? (Is this a prolonged complex partial seizure or prolonged ictal state?)

Examination

Look for the features described below to establish the diagnosis of delirium. When possible (after sedation if necessary), perform a full physical examination, looking for evidence of any of the conditions listed in Table 1.

Appearance

The patient generally appears more frightened than hostile although may act aggressively in self defence against an imaginary enemy. In some cases the patient will appear apathetic and withdrawn rather than agitated.

Behaviour

The patient is commonly restless and may pluck at the bedclothes. The patient may attempt to escape from the ward. By contrast with this picture of 'noisy' delirium, the patient may be withdrawn and underactive, and it might only be on close questioning that the clinician learns that the patient is disorientated and unable to grasp what is going on around him.

Talk

Speech may be incoherent.

Thinking

Ideas of reference (e.g. the ward television is showing a police drama which the patient interprets to mean that he is about to be arrested) and ideas of persecution, but these tend to be fleeting and sketchy. Delusional themes might include the patient being convinced that he is being held in prison, or that staff are trying to poison him. The patient's thinking may become incoherent.

Mood

Mood is often changeable and can fluctuate from intense fear and agitation to milder forms of anxiety, depression and irritability.

Perceptual disturbance

There are illusions and hallucinations. The latter are mainly visual but can also be auditory and tactile. A telephone wire may be perceived as a snake, while the ringing of a telephone might sound like a fire alarm.

Cognitive function

There is disorientation in both time and place and mis-identification of members of staff or members of his own family. The patient is likely to appear dazed and unclear about his surroundings: he has difficulty in grasp-ing what is happening around him and his attention is greatly shortened and he tends to drift off. Attention span is decreased (unable to correctly repeat seven digits). Test attention and concentration further by asking the pati-ent to recite the days of the week and then the months of the year in reverse order, and then to subtract seven from 100 or three from 20.

Insight

This fluctuates with the patient's level of consciousness. After the episode the patient will have little recollection of what he thought, how he behaved and how he was treated.

> **!** Exclude the agitation of severe depression or the excitement of mania by the absence of clouding of consciousness in the affective disorders.

Approach to investigations and management

Investigations

When possible (after sedation if necessary), these should be performed to establish the diagnosis of any of the conditions listed in Table 1. In the absence of obvious clinical clues, the following would be appropriate: electrocardiogram (ECG) (has he had an infarct?); glucose (BM stix plus lab), electrolytes, renal and liver function, full blood count; culture of urine, blood and sputum (if any); pulse oximetry and arterial blood gases; chest radiograph. Other tests may also be required if specifically indicated.

Management

The patient in delirium is unable to co-operate with nursing and medical care. He might refuse medication, become dehydrated or sustain an injury when falling or fighting.

The priorities are:
• Establish and treat the cause of the delirium, e.g. electrolyte imbalance, dehydration, infection, anaemia.
• Review all current medication and withdraw any that can be stopped.
• Keep the patient in touch with his surroundings: a window increases awareness of the contrast between day and night.
• Twenty-four-hour nursing care is indicated, preferably with a single nurse on each shift rather than a succession of nurses 'dropping in'.

For severe agitation haloperidol in a dose of 5–10 mg (p.o. or i.m.) is a useful major tranquillizer. In delirium tremens, to relieve the agitation and prevent withdrawal fits, administer chlordiazepoxide 30 mg four times a day or chlormethiazole 1 g every 6 h (reducing doses) plus Pabrinex (see Section 1.7 and *Emergency medicine*, Section 1.14).

> The course of delirium will obviously vary according to the underlying cause. For example, if the patient has had a stroke the confusional state will clear but the patient might be left with permanent neurological deficit.

> The patient clearly lacks the capacity to give meaningful consent or refusal of potentially life-saving treatment. This is an urgent situation and the staff have a clear duty of care. Emergency measures are covered by common law but it would be advisable to call in the duty psychiatrist to discuss the use of the Mental Health Act [2].

See *Medicine for the elderly*, Section 1.2; *Emergency medicine*, Sections 1.14 and 1.28.

Lishman WA. *Organic Psychiatry: psychological consequences of cerebral disorder* (3rd edn). Oxford: Blackwell Science, 1998.

Moore DP, Jefferson JW. *Handbook of Medical Psychiatry*. London: Mosby, 1996.

1 Mayou R. The psychiatric and social consequences of coronary artery surgery. *J Psychosom Res* 1986; 30(3): 255–271.

2 Feldman E. Medico-legal aspects of liaison psychiatry. *Adv Psychiatr Treat* 1998; 4: 243–249.

1.2 Panic attack and hyperventilation

Case history

A 35-year-old manager presents at accident and emergency (A&E) complaining of intense discomfort in his chest. This had developed as he was driving to work. Over the previous few weeks, since his firm had been taken over by a larger company, he has felt tense, sweaty, shaky and light-headed just before meetings and has been increasingly aware of his heart beating rapidly. New management have imposed stringent targets but he has lost half of his administrative and secretarial staff.

Clinical approach

Is this an organic state presenting with secondary anxiety or a primary anxiety-based disorder?

Consider the following possible common organic causes of anxiety:
• alcohol withdrawal—restless, overactive, disorientated, cannot register new information, fearful, sweating, tremulous, visual hallucinations and illusions. Look for evidence of chronic liver disease and check liver function tests, especially gamma-glutamyl transpeptidase (γ-GT), and also mean corpuscular volume (MCV) (see *Emergency medicine*, Section 1.14; and *Gastroenterology and hepatology*, Section 1.7)
• drug intoxication—restless, overactive, disorientated, cannot register new information, preoccupied with internal experience, lability of mood
• drug withdrawal—look for evidence of drug use— injection sites, abscesses.

Consider also the following possible, rare or very rare organic causes of anxiety:
• thyrotoxicosis—history of heat intolerance and weight loss. Look for goitre, eye signs, tremor, tachycardia. Check thyroid function (see *Endocrinology*, Section 1.13)

• hypoglycaemia—history of diabetes. Check BM stix (see *Endocrinology*, Section 1.4)
• paroxysmal supraventricular tachycardia—check ECG (see *Cardiology*, Section 1.1)
• phaeochromocytoma—episodic sweating, headache, tremor, high blood pressure (see *Endocrinology*, Section 2.2.5).

In your assessment it is important to distinguish the different types of anxiety-based disorders.

International Classification of Diseases (ICD) 10 classification of the neurotic and stress-related disorders

• Generalized anxiety disorder (see Section 2.7.1, p. 189)
• Mixed anxiety and depressive disorder
• Panic disorder (see Section 2.7.2, p. 190)
• Phobic disorder (see Section 2.7.3, p. 191)
• Obsessive–compulsive disorder (see Section 2.8, p. 193)
• Acute stress reaction (see Section 2.9.1, p. 195)
• Post-traumatic stress disorder (PTSD) (see Section 2.9.2, p. 196)
• Adjustment disorders (see Section 2.6, p. 186).

History of the presenting problem

He has been feeling tense and apprehensive and, as well as having chest pain, he is troubled by a headache like a 'tight band' around his skull. He has been sleeping badly and has had difficulty concentrating. He has been using alcohol to help him calm down when he gets home and to help him to get off to sleep at night. He has been reluctant to take any time off work because the firm is downsizing and he fears redundancy.

Ask him for details of the chest pain: could this possibly be due to cardiac ischaemia (see *Cardiology*, Section 1.5)? Ask also about psychological and physical symptoms of anxiety listed in Table 2.

Relevant past history

Look for predisposing factors by asking for the following:
• Is there a personal or family history of anxiety-based disorder or mood disturbance, especially at times of stress and adverse life events?
• Is there a history of separations and insecurity in childhood?

Examination

Be sure to attempt to exclude any underlying physical problem. Although you suspect an anxiety state it is important to perform:
• a thorough cardiac and respiratory examination, since the primary complaint is of chest pain. Myocardial infarction

165

Table 2 The symptoms and signs of an anxiety state.

Psychological symptoms
Irritability
Intolerance of noise
Poor concentration and memory
Fearfulness
Apprehensiveness
Restlessness
Continuous worrying thoughts
Physical symptoms
Dry mouth
Difficulty in swallowing
Shakiness
Diarrhoea
Urinary frequency
Paraesthesia, especially in fingers and around mouth
Hot flushes
Physical signs
Tense
Sweating
Shaky
Pale
Restless
Sighing

makes people anxious, indeed many think that they are going to die, and it is a very bad mistake to jump to the diagnosis of anxiety-related chest pain too readily!
• a careful examination for evidence of any of the organic causes of anxiety listed above, and for physical signs of anxiety listed in Table 2.

In this case the patient was hyperventilating, but no other abnormalities were found.

Approach to investigations and management

• The presenting feature was chest pain, therefore check an ECG. In a 35-year-old man with no previous cardiac history the ECG is likely to be normal.
• The only finding on examination was hyperventilation. Pulse oximetry should be performed, and most would think it appropriate to check arterial blood gases, with a normal PO_2 and low PCO_2 being the expected result.

Further medical tests may be indicated, but if the clinical diagnosis seems clearly to be that of an anxiety state, if there are no real indications of any of the organic causes of anxiety, and if the ECG and blood gases do not suggest an alternative diagnosis, then it is not helpful to embark on an extensive range of investigations that might actually reinforce the situation and make it worse. It is important to do the following:
• elicit the patient's own 'explanatory model', e.g. his conviction that he is about to have a heart attack which leads to frequent checking and recording his own pulse rate
• give the patient some understanding of the link between his symptoms and his faulty physiological assumptions.

Management

The immediate management includes the following:
• Take the patient to a quiet room (if possible) and reassure him, explaining how anxiety induces the physiological effects of excessive adrenaline release.
• If quiet discussion and encouragement does not lead to the patient's respiratory rate slowing and symptoms improving, then breathing in and out of a paper bag to raise plasma PCO_2 can be helpful. This should not be performed in the middle of an open area, where the patient might think he was being made to look a fool.
• Consider oral diazepam in a dose of 5–10 mg.
• For severe restlessness and panic with loss of control— give slow intravenous diazemuls 5–10 mg.
• Warn about the undesirable effects of long-term benzodiazepines with risk of dependence.
• Discuss precipitating and exacerbating factors.

Further management

• Short-term pharmacological treatment (see Section 2.7.2, p. 190)
• Cognitive–behavioural therapy (see Section 2.7.2, p. 193).

Gelder M, Gath D, Mayou R, Cowen, P. *Oxford Textbook of Psychiatry* (3rd edn). Oxford: Oxford University Press, 1996.

1.3 Neuropsychiatric aspects of HIV and AIDS

Case history

A 40-year-old man presents with a skin lesion. He is not aware that he is human immunodeficiency virus (HIV) positive until he is told by a dermatologist when he presents with Kaposi's sarcoma. He fails to attend for his next appointment at the clinic but a friend telephones on his behalf and reports that the patient has been refusing to leave his room, has not taken his medication, and has given up going to work. Eventually the friend persuades him to come to the clinic.

Clinical approach

Psychiatric and behavioural problems associated with HIV infection (Table 3) might:
• develop as psychological reactions
• reflect underlying organic pathology.
  Psychological reactions, especially adjustment disorders, are most likely to occur at the time of notification of a positive

Table 3 Psychological problems associated with human immunodeficiency virus infection.

Psychological causes
As a reaction to diagnosis
As a reaction to progression of acquired immune deficiency syndrome
As maladjustment to unexpected survival
Non-compliance and passive suicide

Organic causes
Direct infection of the brain
Secondary process in the brain
Side effects of antiretroviral medication

Table 4 Organic brain syndromes.

Brain disorder	Symptoms
Primary HIV-related brain disorder	Dementia and minor cognitive disorder
Secondary HIV-related brain disorder	Toxoplasmosis Progressive multifocal leucoencephalopathy Tumour, e.g. lymphoma
Acute and subacute syndromes (delirium)	Systemic disorder Secondary infections

HIV test, the diagnosis of acquired immunodeficiency syndrome (AIDS) or following a sudden progression of AIDS. Physical symptoms that are especially likely to cause distress include dyspnoea, weight loss, diarrhoea, blindness and disfigurement due to facial Kaposi's sarcoma.

There can also be a maladaptive response to unexpected survival ('Lazarus syndrome') while patients may fail to comply with medication, either because of side effects or even as a form of passive suicide. In addition to making a psychiatric diagnosis, it is obviously important to be continuously on the look out for evidence of organic cerebral lesions, including infections and tumours (Table 4). It is also important to watch out for the side effects of antiretroviral medication.

> **!** The order of frequency of psychiatric disorders in patients with HIV and AIDS referred to mental health services is as follows:
> • adjustment disorder (see Section 2.6, p. 186)
> • severe depression (see Section 2.11, p. 198)
> • HIV-associated dementia
> • mania—the exact frequency of mania is unknown but this is the commonest reason for emergency psychiatric hospitalization in AIDS .

The other psychiatric disorders most commonly seen in patients with HIV and AIDS are organic brain syndromes (see Section 2.2, p. 180) and hypochondriacal disorder (see Section 1.6, p. 172).

History of the presenting problem

Try to obtain the following information from the patient and from his friend.
• Did the change in his behaviour follow the diagnosis or did the disturbance predate this event?
• What symptoms has the patient himself complained of, e.g. low mood, panic attacks, sleep disturbance, forgetfulness, poor concentration and slowing of thought?

Relevant past history

Does the patient have any previous or family history of psychiatric disorder?
• Has he suffered bereavements due to AIDS or some other cause? How has he coped in the past with loss and with emotional trauma?
• Does he generally rely on avoidance and denial as a coping style?
• Does his occupational and social history suggest a personality disorder?
• Is there a history of substance misuse?
• Is he generally socially isolated or is his reclusiveness of recent origin?

Note the presence of any of these risk factors for psychiatric morbidity associated with HIV and AIDS.

> **Risk factors for psychiatric morbidity associated with HIV and AIDS**
>
> • pre-HIV psychiatric history
> • personality disorder
> • substance misuse
> • bereavements due to AIDS
> • other losses including occupation and relationships
> • social isolation
> • avoidance and denial as a coping style
> • older age increases risk of HIV-associated dementia.

Examination

• First carry out a thorough physical examination with particular emphasis on the central nervous system (CNS). Look for ataxia of gait, weakness of legs and frontal release signs, e.g. snout reflex, dysarthria and peripheral neuropathy.
• During the psychiatric examination look particularly for disturbance of mood and of memory and intellectual function.

Mood disturbance

The patient may show the typical features of a depressive illness or of an anxiety state. Conversely, his mood might be elated, there may be pressure of speech and grandiose ideas, all suggestive of hypomania or mania, although this is unlikely in a patient who has become reclusive.

167

HIV and mania

When HIV infection and mania occur together:
- there might be a chance association of HIV and bipolar affective disorder
- think of illicit drug use, e.g. amphetamine or cocaine
- consider if the mania is iatrogenic, e.g. due to steroids
- remember that 'new-onset' mania might be associated with cognitive impairment and reduced survival.

Assessment of cognitive function

Look for impairment of memory, intellectual decline and psychomotor slowing.

AIDS-related dementia

This develops rapidly and has a poor prognosis. It is associated with the following features:
- older age
- psychomotor slowing
- low body mass index
- constitutional HIV symptoms
- a CD4 count of under 200
- Zidovudine (AZT) might be protective.

Approach to investigations and management

Evidence of impairment of intellect or memory indicates the need for brain imaging—computed tomography (CT) or magnetic resonance imaging (MRI)—and examination of cerebrospinal fluid (CSF). Look for treatable conditions such as opportunistic infections or lymphomas.

The management of the psychiatric syndromes associated with HIV and AIDS is essentially similar to the management of these disorders in other contexts. However, special attention has to be paid to the risk of suicide and the administration of medication. The use of atypical antipsychotic drugs such as olanzapine is less likely to cause extrapyramidal side effects than major tranquillizers such as haloperidol.

HIV and suicide

The suicide rate and preoccupation with suicide in people with HIV infection is much greater than in the general population.

Medication for HIV disease

Efavirenz (Sustiva) can cause an acute confusional state and psychotic reactions, as well as abnormal dreams, fatigue and impaired concentration.

There is the potential for important interactions between medications used to treat HIV diseases and that given for psychiatric disorder.

'All protease inhibitors and non-nucleoside reverse transcriptase inhibitors are substrates of the cytochrome P450 system and possess enzyme-inhibiting and/or

Medication for HIV disease (*continued*)

inducing properties. Psychotropic medications possess similar metabolic characteristics and may interact with antiretrovirals. Modifications in drug selection, dose or dosing regimen may be needed to ensure adequate antiretroviral concentrations and thus minimize the risk of incomplete viral suppression and/or development of drug resistance ...' [1].

See *General clinical issues*, Section 3.
See *Infectious diseases*, Sections 1.24–1.29, and 2.11.
Catalan J (ed.). *Mental Health and HIV Infection: psychological and psychiatric aspects*. London: UCL Press, 1999.
Lishman WA. *Organic Psychiatry: the psychological consequences of cerebral disorder* (3rd edn). Oxford: Blackwell Science, 1998.
McArthur JC, Hoover DR, Bacellar H, Miller EN, Cohen BA, Becker JT. Dementia in AIDS patients: incidence and risk factors. *Neurology* 1993; 43: 2245–2252.
1 Lin-in Tseng A, Foisy M. Significant interactions with new antiretrovirals and psychotropic drugs. *Ann Pharmacother* 1999; 33: 461–473.

1.4 Deliberate self-harm

Case history

A 30-year-old woman is brought into A&E after taking an unknown quantity of paracetamol 90 min earlier. She is alert and tearful.

Clinical approach

Deliberate self harm (DSH) leads to 100 000 hospital admissions in England and Wales every year and its incidence is increasing. A major concern is that an episode of DSH indicates a greatly increased risk of suicide, and it is this factor that governs the psychiatric approach.

For 10 years after an episode of DSH the risk of suicide is increased to 30-fold higher than that expected, with the first 6 months being the period of greatest risk.
- One per cent of patients kill themselves in the year after an episode of DSH.
- One-fifth to one-quarter of patients who die by suicide have presented to a general hospital after episodes of DSH in the year before their death.

To evaluate short-term risk after an episode of DSH assess:
- patient's state of mind
- recent adverse life events
- quality of social support network.

The highest suicide rate occurs in people aged over 75 but the rate among young men has increased greatly over the past 15 years [2]. Men tend to use asphyxiation with car exhaust fumes and hanging; women tend to use self poisoning with drugs. Most people who commit suicide have a psychiatric disorder:

- depression (15% lifetime risk of suicide)
- schizophrenia (10%)
- alcohol addiction (3.4%).

The following sociodemographic and personal factors are correlated with suicide:

- divorce
- loss of job
- unemployment/retirement
- social isolation
- recent bereavement
- chronic painful or terminal illness
- history of mood disorder, alcoholism or attempted suicide
- loss of a parent in childhood.

History of the presenting problem

Some patients who have taken overdoses will be unable to give a history, often because their conscious level will be impaired by the effects of the drugs or alcohol that they have taken. However, when they are able to talk about things, the main aim of psychiatric assessment is to establish the risk of suicide, bearing in mind the factors detailed above. Ask the following:

- Did she take the overdose on impulse or had she planned it for some time?
- Had she hoarded the pills?
- Was anybody present or nearby, or had she taken precautions to make sure that she was alone and undisturbed?
- Did she leave a suicide note?
- Had she given away her most treasured possessions?
- Had she arranged for the children to be sent away or had her pet dog or cat put down?
- Did she try more than one means of killing herself, e.g. overdose plus jumping out of a window or in front of a lorry?

- Has she been suffering from severe insomnia, panic attacks, agitation or impaired memory?

Relevant past history

Enquire about the following:

- Is there a past history of DSH or a family history of suicide?
- Is she known to suffer from affective disorder, schizophrenia, alcoholism or drug dependence?
- Is she suffering from a chronic, painful, disabling or life-threatening illness?
- Is she socially isolated or recently separated?
- Have there been any other recent adverse life events?
- Is there a history of impulsive or aggressive behaviour?

Examination

The immediate priority in any patient presenting with DSH is physical examination—beginning with airway, breathing, circulation. The clinical approach to the patient who is unconscious is described in *Emergency medicine*, Section 1.26.

When it is possible to examine her mental state the important aspects are:

- Does she exhibit self neglect, anhedonia, pessimism, guilt, remorse and self recrimination?
- Does she convey a feeling of helplessness and despair?
- Are there depressive or nihilistic delusions?
- Has she experienced command hallucinations?
- Does she wish that she had not survived the overdose?

Approach to investigations and management

Notes on the medical management of overdoses are found in *Emergency medicine*, Section 2.1.

> Patients who discharge themselves from A&E before psychosocial screening have three times the rate of repetition of DSH [4].

If the patient refuses life-saving treatment then you should:
• explain risks
• evaluate capacity to make an informed decision.

To decide whether the patient can make an informed decision you need to determine whether they can:
• appraise information provided
• understand the nature and consequences of their choice.
  After this, proceed as follows:
• record assessment of capacity
• if capacity lacking, treat under common law
• enlist support of family or friends to persuade patient
• admit high suicide risk patients either voluntarily or under Mental Health Act (see Section 2.14, p. 203).

The following factors indicate high risk and argue against early discharge after an episode of DSH:
• lack of adequate support and failure to resolve precipitating circumstances
• history of impulsive behaviour
• current substance misuse
• regret that they have survived
• failure to establish rapport with staff.

> See *Emergency medicine*, Sections 1.26 and 2.1.
> 1 Kerkhof AJFM, Arensman E. Attempted suicide and deliberate self-harm: epidemiology and risk factors. In: Gelder MG, Lopez-Ibor JJ, Andreasen N, eds. *New Oxford Textbook of Psychiatry*. Oxford: Oxford University Press, 2000.
> 2 Hawton K, Fagg J, Simkin S, Bale E, Bond A. Trends in deliberate self harm in Oxford, 1985–95. *Br J Psychiatry* 1997; 171: 556–560.
> 3 Dennis M, Beach M, Evans PA, Winston A, Friedman T. An examination of the accident and emergency management of deliberate self harm. *J Accident Emerg Med* 1997; 14: 311–315.
> 4 Crawford MJ, Wessely S. Does initial management affect the rate of repetition of deliberate self harm? Cohort study. *BMJ* 1998; 317: 985.

1.5 Eating disorders

Case history

You are called to A&E where a painfully thin 17-year-old girl appears physically ill, but she is uncooperative with staff. Her parents are there and report that she has not been eating.

Clinical approach

Control and self esteem, or lack thereof, are the issues that patients with eating disorders are usually struggling with [1]. Eating and weight are things they sometimes feel in control of, although a lot of the time even that feels out of control. If they have suffered abuse then these feelings may be even stronger. Anyone telling them to eat and gain weight will be met with considerable hostility, and putting undue pressure on them may arouse feelings of abuse. Their beliefs about their weight and appearance are very strong so they are unlikely to accept the severity of their situation or advice from well-meaning doctors.

Approach the situation with empathy and understanding, concentrating on winning her trust. In this acute setting you largely address urgent medical complications, not the eating disorder itself. It is important to differentiate between anorexia nervosa and bulimia nervosa, as management is different.

> **ICD-10 criteria for anorexia nervosa**
>
> • Body mass index (BMI) ≤17.5 or body weight ≤15% below expected, where BMI = weight (kg)/height^2 (m^2)
> • Self-induced weight loss
> • Body image distortion
> • Abnormalities of the hypothalamic–pituitary–gonadal axis
> • If onset prepubertal, then delayed puberty.
>
> ***Diagnostic and Statistical Manual for Mental Disorders* (DSM)-IV criteria for bulimia nervosa**
>
> • Recurrent episodes of binge eating
> • Recurrent inappropriate compensatory behaviour to prevent weight gain
> • The above occurring ≥ twice weekly for 3 months.

History of the presenting problem

Anorexia nervosa is a clinical diagnosis (see above) and other general medical conditions that may account for the weight loss must be excluded.

> **Other conditions to consider**
>
> Other conditions that may present like anorexia nervosa [2] are:
> • inflammatory bowel disease
> • malabsorption
> • infection—tuberculosis, HIV
> • thyrotoxicosis
> • hypopituitarism
> • diabetes
> • Addison's disease
> • malignant disease
> • depression
> • psychosis
> • obsessive–compulsive disorder.

In most cases the diagnosis is clear and never in substantial doubt, but take care not to rush to conclusions immediately, and enquire regarding bowel habit, abdominal bloating and other symptoms that might indicate malabsorption (see *Gastroenterology and hepatology*, Section 1.10), also for symptoms that might indicate one of the diseases listed above.

Focusing on anorexia nervosa and bulimia nervosa, explore if she relates to these common behaviours/symptoms [3]:
- intense fear of putting on weight
- constantly thinking about food
- hoarding food
- does not eat with family or in public places
- binge eating and self-induced vomiting
- laxative and diuretic abuse
- ritualistic, excessive and possibly abnormal exercise
- amenorrhoea.

Collateral history

She may feel ashamed of her eating pattern and therefore unwilling to divulge information. Her parents can provide information; however, beware of making her feel colluded against.

Relevant past history

Establish from the patient:
- How old was she when the eating disorder started?
- What does she believe set it off?
- How does it affect her life?
- Has she had previous medical complications?
- Has she been abused physically, sexually or emotionally?
- Has she received treatment in the past?

> ! Asking about abuse should only be done when you are alone with her and you perceive that your relationship with her is such that she will not find such a question overwhelmingly intrusive. Assure confidentiality. You may be the first person she has ever told.

Examination

Have someone the patient trusts present during physical examination. Explain to her exactly what you are going to be doing. Take extra precaution to be discreet during the examination, remembering how she is likely to feel about her body.

Establish her height and weight to calculate her BMI.

Look for signs of starvation [4]:
- hypothermia
- lanugo
- loss of muscle mass
- dependent oedema
- bradycardia
- hypotension
- neuropathy.

If she is inducing vomiting, telltale signs are:
- salivary gland enlargement
- dental erosion
- calluses on the fingers/knuckles.

Look for evidence of any other conditions that may present like anorexia nervosa (see above).

Approach to investigations and management

Investigations

Investigations are necessary to identify medical complications and exclude other causes for weight loss rather than to aid in making the diagnosis. Those in Table 5 should be performed as soon as possible to identify urgent problems; those in Table 6 are less urgent, not required in all patients, and should be dictated by clinical need.

Table 5 Urgent investigations required in patients presenting with probable anorexia nervosa [5].

Investigation	Possible abnormalities
Electrolytes	Hypokalaemia Hypochloraemic alkalosis Renal failure
Calcium	Low
Phosphate	Low
Magnesium	Low
Liver function test	Low proteins Raised liver enzymes
Glucose	Low
Full blood count	Low white cell count Normochromic or iron-deficient anaemia
Erythrocyte sedimentation rate	Should be normal
Electrocardiogram	Dysrhythmias T-wave changes, ST depression and lengthened QT interval
Chest radiograph	Small heart Osteoporosis

Table 6 Other investigations that should be considered in patients presenting with probable anorexia nervosa [5].

Investigation	Possible abnormality
Thyroid function test	Low tri-iodothyronine
Amylase	Raised
Iron, folate, B$_{12}$	Low
Cholesterol	Raised
Luteinizing hormone and follicle-stimulating hormone	Low
Growth hormone and cortisol	Raised
Electroencephalogram	Non-specific abnormalities, seizures
Bone scan	Osteoporosis
Computed tomography brain scan	'Pseudoatrophy'

Management

There is no agreed 'best' treatment for anorexia nervosa and outcome is variable. Twenty-year mortality rates are reported between 4 and 20%.

Management of anorexia nervosa

- Treat medical complications
- Restore state of nutrition
- Provide information
- Refer to psychiatric services or general practitioner so psychotherapy and family counselling can be initiated.

Anorexia nervosa—refusal of treatment

If the patient's situation is life threatening and she adamantly refuses treatment, she must be assessed by a psychiatrist for treatment under the Mental Health Act of 1983 (see Section 2.14, p. 203).

See *Gastroenterology and hepatology*, Sections 1.10 and 2.14.
1 Garner DM. Pathogenesis of anorexia nervosa. *Lancet* 1993; 341: 1631–1635.
2 Kaplan HI, Saddock BJ. *Synopsis of Psychiatry* (8th edn). Baltimore, MD: Williams and Wilkins, 1998: 720–726.
3 Freeman C. *Eating Disorders: a Guide for Primary Care.* Edinburgh: Royal Edinburgh Hospital, 1999: 1–28.
4 Treasure J. Anorexia nervosa and bulimia nervosa. *Prescriber's J* 2000; 39(4): 227–233.
5 Beaumont PJV, Russell JD, Touyz SW. Treatment of anorexia nervosa. *Lancet* 1993; 341: 1635–1640.

1.6 Medically unexplained symptoms

Case history

A 45-year-old woman is referred by her general practitioner with an 8-month history of feeling exhausted, unable to engage in any activity that requires physical exertion, and sleeping up to 15 h a day. She feels miserable because of not being able to do what she could previously. Her general practitioner cannot find any explanation for her symptoms.

Clinical approach

Medically unexplained physical symptoms, the somatoform disorders (Table 7), are often dismissed and patients feel they are not being taken seriously despite feeling very ill indeed. These symptoms are difficult to treat and may make doctors feel impotent and frustrated. Obviously psychological aspects are enormously important, but patients

Table 7 Somatoform disorders [1].

Disorder	Characteristic features
Somatization disorder	Many symptoms including gastrointestinal, sexual and neurological. Pain is common
Conversion disorder	One symptom simulating a disease, e.g. motor or sensory symptoms, seizures
Hypochondriasis	Preoccupation with having a particular disease
Body dysmorphic disorder	Subjective feelings of a body defect
Pain disorder	Pain syndrome

rarely accept a purely psychological explanation. A sensible approach is for physician and psychiatrist to work collaboratively. One physician with an interest should investigate possible medical causes and co-ordinate all investigations and care. An empathic but firm and sensible approach is essential. The involvement of a large number of doctors is likely to do more harm than good.

History of the presenting problem

A full medical history and functional enquiry is required, with any leads followed appropriately, but it is very likely that nothing obvious will emerge.

Ask the patient:
- When did the symptoms start?
- When did her mood change?
- What was the first symptom?
- What is her explanation?
- How did other symptoms develop?
- Did anything happen to her just prior to the onset?

Can a diagnosis of chronic fatigue syndrome be made? Are the criteria for chronic fatigue syndrome satisfied?

Diagnostic criteria for chronic fatigue syndrome

Clinically evaluated, medically unexplained fatigue of at least 6 months' duration that is [2]:
- of new onset
- not a result of ongoing exertion
- not substantially alleviated by rest
- a substantial reduction in previous levels of activity.

The occurrence of four or more of the following symptoms:
- subjective memory impairment
- tender lymph nodes
- muscle pain
- joint pain
- headache
- unrefreshing sleep
- postexertional malaise.

Relevant past history

The following need to be excluded [3]:
- any medical illnesses that may explain fatigue

- previously established cognitive, psychotic or mood disorders
- eating disorder
- alcohol or other substance misuse.

> **Chronic fatigue**
>
> Remember to ask about travel to foreign countries to exclude unusual infections (see *Infectious diseases*, Sections 1.20–1.23).

Examination

A full and thorough examination must be performed, but resist repeating examinations excessively unless new circumstances warrant it. Any leads that emerge must obviously be followed.

Approach to investigations and management

Investigations

A thorough, well thought out battery of investigations early on will reassure you, the patient and other doctors involved in her care that there is nothing that needs urgent medical intervention. Routine tests should include [3]:
- full blood count and white cell differential
- erythrocyte sedimentation rate (ESR) and C-reactive protein (CRP)
- urea, creatinine and electrolytes
- calcium
- liver function tests
- glucose
- creatine phosphokinase (CPK)
- thyroid function tests (TFT)
- autoantibodies profile, including antinuclear factor (ANF)
- urine dispstick for protein and sugar
- chest radiograph
- ECG
- anything else guided by findings on history and examination.
Once these have been done, further investigations should not be performed without clear clinical indication. The intelligent mind can always think of 'just one more test': this temptation is to be avoided.

> **Investigations in the chronic fatigue syndrome**
>
> Repeated investigations confirm the patient's belief, often strongly held, that his or her symptoms have a purely physical basis, and hinders the patient exploring psychological coping strategies.

Management

A holistic approach should be taken in treating physical and psychological symptoms.

Illness behaviour often has some secondary gain. Establishing this is helpful in understanding and resolving the situation.

The following are management strategies that have been investigated [2]:
- graded exercise programmes and cognitive–behavioural therapy [4] are the only two treatments shown to be of definite benefit
- corticosteroids, antidepressants, dietary supplements and NADH have limited or unknown effectiveness
- immunotherapy is unlikely to be beneficial
- prolonged rest is ineffective and tends to be harmful.

1 American Psychiatric Association. *Diagnostic and Statistical Manual of Mental Disorders* (4th edn). Washington: American Psychiatric Association, 1994.
2 Fukuda K, Straus S, Hickie I, Sharpe M, Dobbins J, Komaroff A. The chronic fatigue syndrome: a comprehensive approach to its definition and study. *Ann Intern Med* 1994; 121: 953–959.
3 Reid S, Chalder T, Cleare A, Hotopf M, Wessely S. Chronic fatigue syndrome. *BMJ* 2000; 320: 292–296.
4 Sharpe M. Cognitive behaviour therapy for chronic fatigue syndrome: efficacy and implications. *Am J Med* 1998; 105(3A): 104S–109S.

1.7 The alcoholic in hospital

Case history

A 54-year-old man is admitted to hospital in a neglected state. He appears anxious, agitated, shaky and sweaty. He reports that he stopped drinking alcohol 2 days previously.

Clinical approach

Alcohol withdrawal is distressing to the patient and can be fatal, especially in older people. Alcoholics frequently neglect themselves and may have added problems such as malnutrition and infections. Withdrawal symptoms need to be controlled with an adequate dose of benzodiazepine. Other issues can then be addressed, such as social factors that perpetuate the habit and plans for stopping drinking. Alcohol dependence is never a problem in isolation.

History of the presenting problem

Is he dependent on alcohol?

You need to determine if alcohol dependence is the problem and its extent.

DSM-IV criteria for alcohol dependence [1]

- Inability to cut down
- Repeated efforts to control drinking
- Amnesic periods
- Drinking increasing amounts
- Ongoing drinking despite detrimental consequences
- Withdrawal symptoms.

Withdrawal symptoms

- Sweating
- Tachycardia
- Raised blood pressure
- Tremor
- Insomnia
- Nausea and vomiting
- Hallucinations—tactile, visual and auditory
- Agitation and anxiety
- Grand mal seizures.

What, when, why and with whom?

The important aspects to establish are:
- What is he drinking?
- What is the strength?
- How much?
- How often?
- When in the day?
- When was his last drink?
- Does he relate drinking to any particular pattern or situation?
- Alone or with people?

How many units per week is he drinking (Table 8)? The Royal College of Physicians (1995) recommended maximum total units per week for safe use are 21 in men and 14 in women [2]. The Department of Health recommends that women consistently consuming between 2 and 3 units daily and men between 3 and 4 units daily will not accrue any significant health risk. Haemorrhagic stroke, cancer, accidents and hypertension are all associated with alcohol consumption above recommended levels [3].

Table 8 Units of alcohol in common beverages, where 1 unit of alcohol contains 8 g of ethanol.

Type of drink	Units of alcohol
Pint of lager	2
Pint of extra-strong lager	5
150-mL glass of wine	1
1 shot of spirits (25 mL)	1

Is there comorbidity?

One-third of people with alcohol dependence also have another mental illness, most commonly a mood disorder, an anxiety disorder or antisocial personality disorder. Suicide is commonly associated with alcohol [4].

A quick way to screen for alcohol dependence is by the CAGE mnemonic [5]:
C—cutting down: has been trying
A—annoyed by someone commenting on their drinking
G—guilty feelings about drinking
E—eye openers: drinks first thing in the morning.

Social issues

A grasp of his current social circumstances and supports will help him feel understood as a person and will give you an insight into why he continues to drink.

A blaming, moralistic attitude focusing exclusively on alcohol abuse will result in a frustrating, ineffective therapeutic relationship.

Relevant past history

Ask the patient:
- When did he start drinking and why?
- How long has his drinking been a problem?
- Has he experienced withdrawal symptoms in the past and what happened?
- Has he been in an alcohol treatment programme before?
- What precipitated previous relapses?
- Any past medical complications? (see below)
- Has he a family history of alcohol abuse?
- Has he been in fights, had falls or head injuries related to drinking?
- Has he had any drinking and driving offences?
- Has he lost jobs or partners because of his drinking?

Medical conditions associated with alcohol abuse

- Oesophagitis
- Gastritis
- Gastric ulcer
- Alcoholic hepatitis and cirrhosis
- Oesophageal varices
- Pancreatitis
- Cardiomyopathy
- Thiamine deficiency—Wernicke/Korsakoff syndrome
- Neuropathy
- Cerebellar atrophy.

Examination

General physical examination looking for signs of:
- withdrawal (see above)
- infection (especially pneumonia)
- malnutrition
- possible medical complications of alcohol abuse (see above).

Is he confused? Delirium tremens can occur within 72 h of his last drink, but there is a wide differential diagnosis of confusion in the alcoholic. Is there any evidence of the following?

- delirium tremens
- Wernicke's encephalopathy
- postictal state
- delirium due to infection, hepatic failure or other general medical condition
- hypoglycaemia.

Wernicke's encephalopathy classically presents with:
- ophthalmoplegia (horizontal and vertical nystagmus, weakness/paralysis of lateral rectus muscles, weakness/paralysis of conjugate gaze)
- ataxia
- confusion.

Fits in the alcoholic

Before attributing seizures to alcohol withdrawal, exclude other causes:
- hypoglycaemia
- hyponatraemia
- hypomagnesaemia
- other CNS pathology, e.g. subdural haematoma.

Approach to investigations and management

Any of the medical complications of alcohol abuse (listed above) will require appropriate investigation and treatment.

Management of alcohol withdrawal

The important aspects are as follows:
- Benzodiazepines—treat withdrawal symptoms with a 7–10-day course of, for example, diazepam or chlordiazepoxide; usually orally, occasionally intravenous injection (seizures), virtually never intramuscular injection due to erratic absorption. Initially titrate dose until symptoms are controlled, then taper dose until stopping
- Nurse in well-lit, quiet environment
- Give thiamine supplementation
- Monitor for and prevent hypoglycaemia
- Rehydration
- High-calorie, high-carbohydrate diet
- Avoid antipsychotics as they lower seizure threshold
- Refer to alcohol services for follow-up, support, advice, cognitive and behavioural therapy; to psychiatrist if comorbid mental illness is present.

1 American Psychiatric Association. *Diagnostic and Statistical Manual of Mental Disorders* (4th edn). Washington: American Psychiatric Association, 1994.
2 *Alcohol and the heart in perspective—sensible limits reaffirmed.* Joint report with the Royal Colleges of Psychiatrists and General Practitioners. Royal College of Physicians, London, 1995.
3 Department of Health. *Sensible drinking.* The report of an Inter-Departmental Working Group, 1995.
4 Regier DA, Farmer ME, Rae DS. Comorbidity of mental disorders with alcohol and other drug abuse: results from the Epidemiologic Catchment Area (ECA) Study. *JAMA* 1990; 264: 2511–2518.
5 Ewing JA. Detecting alcoholism: the CAGE questionnaire. *JAMA* 1984; 252: 1905–1907.

1.8 Drug abuser in hospital

Case history

A 29-year-old woman has been admitted to a surgical ward for drainage of an abscess on her forearm. She uses heroin intravenously, says that she is about to go into opioid withdrawal, and your opinion is sought.

Clinical approach

Drug users will only be managed successfully if they are treated in an understanding but firm manner. Look beyond the drug abuse. The golden rule is always question the fact when someone says they are dependent on opioids and never accept the dose they report. People have died from being inadvertently overdosed during opioid replacement therapy. If they claim to be having withdrawal symptoms, look for objective evidence. Drug users will go to great lengths for a fresh supply and may present with challenging behaviour. Ask open-ended questions as a way of determining the consistency of their history.

History of the presenting problem

What and when?

The most important points are:
- What substances is she using? (this list may be extensive)
- Since when?
- By what method?
- How much?

Heroin can be smoked, injected or snorted, and may be used in conjunction with other opioids. Ask her to describe any withdrawal symptoms she may be experiencing or have experienced in the past. Has she developed tolerance? Does she have any plans to kick her habit?

Symptoms of opioid withdrawal [1]

- Dysphoric mood
- Nausea or vomiting
- Muscle aches
- Lacrimation or rhinorrhoea
- Pupillary dilation, piloerection or sweating
- Diarrhoea
- Yawning
- Fever
- Insomnia.

Features that indicate drug dependence [2]

- Tolerance
- Withdrawal symptoms upon cessation
- Greater use than initially intended
- Time spent on drugs at the expense of other daily activities
- Unsuccessful attempts to cut down
- Continued use despite physical and psychological complications.

Social issues

Check with the patient:
- What are her current social circumstances and social supports?
- Does she have children?
- Might she be pregnant?
- Does she have a safe place to live?
- How does she fund her drug habit?

Understanding these issues will help establish a therapeutic alliance as well as giving you a more holistic view of her problems.

Polysubstance abuse

- Common among heroin users
- Withdrawal symptoms may be altered
- Does not necessarily mean dependence on all substances.

Relevant past history

- When did her drug abuse start and what was happening in her life at that time?
- Establish if she has had or has any other mental health problems. Comorbidity of drug abuse and psychiatric illness is common (about 50% of people with drug dependence have a current psychiatric illness).
- Has she got any of the medical complications of drug abuse? Ask in particular about chronic liver disease and its complications, endocarditis and HIV. Has she ever been tested for HIV and hepatitis [3]?

Examination

People with drug-dependence problems may present in a demanding and overwhelming manner, but do not let this put you off from establishing objective evidence of drug withdrawal symptoms [3].

Signs of drug use include:
- needle track marks
- discoid scars from subcutaneous injection
- burn marks on fingers
- neglected self care.

Look for the signs of opioid withdrawal (see above), also for hypertension, tachycardia and temperature dysregulation. If, by contrast, the patient is hypotensive with septic shock, proceed as described in *Emergency medicine*, Section 1.28.

Approach to investigations and management

Investigations

Urine test kits are now freely available that will tell you within 10 min whether any drug or its metabolites are present in the urine. These kits usually just indicate the presence or absence of a drug, not the amount. Most A&E departments stock them.

In this woman with an obvious septic focus it will be appropriate to check full blood count, glucose, electrolytes, renal and liver function tests, clotting and blood cultures; also to swab the abscess. These tests should be performed routinely on any drug user admitted to hospital since they are at risk of malnutrition and infections. Further tests may be required if there are specific indications, e.g. echocardiography if suspicion of endocarditis.

Discuss with her whether she would like to be tested for hepatitis B and C, HIV and syphilis.

Management

Aside from drainage of the abscess, appropriate antimicrobial therapy and treatment of any other medical problems, the question to be tackled is 'how should opioid withdrawal be prevented or treated?'

- Never give a methadone dose equivalent to what the patient reports they are using (Table 9).
- Never prescribe methadone to occasional opioid users.

If you have determined that she is dependent on opioids and in withdrawal, she will need methadone substitution to relieve her symptoms. If she is pregnant this is mandatory as opioid withdrawal is associated with spontaneous abortion and fetal death.

Initially give 10 mg of methadone syrup and wait about 60 min to determine its effect. Continue administering 10-mg increments until symptoms are in control. It is rare to exceed a total dose of 40 mg over 24 h. Determine how much methadone is required over a 24-h period and

Table 9 Equivalent opioid doses [5].

Drug	Dose	Methadone equivalent
Street heroin	*	*
Pharmaceutical heroin	10-mg tablet or ampoule	20 mg
Morphine	10-mg ampoule	10 mg
Dihydrocodeine (DF 118)	30-mg tablet	3 mg
Buprenorphine hydrochloride	200-µg tablet	5 mg
	300-µg ampoule	8 mg
Codeine phosphate	15-mg tablet	1 mg
J. Collis Brown 100 mL	10-mg extract of opium	10 mg

* Purity varies, hence it is impossible to make an accurate estimate.

then that dose can be given as a single or divided dose. Beware of overdosing her as this could result in respiratory arrest. Remember that she may be getting opioids from an alternative source whilst in hospital so look for signs of intoxication.

Clonidine and lofexidine are centrally acting agents used to dampen down sympathetic tone, thereby reducing the severity of withdrawal symptoms. Try to avoid the use of benzodiazepines as these are frequently also abused.

Also note the following:
• An acute admission is not a suitable setting to embark on an opioid withdrawal programme. Aim to stabilize the dose of methadone and then refer to a drug rehabilitation unit. If withdrawal is deemed appropriate, this should take 10–14 days and it is then imperative to refer to a drug service for ongoing rehabilitation.
• This may be the only contact she has with medical services so try to provide her with some information about safer drugs use, the availability of services, HIV and hepatitis.
• Refer to a psychiatrist if comorbidity is suspected or behaviour is very challenging.
• Encourage attendance at a drug rehabilitation unit. Strategies used here include motivational interviewing, cognitive–behavioural therapy, methadone maintenance [4] or withdrawal programmes, inpatient treatment programmes, drug substitution and assistance with social problems. Naltrexone may be used to prevent relapse.

1 American Psychiatric Association. *Diagnostic and Statistical Manual of Mental Disorders* (4th edn). Washington: American Psychiatric Association, 1994.
2 Kaplan HI, Saddock BJ. *Synopsis of Psychiatry* (8th edn). Baltimore, MD: Williams and Wilkins, 1994: 436–442.
3 Seivewright N, Daly C. Personality disorder and drug use: a review. *Drug Alcohol Rev* 1997; 16: 235–250.
4 Farrel M, Ward J, Mattick R *et al*. Methadone maintenance treatment in opiate dependence: a review. *BMJ* 1994; 309: 997–1001.
5 Strang J, Farrell M. Illicit drug use: clinical features and treatment. In: Chick J, Cantwell R, eds. *Seminars in Alcohol and Drug Misuse*. London: Gaskell, 1994: 33–52.

1.9 The frightening patient

Case history

A tall and physically intimidating man is brought to A&E by the police. He appears dishevelled. He is shouting abuse and lashing out at anyone who approaches him.

Clinical approach

When dealing with aggressive people in hospital, the first distinction you need to make is between people who are:
• aggressive as a result of mental illness or distress
• habitually violent.

The approach and management will be different in each. Some people react in an angry and blaming way to the feelings of uncertainty and loss of control that may accompany an illness. People with mental illness might be aggressive because they are very frightened by their symptoms. Understanding and reassurance go a long way to resolve these situations, while being rigidly authoritarian will just escalate matters. The more information you can gather about the person the better you will be equipped to make good decisions in a calm and rational manner. Habitually violent people need to be dealt with by the police service.

> Only boxers are paid to get beaten up!

If you are concerned that a patient might be violent:
• do not take any risks
• never see him alone
• call back-up, e.g. hospital security and/or police
• remove your necktie or scarf
• make sure that you and other staff always have easy access to an exit door
• remove other patients from the area
• remove potential weapons from the area
• do not let back-up, e.g. hospital security and/or police, leave until you feel the situation is safe.

History of the presenting problem

The information you are able to gain from the patient may be sparse. Obtain collateral information from family, friends, police, medical notes, etc.

If possible, find out:
• What is he normally like?
• When did this behaviour start?

- Did anything precipitate it?
- What was he doing when he was found by the police?
- Has he threatened or injured anyone?
- Has he destroyed property?
- Has he used drugs or alcohol?
- What has he been saying?
- Has he been making sense?

> Violent behaviour is most often linked to [1]:
> - men
> - age under 30 years
> - access to weapons
> - drug and alcohol abuse.

Relevant past history

If possible, establish the following:
- What past medical conditions has he had?
- Is he normally on medication and is he compliant?
- Has he received treatment for a mental illness?
- Does he have a history of aggressive behaviour?
- Does he have a history of drug and alcohol abuse?
- Has he been arrested or convicted in the past?

> **Mental disorders that may present with violence**
> - Delirium (see Section 1.1, p. 163)
> - Mood disorders (see Sections 2.11, p. 198 and 2.12, p. 201)
> - Psychotic disorders (see Section 2.3, p. 182).

Examination

If possible:
- Check for concealed weapons.
- Does his general appearance give clues to an underlying condition?
- Listen to what he is saying. Is he confused? Is he deluded?
- Is his behaviour bizarre?
- Is he responding to hallucinations?
- Try to get his co-operation to do a physical examination or as much of one as he can tolerate.

Approach to investigations and management

Investigations

This depends on what you suspect the underlying cause of aggression is. It may not be possible to perform any investigations before sedation is administered: if it is possible to do something, then only do what is absolutely necessary as excessive demands may irritate him.
- Drug abuse—urine drug screen (see Section 1.8, p. 175)
- Alcohol abuse—breathalyser test or saliva alcohol test
- Delirium—check BM stix: perform those tests listed in Section 1.1, p. 163, that are indicated and possible.

Management

Remember not to risk your safety or that of other hospital staff.

Interpersonal issues

The following are important:
- keep a calm appearance
- be pleasant, clear and firm
- do not bargain with, argue with or threaten him
- minimize eye contact
- maintain a safe distance
- offer food and drink (cooled tea, not hot!)
- reassure the patient and let him know you appreciate how frightened or angry he must be and you would like to help
- praise any attempts at self control, no matter how minor
- try to establish an emotional relationship.

Treatment and disposal

Remember:
- physical restraints should not be used and may be construed as assault
- the police or staff trained in control and restraint may restrain him if necessary, but beware of positional asphyxia if a patient's movement or breathing is in any way restricted
- offer oral sedation
- in extreme situations, sedation can be administered *once* as an emergency treatment under common law
- treat any underlying medical condition
- decide if psychiatric admission is necessary
- consider admission under Mental Health Act (see Section 2.14, p. 203)
- if he is not ill, ask police to remove him.

> **Emergency sedation** [2]
>
> First try:
> - lorazepam 1–4 mg p.o. or i.m.
> - haloperidol in an initial dose of 2.5 mg p.o. or i.m., rising to 5 mg or 10 mg if necessary. In view of the cardiotoxicity of droperidol (prolongation of the cardiac QT interval), haloperidol is preferred.
>
>   If the patient cannot take or be given these and you think it essential to sedate, e.g. to give urgent medical treatment, then:
> - request four people trained in control and restraint: one for each arm and one for each leg
> - request an anaesthetist and ensure that resuscitation equipment and antidote (flumazenil) is available
> - draw up several syringes, each containing an intravenous benzodiazepine, e.g. diazemuls 10 mg
> - restrain the patient
> - insert a butterfly cannula into a large vein
> - inject 10 mg diazemuls, wait 60 s, repeat as necessary until sedation is achieved (lower doses would be appropriate for those who are elderly, intoxicated, delirious or have not had these drugs before).

Preventing aggression in hospitals

- Do not keep agitated patients waiting
- Encourage patients to air their grievances
- Keep patients informed about what you are doing
- Staff in high-risk areas should receive training in control and restraint
- Better security measures, e.g. video surveillance, security staff
- Design and layout of clinics should be relaxing and pleasant, but with security in mind.

Do not use antipsychotics in patients with heart disease (see Section 2.3, p. 182).

1 Kuhn W. Violence in the emergency department. *Postgrad Med* 1999; 105: 143–154.
2 Atakan Z, Davies T. Mental health emergencies. *BMJ* 1997; 314: 1740–1742.

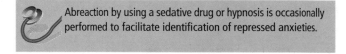

2 Diseases and treatments

2.1 Dissociative disorders

Psychopathology

There is a temporary but drastic modification of a person's character or sense of personal identity, usually to avoid emotional distress, but also occurring at times of extreme emotion, e.g. religious experiences, drug intoxication.

Epidemiology

The exact prevalence is unknown. They are more common in women and adolescents/young adults. They may occur in epidemics, especially in children. Dissociative amnesia is the most common, fugue is rare. The prevalence of dissociative identity disorder among psychiatric admissions in the USA has been reported as high as 0.5–2% [1]. In the UK it is rarely diagnosed and the symptoms are often felt to fit in better with the concept of personality disorder.

As an isolated symptom, depersonalization is very common, but as a recurrent persistent problem it is rare.

Clinical presentation

Dissociative disorders present in different ways [1] and the features of recognizable syndromes are described in Table 10.

Differential diagnosis

Conditions that may present with dissociative symptoms include [2]:
* schizophrenia
* temporal lobe epilepsy
* depression

Table 10 Types of dissociative disorders.

Type	Characteristics
Amnesia	Sudden inability to recall periods of their lives or identity
Fugue	Travel away from usual surroundings, amnesia for past identity and may even assume new identity
Identity disorder	Presence of two or more distinct identities/personality states
Depersonalization	Mental processes or body are perceived as unreal, remote or automatized—'dream-like state'

* head injury
* delirium
* dementia
* drugs
* acute stress disorder.

Treatment

Treatment needs to be tailored to the individual and the following are guiding principles.
* Treat any underlying medical and psychiatric illnesses that may be the primary problem.
* Identify and address stressors.
* Use psychological interventions to help the person process and integrate stressful feelings [2].

> Abreaction by using a sedative drug or hypnosis is occasionally performed to facilitate identification of repressed anxieties.

Prognosis

Dissociative amnesia and fugue usually recover as abruptly as they started and recovery is usually complete with few relapses. Dissociative identity disorder is often associated with borderline personality disorder and usually has a chronic course, seldom with complete resolution of symptoms [1].

Frankel FH. Dissociation: the clinical realities. *Am J Psychiatry* 1996; 153: 64–70.
1 Gelder M, Gath D, Mayou R, Cowen P (eds). *Oxford Textbook of Psychiatry* (4th edn). Oxford: Oxford University Press, 2000: 160–196.
2 Kaplan HI, Saddock BJ. *Synopsis of Psychiatry* (8th edn). Baltimore, MD: Williams and Wilkins, 1998: 660–676.

2.2 Dementia

Psychopathophysiology

Dementia is characterized by:
* memory impairment
* multiple other cognitive impairments
* a decline from previous levels of functioning
* mood and behaviour changes
* no impairment of consciousness.

Epidemiology

In community residents, 5% over 65 years and 20% over 80 years have dementia, comprising [1]:
- 50% due to Alzheimer's disease
- 5–25% due to dementia with Lewy bodies
- 10–20% due to vascular dementia.

Huntington's disease affects women and men equally, usually diagnosed in late 30 s and 40 s, but can occur between 4 and 85 years. Prion diseases, e.g. Creutzfeldt–Jakob disease (including new variant), are rare, and age of onset depend on age at exposure to the prions and incubation period. HIV and head injury affect a younger population. Minor cognitive problems due to HIV are common [2] and AIDS dementia complex is the AIDS-defining illness in about 4.5% of cases [3].

Clinical presentation

The typical clinical presentations of the different types of dementia are shown in Table 11.

Table 11 Clinical presentation of dementia.

Alzheimer's disease [4]
Gradual onset and decline. Forgetfulness, lack of spontaneity, disorientation, depressed mood, deterioration in self care, dysphasia, apraxia, agnosia and executive dysfunction

Vascular dementia [1]
Presence of vascular disease elsewhere. Course is typically fluctuating with stepwise progression. Similar to Alzheimer's disease and differentiation difficult, although presence of strokes or localizing signs are highly suggestive

Lewy body dementia [1]
Fluctuating cognition, visual hallucinations, parkinsonism, neuroleptic sensitivity, falls/transient loss of consciousness/syncope, delusions

Frontal lobe dementia [1]
Personality changes, executive dysfunction, deterioration in social skills, emotional blunting, disinhibition and language problems

Human immunodeficiency virus [4]
Forgetfulness, slowness, poor concentration, problem-solving difficulty, apathy, neurological abnormalities

Head injury [4]
Depends on location and extent of brain injury. Memory impairment, attention problems, irritability, lability, apathy

Huntington's disease [4]
Depression, irritability, anxiety, choreoathetosis, memory impairment, executive functioning problems (single autosomal dominant gene on chromosome 4)

Prion diseases [4]
Fatigue, anxiety, poor concentration, involuntary movements, periodic electroencephalogram activity and progressive cognitive impairment

Executive dysfunction = problems with planning, organization, sequencing and abstraction; all functions of the frontal lobe.

Differential diagnosis

Exclude reversible cause of cognitive dysfunction:
- 'pseudodementia' due to depression
- delirium
- alcohol
- hypothyroidism
- syphilis
- vitamin B_{12} deficiency
- normal pressure hydrocephalus.

Treatment

Consider the following [5]:
- Social support
- Behavioural problems managed through behavioural and environmental modifications. Rarely a short course of low-dose neuroleptics (e.g. risperidone) may be used as an adjunctive. Also antidepressants to treat low mood and regulate sleep
- Cholinesterase inhibitors in Alzheimer's disease, e.g. donepezil, rivastigmine
- Insufficient evidence as yet to recommend vitamin E or ginko biloba.

Complications

Be aware that complications of dementia are not only medical, but also social and behavioural problems that include:
- distress of caregivers [5]
- social isolation
- self neglect
- risk of personal injury, e.g. accidents, falls, wandering
- vulnerability to exploitation
- aggression and other behavioural problems.

Prognosis

Alzheimer's disease has a variable course, but death usually occurs within 5–8 years of onset [2]. Except for dementia due to head injury, all dementias are progressive, but in some progression can be halted temporarily (e.g. HIV, Alzheimer's disease) or permanently (e.g. hypothyroidism, syphilis).

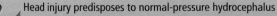
Head injury predisposes to normal-pressure hydrocephalus
- Enlarged ventricles
- Progressive dementia
- Urinary incontinence
- Gait disturbance.

Prevention

Consider the following [5]:
- genetic counselling (Huntington's)
- cardiovascular disease prevention and treatment
- antioxidants, e.g. vitamin E, selegiline
- hormone replacement therapy in Alzheimer's disease
- non-steroidal anti-inflammatory drugs (NSAIDs) in Alzheimer's disease.

Important information for patients

People with dementia should be encouraged to plan early for eventual cessation of driving [5].

See *Medicine for the elderly*, Section 2.7; *Neurology*, Section 2.4.
1. Jones RW. Dementia. *Scott Med J* 1997; 42: 151–153.
2. Gelder M, Gath D, Mayou R, Cowen P (eds). *Oxford Textbook of Psychiatry* (3rd edn). Oxford: Oxford University Press, 2000: 308–341.
3. Khouzam HR, Donnelly NH, Ibrahim NF. Psychiatric morbidity in HIV patients. *Can J Psychiatry* 1998; 43: 51–56.
4. American Psychiatric Association. *Diagnostic and Statistical Manual of Mental Disorders* (4th edn). Washington: American Psychiatric Association, 1994.
5. Patterson CJS, Gauthier S, Bergman H, *et al*. The recognition, assessment and management of dementing disorders: conclusions from the Canadian consensus conference on dementia. *Can Med Assoc J* 1999; 160 (12 Suppl.): S1–S15.

2.3 Schizophrenia and antipsychotic drugs

2.3.1 SCHIZOPHRENIA

Aetiology/psychopathology

Schizophrenia is currently believed to be a neurodevelopmental disorder. There is strong evidence of genetic risk, e.g. identical twins have a 48% chance of concordance. Structural changes seen in MRI studies include decreased volume of areas such as the parahippocampus, thalamus, superior temporal gyri and frontal lobes. Older neurotransmitter theories focused on defects in the dopamine system, but newer theories include defects in glutaminergic neurotransmission involving the hippocampal N-methyl-D-aspartate receptors.

Epidemiology

Statistics are [1]:

Table 12 Core symptoms of schizophrenia.

Symptoms	Characteristics
Delusions	Firmly held beliefs, often bizarre, on inadequate grounds, inconsistent with person's intelligence and cultural background, that cannot be altered through reasoning
Hallucinations	A perception experienced in the absence of an external stimulus to the sense organ involved
Disorganized speech	Loss of normal structure of thinking
Negative symptoms	Blunted affect, apathy, poverty of speech, attentional impairment, poor motivation
Disorganized behaviour	

- prevalence—0.5–1% of the general population
- incidence—15–20 per 100 000 per year
- median age at onset—males 28 years, females 32 years.

Clinical presentation

An important aspect of schizophrenia is its devastating effect on a person's interpersonal relations, work, self care and other goal-directed behaviours. The diagnosis of schizophrenia requires the presence of at least two symptoms in Table 12 for at least 6 months' duration, including prodromal and residual symptoms, with 1 month of active symptoms [2]. Exclude mood disorders, substance abuse and general medical conditions.

Differential diagnosis

Other disorders presenting with schizophrenia-like symptoms include the following [2]:
- schizophreniform disorder—symptoms present for 1–6 months' duration
- schizoaffective disorder—concurrent mania or severe depression
- delusional disorder—encapsulated delusions with minimal hallucinations
- brief psychotic disorder—less than 1 month's duration
- shared psychotic disorder—an individual influenced by someone else
- due to general medical condition
- substance induced.

Treatment

This is a complex illness that needs a comprehensive treatment approach. Always obtain collateral information. Physical examination and special investigations are needed to exclude concurrent medical problems. A useful approach to treatment is to use the 'biological, psychological, social' guidelines in Table 13.

Table 13 'Biological, psychological, social' approach for the treatment of schizophrenia.

Biological
Antipsychotic medication

Psychological
Cognitive therapy
Crisis management
Social skills training

Social
Family therapy
Vocational rehabilitation
Education

 High expressed emotion, i.e. criticism, hostility and overinvolvement of parents or caregivers, towards people with schizophrenia is a significant risk factor for relapse.

Complications

Suicide
Ten per cent of patients with schizophrenia die by suicide, and up to 50% attempt suicide.

Prognosis

Prognosis is variable and difficult to predict for any individual [3]. Estimates are as follows:
• 20–30% good prognosis
• 20–30% continue to experience mild symptoms
• 40–60% significantly impaired for the rest of their lives.

Predictors of poor outcome [3]:
• male
• obstetric complications
• abnormal premorbid personality
• low IQ
• single
• early age at onset
• insidious onset
• substance abuse
• family history of schizophrenia
• absence of obvious precipitant.

2.3.2 ANTIPSYCHOTICS

Principle

About 70% of patients with schizophrenia respond to standard antipsychotic drugs, and a further 10% respond

Table 14 Subgroups of antipsychotics.

Subgroup	Examples	Discussion
Low-potency drugs	Chlorpromazine, thioridazine	Generally associated with more anticholinergic, antihistaminergic and α-adrenergic blocking side effects. Therefore more epileptogenic and cardiotoxic (prolonged QT interval)
High-potency drugs	Haloperidol, droperidol, trifluoperazine	Associated with greater extrapyramidal side effects
Atypical drugs [6]	Clozapine, risperidone, olanzapine, quetiapine	Far fewer side effects. Agranulocytosis is a serious problem with clozapine Weight gain and sedation can be problematic

to atypical antipsychotics. Antipsychotics also significantly reduce relapse rates [4].

The main mechanism of action of antipsychotics is through blocking dopamine receptors. The atypicals also act by blocking serotonin receptors in the striatal system and the frontal cortex, hence fewer extrapyramidal side effects and greater efficacy for negative symptoms [5].

Antipsychotics can be divided into low-potency, high-potency and atypical drugs (Table 14).

Indications

The main indication is for psychosis, and use in any other condition (Table 15) must be carefully considered because these drugs have severe side effects that can be permanent, most notably tardive dyskinesia.

Use antipsychotics judiciously because of the risk of tardive dyskinesia.

Table 15 Other conditions in which antipsychotics are used [3].

Condition	Example of antipsychotic
Anxiety	Low doses used
Impulsivity	Low doses used
Tourette's syndrome	Haloperidol
Nausea	Prochlorperazine
Chronic hiccoughs	Chlorpromazine
Infant opioid withdrawal	Chlorpromazine
Emergency sedation	Haloperidol, droperidol, risperidone (elderly)

Antipsychotics

- Always use the lowest dose possible.
- Start with a low dose and slowly titrate up until therapeutic effect is achieved.
- Always be aware of side effects.
- Do not use more than one antipsychotic at a time.

Contraindications

- Drowsiness, confusion, coma due to CNS depressants
- Bone-marrow suppression
- Phaeochromocytoma
- If at all possible avoid in pregnancy and breast feeding.

Complications

Side effects

Side effects to antipsychotics are common, and they can be severe and even life threatening. These are listed and briefly described in Table 16.

Most important adverse effects of antipsychotics

- Agranulocytosis
- Neuroleptic malignant syndrome
- Acute dystonia
- Tardive dyskinesia
- Akathisia.

Table 16 Side effects of antipsychotics.

Side effect	Characteristic
Extrapyramidal symptoms	Stiffness, tremor, hypersalivation, acute dystonia, akathisia, tardive dyskinesia
Anticholinergic symptoms	Blurred vision, constipation, urinary retention, dry mouth, confusion, agitation, seizures
Antihistaminergic symptoms	Sedation
α-adrenergic blocking	Orthostatic hypotension
Leucopenia	Agranulocytosis can occur with all antipsychotics, but high incidence with clozapine
Increased prolactin secretion	Amenorrhoea, galactorrhoea, sexual dysfunction
Weight gain	—
Obstructive jaundice	Thought to be due to additives in old phenothiazine preparations
Retinitis pigmentosa	Associated with thioridazine at doses above 600 mg/day
Allergic dermatitis and photosensitivity	—
Neuroleptic malignant syndrome [2]	Muscle rigidity, hyperthermia, fluctuating level of consciousness and autonomic dysfunction, leucocytosis, elevated creatine phosphokinase

1 Gelder M, Gath D, Mayou R, Cowen P (eds). *Oxford Textbook of Psychiatry* (4th edn). Oxford: Oxford University Press, 2000: 246–293.
2 American Psychiatric Association. *Diagnostic and Statistical Manual of Mental Disorders* (4th edn). Washington: American Psychiatric Association, 1994.
3 Kaplan HI, Saddock BJ. *Synopsis of Psychiatry* (8th edn). Baltimore, MD: Williams and Wilkins, 1998: 1019–1042.
4 Kane JM. Management strategies for the treatment of Schizophrenia. *J Clin Psychiatry* 1999; 60 (Suppl. 12): 13–17.
5 Schultz SK, Andreasen NC. Schizophrenia. *Lancet* 1999; 353: 1425–1430.
6 McGrath J, Emmerson WB. Treatment of schizophrenia. *BMJ* 1999; 319: 1045–1048.

2.4 Personality disorder

Psychopathology

Personality disorder (PD) is defined in DSM-IV [1] as an enduring pattern of inner experience and behaviour that:
- deviates markedly from the expectations of the individual's culture
- is pervasive and inflexible
- has an onset in adolescence or early adulthood
- is stable over time; and
- leads to distress or impairment.

PD is often accompanied by a history of being abused or having behavioural disturbances during childhood. There are different types of PD (Table 17).

Table 17 Classification of personality disorders.

Cluster	Types	Characteristics
A	Paranoid, schizoid and schizotypal	Often appear odd or eccentric
B	Antisocial, borderline, histrionic and narcissistic	Often appear dramatic, emotional and erratic
C	Avoidant, dependent and obsessive–compulsive [1]	Often appear anxious or fearful

Epidemiology

The prevalence ranges between 2 and 13% in the general population [2]. There are gender differences:
- antisocial PD diagnosed more frequently in men
- histrionic, borderline and dependent PD diagnosed more frequently in women.

Clinical presentation

Diagnosis needs a longitudinal view of a person's lifelong behaviour patterns. Difficult and odd behaviour in reaction to a stressful situation can easily be confused with a personality disorder [2,3].

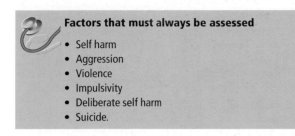

Factors that must always be assessed

- Self harm
- Aggression
- Violence
- Impulsivity
- Deliberate self harm
- Suicide.

Comorbid mental illness is frequently present, e.g. depression, drug dependence, alcohol dependence, anxiety disorders [3].

Treatment

Psychotherapy remains the mainstay of treatment. The success rate can be as high as 52% of patients recovering sufficiently to no longer meet the diagnostic criteria for PD [4]. Types of psychotherapy used include:
- psychodynamic therapy
- cognitive–behavioural therapy
- interpersonal therapy
- group therapy.

Certain PDs tend to be resistant to treatment, e.g. antisocial PD.

Drug treatments are only occasionally effective in reducing problematic behaviours and should be prescribed in a specialist setting only. The following have been found to have some limited efficacy [2]:
- antipsychotics and selective serotonin reuptake inhibitors (SSRIs) at low doses for impulsive deliberate self harm behaviour
- carbamazepine for aggressive behaviour.

> **!** Drug treatments can be effective when they are used to treat a comorbid illness, e.g. depression, and problem behaviours may abate.

Prognosis

The course of PD is variable, but as a general rule it ameliorates with age and may even remit.

1 American Psychiatric Association. *Diagnostic and Statistical Manual of Mental Disorders* (4th edn). Washington: American Psychiatric Association, 1994.
2 Marlowe M, Sugarman P. Disorders of personality. *Br J Psychiatry* 1997; 315: 176–179.
3 Dhossche DM, Shevitz SA. Assessment and importance of personality disorders in medical patients: an update. *South Med J* 1999; 92(6): 546–556.
4 Perry JC, Banon E, Ianni F. Effectiveness of psychotherapy for personality disorders. *Am J Psychiatry* 1999; 156(9): 1312–1321.

2.5 Psychiatric presentation of physical disease

Epidemiology

Psychiatric symptoms are common in general medical conditions: on general medical wards 15–25% of patients experience delirium [1], and 30–50% of patients with epilepsy have a psychiatric difficulty at some time.

Clinical presentation

When medical conditions have psychiatric symptoms as part of their presentation, it is necessary to decide whether psychiatric symptoms are:
- a result of the medical illness
- part of a separate mental disorder
- a psychological reaction to having an illness (see Section 2.6, p. 186).

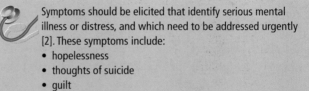

Symptoms should be elicited that identify serious mental illness or distress, and which need to be addressed urgently [2]. These symptoms include:
- hopelessness
- thoughts of suicide
- guilt
- loss of interest
- severe insomnia
- psychosis.

Common mental disorders that may be the result of an underlying medical condition or medication are as follows [1]:
- delirium
- dementia
- amnesia
- mood disorders
- anxiety disorders
- eating disorders
- sleep disorder
- sexual disorders.

Medical conditions that commonly present with symptoms and signs of mental disorder:
- epilepsy
- degenerative disorders, e.g. Parkinson's, Huntington's, Wilson's diseases
- brain tumours
- head trauma
- demyelinating disorders
- infectious disease, e.g. syphilis, encephalitis, meningitis, Creutzfeldt–Jakob disease, HIV (AIDS)

- autoimmune immune disorders, e.g. systemic lupus erythematosus (SLE)
- endocrine disorders, e.g. thyroid, pituitary, adrenal disease
- metabolic disorders, e.g. hepatic, uraemic, hypoglycaemic encephalopathies, porphyria
- nutritional disorders, e.g. thiamine, niacin deficiencies
- toxins, e.g. organophosphates, heavy metals.

> **Other comorbid problems that may complicate the picture**
>
> - Alcohol and drug abuse
> - Personality disorders
> - Malingering.

Treatment

A general principle is to address medical problems as far as possible before attempting to treat any psychiatric symptoms or suspected mental disorders, because these may resolve. However, circumstances may be such that recovery from the medical condition is dependent on the person's mental health and then the mental disorder should be treated early. For example, a person with diabetes may find their motivation to remain compliant with treatment is poor because they are depressed. Very severe psychiatric problems clearly warrant symptomatic treatment.

> **Psychiatric treatments in physical illness**
>
> Treatments are the same as would be used in patients who did not have concurrent physical illness, but be aware of drug interactions.

Treatment strategies to help alleviate psychiatric symptoms are as follows:
- Use an empathic, reassuring approach.
- Ensure physical needs are met.
- Provide information about illness, investigations, treatment and their likely effects to help allay fears and anxieties.
- The nursing environment should be well lit, quiet and tranquil.
- Invite family or other people who are familiar to visit.
- Hypnotics and anxiolytics should only be used if the patient is not responding to the above treatment strategies.

If there is concern that the patient is severely depressed, or psychotic, a psychiatric opinion should be sought immediately. Otherwise a psychiatric assessment may be helpful in identifying the psychological processes that are affecting recovery and compliance.

> 1 Kaplan HI, Saddock BJ. *Synopsis of Psychiatry* (8th edn). Baltimore, MD: Williams and Wilkins, 1998: 350–364.
> 2 Gelder M, Gath D, Mayou R, Cowen P. *Oxford Textbook of Psychiatry* (3rd edn). Oxford: Oxford University Press, 2000: 342–413.

2.6 Psychological reactions to physical illness (adjustment disorders)

Aetiology/psychopathology

When considering psychiatric disorder in a physically ill person, think of the possible interactions between mind, body and behaviour (Table 18).

The commonest reactions to physical illness and disability are adjustment disorders. These are generally seen in primary care, but 5–20% of psychiatric outpatients may present with this clinical picture. The stressor is usually much less intense and severe than in cases of post traumatic stress disorder. The onset should be within 1 month or so of the stressful event. Predisposing factors include PD or immature personality.

Table 18 Possible interactions between mind, body and behaviour.

Coincidental
A person with schizophrenia contracts pneumonia

Causal
Physical illness causing psychiatric disorder, e.g. hypothyroidism causing depression

Reactive
Anxiety and depression are the commonest reactions to threatening or progressive illness

Iatrogenic
Treatment of physical illness causes psychiatric disorder, e.g. L-dopa causing delirium

Reciprocal
Failure to mobilize after a stroke causing and/or caused by depression

Compliance
Poor compliance, e.g. in the depressed diabetic or hypertensive, or abuse of prescribed medication, e.g. analgesics and hypnotics

Somatization
Psychiatric illness presents as a physical one

Denial
A psychological defence mechanism by which frightening news, e.g. a diagnosis of cancer, is excluded from conscious awareness and the patient behaves as if they are unaware of the distressing facts

Epidemiology

Males and females are equally affected.

Clinical presentation

- Usually severe subjective distress and emotional disturbance (this is based on the clinician's own subjective judgement)
- Impairment of social functioning and performance
- Onset within 1 month of a significant life change leading to continued unpleasant circumstances.

Symptoms include:
- depressed mood
- tearfulness and/or hopelessness
- nervousness
- anxiety
- worry
- inability to cope or plan ahead
- disability in performance of daily routine.

The symptoms are not sufficiently severe to justify a more specific diagnosis such as major depression. Usual duration is a maximum of 6 months. Symptoms can last longer in a chronic disabling medical condition.

Diagnosing depression in physical illness

Approximately 30% of cancer patients develop depression, a generalized anxiety disorder or an adjustment disorder within the first 2 years of diagnosis, but only a small proportion of this morbidity is recognized and treated.

Depression in physical illness

Be aware:
- of dismissing depression as an understandable reaction to severe illness
- that biological symptoms are unreliable, therefore use the Hospital Anxiety and Depression (HAD) Scale (see below)
- of depressive cognitions, e.g. 'I deserve to be ill', or 'I am not worth treating', also loss of interest in other people
- of suicidal ideas
- of tearfulness (especially in men)
- of indecisiveness
- of past history of depression.

The diagnosis of depression in patients with physical illness can be complicated by the presence of:
- fatigue
- loss of appetite and sex drive
- insomnia.

These symptoms can also be the typical biological symptoms of depression. It is helpful to use the HAD Scale that excludes somatic symptoms and concentrates on the psychological symptoms of depression and anxiety (Fig. 1). This self-rating scale has only 14 items and is easy to complete and to score. It was designed specifically for use in non-psychiatric hospital departments [1]. A score of 11 or more on either the anxiety or the depression subscale indicates 'caseness' (the range on each subscale is 0–21).

Treatment

- Encourage discussion and ventilation of feelings to help overcome denial and avoidance.
- Teach a problem-solving technique.

Problem-solving technique

Problem solving is a straightforward counselling technique with the following components:
- listing the problems
- selecting one specific problem to focus on
- listing alternative courses of action
- evaluating each action plan
- selecting and implementing the most promising course of action
- evaluating results of the trial
- repeating the process until positive results are obtained.

This technique is applied collaboratively with the patient, who takes responsibility for the process, thereby enhancing their sense of autonomy and control.

Complications

Complications of adjustment disorders include:
- decreased compliance with medical treatment
- increased length of hospital stay
- impaired performance at work
- disruption of social relationships
- increased risk of suicide attempts and suicide.

House A, Mayou R, Mallinson C (eds). *Psychiatric Aspects of Physical Disease.* London: Royal Colleges of Physicians and Psychiatrists, 1995.

Murray Parkes C, Markus A. *Coping with Loss: helping patients and their families.* London: BMJ Publishing Group, 1998.

van der Molen B. *Communication and Cancer: how to give and receive information.* London: The Cancer Resource Centre, 1999.

1 Zigmond AS, Snaith RP. The Hospital Anxiety and Depression Scale. *Acta Psychiatr Scand* 1983; 67: 361–370.

This questionnaire will help you to let us know how you are. Read each item and underline the response which comes closest to how you have felt in the last few days. Don't take too long over your replies, your immediate reaction will probably be more accurate than a long thought-out response.

I feel tense or 'wound up'

Most of the time

A lot of the time

From time to time, occasionally

Not at all

I still enjoy the things I used to enjoy

Definitely as much

Not quite as much

Only a little

Hardly at all

I get a sort of frightened feeling as if something awful is about to happen

Very definitely and quite badly

Yes, but not badly

A little, but it doesn't worry me

Not at all

I can laugh and see the funny side of things

As much as I always could

Not quite so much now

Definitely not as much now

Not at all

Worrying thoughts go through my mind

A great deal of the time

A lot of the time

From time to time but not often

Only occasionally

I feel cheerful

Not at all

Not often

Sometimes

Most of the time

I can sit at ease and feel relaxed

Definitely

Usually

Not often

Not at all

I feel as if I am slowed down

Nearly all the time

Very often

Sometimes

Not at all

I get a sort of frightened feeling like 'butterflies' in my stomach

Not at all

Occasionally

Quite often

Very often

I have lost interest in my appearance

Definitely

I don't take as much care as I should

I may not take quite as much care

I take just as much care as ever

I feel restless as if I have to be on the move

Very much indeed

Quite a lot

Not very much

Not at all

I look forward with enjoyment to things

As much as ever I did

Rather less than I used to

Definitely less than I used to

Hardly at all

I get sudden feelings of panic

Very often indeed

Quite often

Not very often

Not at all

I can enjoy a good book or radio or TV programme

Often

Sometimes

Not often

Very seldom

Fig. 1 Hospital Anxiety and Depression (HAD) Scale [1]. Four options follow each statement: the best response (least anxious or depressed) scores 0; the worst response (most anxious or depressed) scores 3. See text for further discussion.

2.7 Anxiety disorders

Anxiety is familiar to everyone as an adaptive response to external threat. Normal fear and apprehension are accompanied by increased activity of the sympathetic nervous system in preparation for 'fight or flight'. Anxiety becomes pathological when it is excessive, prolonged or recurrent, and inward-looking (Table 19).

Morbid anxiety can be either:
- generalized (generalized anxiety disorder—see below)
- episodic (panic disorder—see Section 2.7.2, p. 190)
- situational (phobias—see Section 2.7.3, p. 191).

The distinction between these is shown in Table 20. See also Section 1.2, p. 165.

2.7.1 GENERALIZED ANXIETY DISORDER

Aetiology/psychopathology

A genetic contribution to generalized anxiety disorder (GAD) has not yet been established.

Biology of anxiety

- Release of noradrenaline (NA), e.g. by yohimbine, increases anxiety.
- Gamma amino butyric acid (GABA) inhibits anxiety.

There may be an underlying anxious personality disorder (see Section 2.4, p. 184) with long-standing persistent and pervasive feelings of tension, apprehension

Table 19 Comparison of normal and morbid anxiety.

	Normal anxiety	Pathological anxiety
Reaction to a threat	Proportionate	Excessive
Duration	Brief	Prolonged
Focus of attention	Towards the external world	Inwardly directed; morbid preoccupation with physiological response, e.g. rapid heart beat means imminent heart attack

Table 20 Distinction between generalized anxiety disorder (GAD), panic disorder and phobias.

Diagnosis	Characteristics of morbid anxiety
GAD	Continuous pervasive and persistent ('free floating')
Panic disorder	Episodic with intense unpredictable panic attacks lasting about 15 min. Can occur in any situation
Phobias	Situation specific

and inferiority with an intense fear of disapproval and rejection.

The precipitating event is generally a threat to the person's security in a relationship or at work, or being given the diagnosis of a serious physical illness. Thus, 'danger events', i.e. the expectation of loss or deprivation, precede anxiety [1] while depression tends to be preceded by actual loss. Anxiety reactions are more likely to occur where there is lack of social support due to separation, divorce or bereavement. Some physical disorders and drugs are particularly likely to be associated with GAD (Table 21).

Table 21 Medical disorders and drugs causing generalized anxiety.

Medical
Hyperthyroidism
Hypoglycaemia
Cardiac dysrhythmia
Phaeochromocytoma
Respiratory dysfunction

Prescribed drugs
Selective serotonin reuptake inhibitors
Sympatheticomimetics

Recreational drugs
Caffeine
Amphetamine
Cocaine
LSD

Drug withdrawal
Alcohol
Benzodiazepines
Opiates

Epidemiology

- Six-month prevalence is 2.5–6.5%. The OPCS National Survey of Psychiatric Morbidity found that in the week before interview nearly 3% of the population had a GAD and over 7% had a mixed anxiety depression [2].
- More common in females. This might be due to conflict between work and the responsibilities of child care.
- Rates of neurotic disorders such as anxiety are much commoner in those with lower socio-economic status.
- Onset is commonest in late adolescence and early adulthood.

Clinical presentation

Anxiety states are characterized by a combination of psychological and somatic symptoms.

Psychological symptoms

- An inappropriate and excessive sense of apprehensiveness and dread that impairs everyday functioning

Table 22 Somatic symptoms of anxiety.

Somatic symptom	Signs
Autonomic arousal	Palpitations
	Muscle tremor
	Sweating
	Epigastric discomfort
Muscle tension	Constricting headaches
	Backache
Hyperventilation	Paraesthesia
	Headache
	Dizziness
	Faintness

- Excessive fear of loss, illness, death, accident, losing control, going insane
- Irritability, restlessness, worrying, poor concentration, insomnia
- Thoughts of impending personal catastrophe.

Somatic symptoms

These arise from autonomic arousal, muscle tension and hyperventilation (Table 22). Hyperventilation causes a low PCO_2 and alkalosis.
- Cardiac—rapid heart beat, palpitations
- Pulmonary—hyperventilation, tightness in chest, breathlessness
- Gastrointestinal—dry mouth, difficulty in swallowing, 'butterflies in the stomach', nausea, frequent bowel motions
- Urinary—frequency
- Neurological—headache, light-headedness, paraesthesia around mouth and in hands, tremor, muscle aches
- Autonomic—sweating, shakiness, feeling too hot or cold, erectile impotence.

Treatment

- Try to avoid benzodiazepines. Beta-blockers might help to reduce tremor. A sedative antidepressant, e.g. trazodone, reduces insomnia.
- Cognitive–behavioural therapy is the safest and most effective treatment [3].

Complications

- Anxiety disorders are associated with increased mortality due to suicide as well as alcohol and smoking-related disorders [4].
- Dependence on benzodiazepines, hypnotics and alcohol.

Prognosis

Good prognostic indicators:

- a stable premorbid personality
- development of acute symptoms in response to transitory stress.

There is a poor prognosis with:
- chronic or severe symptoms
- agitation, depersonalization or conversion symptoms
- suicidal preoccupations
- persistent social/occupational factors
- inadequate social support.

> **!** Patients with an anxiety disorder:
> - might have a concurrent depressive illness
> - might later develop a depressive illness
> - might present with somatic rather than psychological symptoms
> - might have an underlying medical disorder (see Table 21).

2.7.2 PANIC DISORDER

Aetiology/psychopathology

Panic disorder consists of recurrent bouts of intense and rapidly escalating anxiety associated with the anticipation of imminent personal catastrophe. The condition is probably caused by an interaction between biochemical and psychological events, perhaps from a biochemical abnormality associated with poorly regulated autonomic responses. Patients with panic disorder are more likely than normal subjects to experience panic attacks when given:
- yohimbine, an α-adrenergic antagonist; or
- sodium lactate infusions.

Panic disorder is five times commoner in first-degree relatives than in the general population.

Psychological factors

Patients with panic disorder are more likely than those with GAD to make alarming deductions from the physical symptoms of anxiety. According to this cognitive hypothesis, there is a vicious circle of fear (Fig. 2) which intensifies the autonomic response so that the patient interprets an increase in their heart rate as a sign of an imminent heart attack, which in turns heightens their anxiety and further accelerates their heart rate.

Epidemiology

There is a lifetime prevalence of 1.5%, with the onset usually before the age of 40. There is a female to male ratio of 2 : 1.

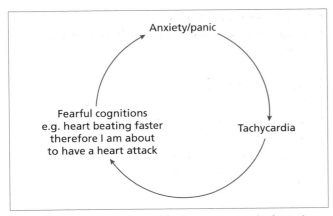

Fig. 2 The vicious circle of emotion, autonomic response and negative thoughts.

Clinical presentation

The patient experiences repeated unexpected bouts of severe anxiety that can occur in any situation and are not restricted to certain places. Physical and psychological symptoms are similar to those of GAD but are episodic and intense. There is an overwhelming fear of loss of control and of imminent death, generally from a heart attack. As the disorder progresses, fear and avoidance of specific situations develops, generally of places such as supermarket checkout queues and public transport where the patient fears they might be trapped and unable to obtain emergency medical assistance. As the patient becomes increasingly house-bound, their disorder might be more appropriately labelled as panic disorder with agoraphobia.

Differential diagnosis

Panic attacks can occur in the course of GAD, agoraphobia, depression and alcohol withdrawal. The diagnosis of panic disorder depends on the characteristics and severity of the panic attacks and on whether their onset precedes one of these other conditions.

Treatment

• Provide reassurance and explanation by describing the interaction between fear and overactivity of the sympathetic nervous system.
• Give the patient a simple diagram of the vicious circle that develops when fear caused by the physical symptoms of anxiety intensifies their thoughts of imminent catastrophe (Fig. 2).
• It might be necessary to give a single dose of a benzodiazepine (e.g. diazepam) to a patient who is just recovering from a panic attack, but benzodiazepines are to be avoided in the longer-term treatment of panic disorder because of the risk of dependence.

• Antidepressants have anti-panic effects.
• Cognitive–behavioural therapy—this is as effective as antidepressants and has a lower relapse rate.
   Antidepressents used include:
• imipramine—low starting dose of 10 mg daily (a higher initial dose can actually exacerbate anxiety and insomnia). The dose is gradually increased over a period of weeks to about 150 mg daily. Be aware of cardiovascular and anti-cholinergic side effects as well as α-adrenoceptor blockade and the risk of seizures. Note that about one-third of patients with panic disorder relapse when imipramine is withdrawn.
• SSRIs—be aware of rebound anxiety when the anti-depressant is withdrawn as well as common gastrointestinal and sexual side effects.

Complications

• Major depressive disorder occurs in at least half of those who have panic disorder.
• Agoraphobia is a common complication.
• Some patients become dependent on alcohol as a form of self medication.
• Benzodiazepine dependence is not uncommon.

Prognosis

The course tends to fluctuate. Even with treatment 20–30% of patients with panic disorder are symptomatic at 6-year follow-up.

Rickels K, Scheweizer E. The clinical presentation of generalized anxiety in primary care settings: practical concepts of classification and management. *J Clin Psychiatry* 1997; 58: 4–10.
Snaith P. *Clinical Neurosis* (2nd edn). Oxford: Oxford University Press, 1991.
1 Finlay-Jones R. Anxiety. In: Brown G, Harris T, eds. *Life Events and Illness*. London: Hyman, 1989: 95–112.
2 Melzer H, Gill B, Petticrew M. OPCS Surveys of Psychiatric Morbidity in Great Britain. Report no. 1. The prevalence of psychiatric morbidity among adults aged 16–64 living in private households in Great Britain. London: HMSO, 1995.
3 Clark DM, Fairburn CG. *Science and Practice of Cognitive Behaviour Therapy*. Oxford: Oxford University Press, 1997.
4 Allgulander C. Suicide and mortality patterns in anxiety neurosis and depressive neurosis. *Arch Gen Psychiatry* 1994; 51: 702–712.

2.7.3 PHOBIC ANXIETY DISORDERS

Aetiology

The cardinal features of phobias are:
• fear
• avoidance.

	Age of onset, general	Male/female ratio	Other features	Prevalence in population (%)
Specific phobias	From childhood	F ≫ M	Might follow traumatic event, e.g. being trapped in a lift	10
Blood/injury/ injection phobia	From childhood	F > M	Vasovagal reaction, positive family history	(not known)
Agoraphobia	Age 20–40	F ≫ M	Often associated with panic attacks	3
Social phobia	Mid-teens	F = M		2.5

Table 23 Epidemiology of phobias.

The fear is disproportionate to the circumstances and the patient recognizes this. Despite this insight, the phobic patient feels intensely anxious at the very thought of a particular situation.

Phobias are classified as:
- specific or simple
- blood/injection/injury
- agoraphobia
- social phobia.

Specific or simple phobias

Simple phobias can sometimes be traced to a single traumatic incident such as being stuck in a lift or underground train, being attacked by a vicious dog or involvement in a road traffic accident. Specific phobias might sound trivial but they can severely impair performance at work and social life (e.g. due to inability to travel by plane). Specific phobias include familiar fears of:
- spiders
- snakes
- heights
- flying
- thunder.

Blood/injection/injury phobia

Blood/injection/injury phobia can occur after a traumatic medical incident, and is the most important phobia in the hospital setting. It includes the sight of blood, injury or medical apparatus, especially syringes and needles. There might also be excessive fear of contamination. A phobia of diseases such as AIDS might lead to total avoidance of physical contact with other people, repeated medical consultations, or multiple requests for HIV testing. This could lead to:
- delay in seeking medical help
- refusal to have blood tests
- reluctance to submit to any invasive medical procedure.

Blood/injection/injury phobia is associated with an unusual physiological response. Whereas other specific phobias are associated with acceleration of heart rate on exposure to the focus of fear and avoidance, blood/injection/injury phobic people have a strong vasovagal response with deceleration of heart rate and a fall in blood pressure.

Agoraphobia

Agoraphobia sometimes follows one or two isolated panic attacks occurring in a public, crowded or confined space. The patient's fear of a further attack encourages them to remain at home. This avoidance behaviour prevents deconditioning and perpetuates the condition, which is reinforced by the conviction that further potentially harmful panic attacks will occur if they venture out again.

Social phobias

Social phobias might develop after an embarrassing incident. Thus, a sensitive person whose credit card is rejected due to a computer error might subsequently be afraid to sign cheques in public because they fear that their anxious tremor will be noticed.

Epidemiology

The epidemiology of various phobias is shown in Table 23.

Clinical presentation

The phobic patient experiences both the psychological and the somatic symptoms of morbid anxiety in specific circumstances. Even the anticipation of those situations provokes anxiety and this leads to avoidance. Patients may postpone seeking treatment until there is a change in their domestic or occupational circumstances which forces them to seek help. For example, the social phobic may be given the responsibility of making a public presentation; an agoraphobic may lose a relative who used to do his or her shopping; whilst a blood/injection/injury phobic might develop severe anaemia and need to have laboratory tests.

Agoraphobia

Agoraphobics fear and avoid any situation from which escape might be difficult or embarrassing. Agoraphobic people are afraid of:
- leaving home
- going into crowded places (e.g. supermarkets)
- using public transport
- collapsing, having a convulsion, fainting
- going mad
- being incontinent in a public place
- having a heart attack without access to immediate help.

Social phobia

Social phobia is the fear and avoidance of social situations (e.g. restaurants, parties, public speaking, committee meetings). In social phobia the fear is that others will regard the person as gauche or will notice his or her anxiety-induced tremulousness or sweating.

Differential diagnosis

A delusional disorder (see Section 2.13, p. 202) has to be excluded in both social phobias and agoraphobia.
- In social phobia, the person retains insight and recognizes that the fear that other people will observe them and judge them critically is excessive and disproportionate. The person is aware that the discomfort derives from his or her own self consciousness. By contrast, the paranoid person suspects that other people regard them with unjustified hatred and malevolence.
- Both agoraphobic and paranoid people will be afraid to venture out of their homes, but the agoraphobic is housebound because he or she fears his or her own anxiety and panic, while the paranoid person locates danger in other people's actions and intentions.

Patients with dysmorphophobia (body dysmorphic disorder) might also eschew social events and public places (see Section 1.6, p. 172).

Treatment

Cognitive–behavioural therapy is the treatment of choice [1,2].

Complications

Dependence on alcohol and benzodiazepines.

Prognosis

Without treatment phobias tend to follow a chronic course.

Clark DM, Fairburn CG (eds). *Science and Practice of Cognitive-Behaviour Therapy*. Oxford: Oxford University Press, 1997.
Marks I. *Fears, Phobias and Rituals*. New York: Oxford University Press, 1987.
Stravynski A, Greenberg D. The treatment of social phobia: a critical assessment. *Acta Psychiatr Scand* 1998; 98: 171–181.
1 Hawton K, Salkovskis PM, Kirk J, Clark DM. *Cognitive-Behaviour Therapy for Psychiatric Problems: a practical guide*. Oxford: Oxford University Press, 1989.
2 Liebowitz MR. Update on the diagnosis and treatment of social anxiety disorder. *J Clin Psychiatry* 1999; 60: 22–26.

2.8 Obsessive–compulsive disorder

Aetiology/psychopathology

There is a possible genetic contribution to obsessive–compulsive disorder. First-degree relatives have increased rates of other psychiatric disorders, but not necessarily of obsessive–compulsive disorder. A significant proportion of sufferers have an anankastic previous personality that is characterized by extreme punctuality, orderliness and cleanliness. Obsessive–compulsive disorder is often accompanied by soft neurological signs. The condition can also occur in a number of organic disorders including Huntington's chorea, and Gilles de la Tourette's syndrome. Obsessive–compulsive disorder can also follow head injury and encephalitis. Studies of cerebral metabolic function show an association between obsessive–compulsive symptoms and striatal and orbitofrontal activity.

Epidemiology

One-week prevalence is 1.3% of the general population. Men and women are equally affected.

Clinical presentation

- Obsessions—unwanted, distressing and intrusive thoughts, images or impulses which the patient recognizes as coming from their own mind. They are involuntary and the sufferer tries to suppress them, but this resistance only heightens their frequency and intensity. Both the obsessions themselves and the attempts to resist them cause severe anxiety.
- Compulsions—stereotyped actions which are carried out either to counteract the anxiety caused by obsessional urges and images or to neutralize their imaginary disastrous consequences.

The clinical features of obsessions are:
- recurrent
- unbidden
- unwelcome

	Obsessive–compulsive disorder	Phobia	Paranoid delusions
Focus of fear	Fear of consequences of obsessions or of failure to carry out compulsive rituals	Fear and avoidance of specific situations which induce marked anxiety	Fear of danger to self from imaginary enemies
Insight	Retained (the patient partly recognizes that their fears are irrational and absurd)	Retained (the patient is aware that their fear is disproportionate to objective danger)	Absent (the patient is absolutely convinced that the danger is real and they do not try to suppress their unusual thoughts)

Table 24 The differential diagnosis of obsessive–compulsive disorder.

- distressing
- resisted
- cannot be got rid of
- accompanied by anxiety
- lead to 'cancelling out' rituals.

Compulsive rituals include repetitive hand washing, cleaning and checking, which provide temporary relief from the anxiety caused by the obsession itself or its feared consequences, e.g. that a blasphemous thought might cause a beloved relative to develop a malignant disease. Compulsive rituals are often performed a specific number of times. Many patients have obsessional doubts (*folie de doute*) which make them feel uncertain about whether they have actually carried out their rituals, so they then feel compelled to repeat this activity.

The content of obsessions is often obscene, sadistic or blasphemous. The patient might have recurrent ruminations about danger, disaster, disease or contamination. Obsessions and compulsions can occur in the course of a depressive illness and might remit on recovery from the depression.

Differential diagnosis

The main differential diagnoses to be considered are phobias and paranoid delusions: consider the characteristics shown in Table 24.

Thirty per cent of patients with major depression have obsessional symptoms while 30% of patients with obsessive–compulsive disorder also suffer concurrently from major depression.

Treatment

This consists of either behaviour therapy and/or pharmacotherapy [1,2].

Behaviour therapy

This treatment [3] consists of exposure to the environmental triggers that provoke compulsive rituals (e.g. contact with dirt), combined with prevention from carrying out the ritual activity such as compulsive hand washing (prolonged exposure and response prevention). This treatment produces long-lasting improvement in up to two-thirds of patients.

Medication

Serotonergic antidepressants such as clomipramine and fluoxetine reduce obsessive–compulsive symptoms, especially where there is concurrent clinical depression [4]. The prognosis is more favourable if obsessive–compulsive disorder is secondary to depression.

Complications

Severe depression.

Prognosis

The course tends to be chronic.

Marks I. *Fears, Phobias and Rituals*. New York: Oxford University Press, 1987.

1 Salkovskis PS. Understanding and treating obsessive–compulsive disorder. *Beh Res Ther* 1999; 37: 29–52.

2 Pigott TA, Seay SM. A review of the efficacy of selective serotonin reuptake inhibitors in obsessive–compulsive disorder. *J Clin Psychiatry* 1999; 60: 101–106.

3 Marks IM, Lelliot P, Basoglu M *et al.* Clomipramine, self-exposure and therapist-aided exposure for obsessive–compulsive rituals. *Br J Psychiatry* 1998; 52: 522–534.

4 Piccinelli M, Pini S, Bellantuono C. Efficacy of drug treatment in obsessive–compulsive disorder: a meta-analytic review. *Br J Psychiatry* 1995; 166: 424–443.

2.9 Acute stress reactions and post-traumatic stress disorder

These conditions are produced by exceptionally stressful and life-threatening events.

Table 25 Three types of reaction to stressful experiences.

	Trigger	Onset	Duration	Clinical features
Acute stress disorder	Exposure to sudden and unexpected danger, e.g. an assault	Immediate	Brief: days	Anxiety Panics Autonomic arousal Denial Numbing
Post-traumatic stress disorder	Extreme event e.g. natural disaster, transport disaster, torture, rape	Immediate or delayed	Prolonged: months/years	Intrusions Avoidance Increased arousal
Adjustment disorder	Major adverse life event, e.g. being informed of life-threatening illness, e.g. AIDS, cancer	Gradual	Prolonged: weeks/months	Denial, intrusions and memories of life event Anxiety Depression

• Acute stress reactions tend to develop rapidly and are short-lived.

• Post-traumatic stress disorder (PTSD) runs a more protracted course.

Adjustment disorders (Section 2.6) are provoked by major adverse life events which are less intense and immediately traumatic than those which cause acute stress reactions and PTSD. The characteristics of acute stress disorders, PTSD and adjustment disorder are shown in Table 25.

2.9.1 ACUTE STRESS REACTION

Aetiology/psychopathology

By definition the necessary and immediate causative factor for this condition is an exceptionally stressful life event. Some individuals might be more prone to developing this disorder than others, and the reaction is more likely to occur in the elderly or if the person is physically exhausted. A previous history of psychiatric disorder also increases vulnerability.

Epidemiology

The prevalence of acute stress reactions depends on the severity of the trauma and the degree of exposure to it. Thus, the incidence of acute stress reactions among the survivors of an industrial explosion and fire at a Norwegian paint factory was directly proportionate to the individual's proximity to the centre of the explosion and conflagration. On the other hand, one-fifth of police officers who had to handle bodies after an aeroplane crash developed a severe stress reaction although there was no direct personal threat.

Clinical presentation and prognosis

This is a short-lived but severe disorder caused by an over-

Table 26 Clinical presentation of acute stress disorder.

Psychological symptoms
Feeling numb and detached, dazed and disorientated
Denial that the event has occurred
Agitation and overactivity
Fear, dejection, irritability and anger
Hypervigilance and enhanced startle response
'Action replays' of the incident in intrusive memories and dreams
Withdrawal and avoidance of reminders of the incident
Irrational guilt about surviving or failing to help others
Poor concentration
Loss of interest

Physical symptoms
Sweating
Shakiness
Rapid heart beat
Fatigue
Insomnia
Nightmares
Loss of appetite
Nausea and diarrhoea

whelming, psychologically traumatic experience [1]. The condition generally subsides within hours or days. Examples of such exceptional stressors include rape, assault, a life-threatening accident, a transport disaster, a domestic fire or multiple bereavement.

The symptoms of an acute stress reaction develop rapidly and tend to vary in character and fluctuate in intensity during the first few hours after exposure to the precipitating event (Table 26). The condition tends to resolve within a matter of days but some survivors will go on to develop PTSD (see Section 2.9.2, p. 196). Some victims might withdraw into a dissociative stupor (see Section 2.1, p. 180) or run away from the scene in a state of fugue.

Treatment

• If there is persistent denial that the event has occurred,

the survivor should be cautiously prompted to recall the facts.
• A very short course of a benzodiazepine tranquillizer and/or hypnotic is indicated for severe agitation or insomnia.

2.9.2 POST-TRAUMATIC STRESS DISORDER

Aetiology/psychopathology

The individual is involved in or witnesses an event which is an extreme threat to themselves or others, such as:
• a large-scale disaster (e.g. Hillsborough Football Stadium in 1989, the Kings Cross fire or the Paddington rail crash)
• a personal trauma such a rape, torture or assault.

The psychological impact of the traumatic event is known to be more severe when the stressor is 'man made' rather than an act of God such as a natural disaster. Vulnerability factors include a previous history or family history of psychiatric disorder. Children and the elderly have an increased risk of developing PTSD. In some cases physical injury might also increase the risk, but in other victims (e.g. civilians exposed to bomb outrages in Northern Ireland) survivor guilt was more frequently encountered in those who were physically unscathed.

Epidemiology

The incidence of PTSD is proportionate to the intensity of the psychological trauma. For example, 70% of rape victims are found to have PTSD at 9-month follow-up. In general about 25% of individuals exposed to traumatic events develop full-blown PTSD, but the frequency can vary. Thus, about 16% of London Underground train drivers who witnessed a train striking a person on the track developed PTSD, while careful psychological preparation of the police officers who handled the bodies of the Piper Alpha victims prevented the occurrence of any post-traumatic illness.

Clinical presentation

PTSD is a protracted psychological and behavioural reaction to an exceptionally threatening or catastrophic event which immediately induces intense fear, horror and/or helplessness.

The onset can be delayed for some years and it might only emerge when the victim is exposed to a new extreme stressor.

The symptoms of PTSD are:
• recurrent, distressing, intrusive images of the event
• dreams and nightmares which do not necessarily depict the incident
• avoidance of reminders of the trauma

• detachment and numbness
• hyperarousal, anxiety, insomnia, poor concentration, enhanced startle response and irritability.

The patient may also experience:
• survivor guilt, which is defined as the irrational sense that one's life was purchased at the cost of another's
• phobic avoidance of any situation that resembles the original traumatic event
• depression
• generalized anxiety disorder
• substance misuse.

Some patients become aggressive while others (surprisingly) behave recklessly.

Treatment

• Psychological—direct exposure therapy, anxiety management training and cognitive therapy all improve PTSD by 20–80%.
• Pharmacological—both tricyclic and SSRI antidepressants may help to suppress flashbacks and nightmares and reduce the frequency of panic attacks in addition to their specific antidepressant effect.

Prognosis

This has not yet been clearly established. About a quarter of rescuers involved in an oil rig disaster were found to have PTSD almost 12 months after the event. There was still a high rate of PTSD in severely abused former prisoners of war 50 years after their release. Prevalence rates for PTSD can range from about 30% among Australian fire fighters [1] to over 80% among Cambodian refugees [2].

Prevention

• Remind the survivor that it is perfectly normal to react emotionally to an abnormal event.
• Gently encourage the survivor to talk about the traumatic event rather than sweep it under the carpet. Go at their own pace and without intrusive pressure.
• Advise them to avoid using alcohol to suppress symptoms, because it can delay resolution.
• Encourage them to keep up usual routine activities.

There have been no large-scale, controlled, prospective studies of the efficacy of early crisis intervention. Psychological debriefing is widely used and involves the disclosure of expectations, facts, thoughts, sensory impressions and emotions about the event. The aim is to promote 'information processing' and integration rather than avoidance and denial of the experience.

Debriefing should include teaching about normal reactions to stress.

Black D, Newman M, Harris-Hendriks J, Mezey G (eds). *Psychological Trauma: a developmental approach.* London: Royal College of Psychiatrists, Gaskell, 1997.

Joseph S, Williams R, Yule W. *Understanding Post-Traumatic Stress: a psychosocial perspective on PTSD and treatment.* Chichester: John Wiley and Sons, 1997.

O'Brien LS. *Traumatic Events and Mental Health.* Cambridge: Cambridge University Press, 1998.

1 McFarlane AC. The longitudinal course of post-traumatic morbidity: the range of outcomes and their predictors. *J Nerv Ment Dis* 1988; 176: 30–40.

2 Bernstein CE, Rosser-Hogan R. Trauma experiences, post-traumatic stress, dissociation and depression in Cambodian refugees. *Am J Psychiatry* 1991; 148: 1548–1561.

2.10 Puerperal disorders

Psychiatric disorders associated with childbirth [1] are:
- maternity blues (see Section 2.10.1)
- depressive disorder (see Section 2.10.2)
- puerperal psychosis (see Section 2.10.3).

2.10.1 MATERNITY BLUES

Aetiology/psychopathology

Biological factors are:
- more common in first pregnancy
- more common with history of premenstrual tension
- not related to complications at delivery
- modestly associated with marked postnatal fall in progesterone levels.

Epidemiology

It occurs in 50–70% of women, mainly on the third to fourth day after delivery.

Clinical presentation

The midwives or husband might report:
- lability of mood
- tearfulness
- irritability.
- There tends to be a rapid and spontaneous resolution.

Treatment

Provide support and reassurance.

2.10.2 POST-NATAL DEPRESSIVE DISORDER

Aetiology/psychopathology

Predisposing factors:

- previous depressions
- recent adverse life events
- marital conflict
- lack of social support
- younger age
- poor relationship with own mother.

Epidemiology

It occurs in 10–15% of women.

Clinical presentation

It usually starts about 2 weeks after childbirth but can start within 3 months. Clinical picture as in non-psychotic depression.

Treatment

- Psychosocial interventions
- Antidepressants for severe or persistent symptoms (see below)
- Counselling and mother and baby groups to reduce isolation.

Prognosis

> **Outcome of postnatal depression**
>
> Untreated postnatal depression can last for up to 2 years with damage to:
> - marriage
> - emotional and cognitive development of the baby
> - any other children.

Risk of further episode is 1 in 6.

2.10.3 PUERPERAL PSYCHOSIS

Aetiology/psychopathology

- Genetic—strong family history of affective disorder
- Environmental—social stress is not implicated (unlike postnatal depression)
- Hormonal—postpartum fall in oestrogen causes supersensitivity of dopamine receptors.

Epidemiology

The frequency is 1 in every 500 births.
 Risk factors are:
- past history or family history of mood disorder
- primipara
- older age
- caesarean section.

Clinical presentation

Usually affective (especially manic) disorder but 20% are schizophrenia-like. Onset tends to be abrupt, in first 2 weeks postpartum.

Management of puerperal psychosis

- Antenatal identification of high-risk mothers
- Move to specialist mother and baby unit with nurses trained in both mental health and baby care
- Attempt to preserve mother–child bonding
- Conventional treatment of depression, mania or schizophrenia including ECT if necessary
- Breast feeding (see below)
- Assess mother–baby interaction before discharge
- Monitor carefully during subsequent child bearing.

Risks of puerperal psychosis

- Suicide
- Neglect of child (and of other children)
- Harm to baby if delusional ideas about the child, and of infanticide followed by suicide.

Prognosis

The prognosis is good for immediate recovery but there is a risk of recurrence in 30–50% in subsequent deliveries and 50% develop non-puerperal depression.

Drug treatment of psychiatric disorders in pregnancy and when breast feeding

Lithium

Avoid lithium in pregnancy and after delivery because:
- in first trimester it can cause atrialization of right ventricle
- renal clearance of lithium falls abruptly after delivery causing dangerous rise in serum lithium
- lithium is secreted in breast milk and if the infant becomes dehydrated, toxic lithium levels develop rapidly.

Other psychotropic drugs and breast feeding [2]

- All psychotropic drugs are secreted in breast milk, therefore use lowest effective dose
- The mother should not breast feed if her dose of haloperidol exceeds 20 mg per day or chlorpromazine 200 mg per day
- Avoid monoamine oxidase inhibitors (MAOIs) and clozapine (risk of agranulocytosis)
- Avoid use of more than one psychotropic drug.

The infant

- Monitor for development, sedation and irritability
- Check hepatic and renal function.

Do

- Use tricyclic antidepressants (except doxepin) because more data are available
- Use chlorpromazine, haloperidol or trifluoperazine for the same reason
- Use carbamazepine or sodium valproate instead of lithium.

Pseudocyesis

Pseudocyesis is a rare condition in which the patient erroneously believes that she is pregnant. She has amenorrhoea and abdominal distension. The conviction that she is pregnant is so strong that the patient prepares for the delivery by buying a cradle and baby clothes, etc. In addition to amenorrhoea and abdominal enlargement there may be swelling and tenderness of the breasts, together with morning sickness and sometimes pica. The majority of patients claim to feel fetal movements.

Hyperprolactinaemia can mimic pseudocyesis since it causes amenorrhoea, galactorrhoea and abdominal enlargement due to obesity or water retention. The psychological basis includes an intense desire for children.

Brockington I. *Motherhood and Mental Health*. Oxford: Oxford Medical Publications, 1998.
Pritchard DB, Harris B. Aspects of perinatal psychiatric illness. *Br J Psychiatry* 1996; 169: 555–562.
1 Altshuler LL, Hendrick V, Cohen LS. Course of mood and anxiety disorders during pregnancy and the postpartum period. *J Clin Psychiatry* 1998; 59: 29–33.
2 Yoshida K, Smith B, Kumar R. Psychotropic drugs in mothers' milk: a comprehensive review of assay methods, pharmacokinetics and of safety of breast-feeding. *J Psychopharmacol* 1999; 13: 76–92.

2.11 Depression

Aetiology/psychopathology

Impaired neurotransmission in depression has been explained by the catecholamine and indoleamine hypotheses, i.e. low mood is associated with reduced synaptic NA or 5-hydroxytryptamine (5HT; serotonin). Reserpine, a monoamine-depleting drug can cause depression. Conversely, tricyclic and MAOI antidepressants increase synaptic availability of NA and 5HT in the synaptic cleft. However, there is a delay between antidepressant-induced rise in synaptic NA and 5HT and improvement in mood. Furthermore, depressed patients do not have decreased NA, 5HT or their metabolites in blood, urine or cerebrospinal fluid (CSF). There is an excess of 5HT reuptake receptors in the frontal cortex of people who have committed suicide.

Some common exogenous causes of depression are shown in Table 27.

Vulnerability factors in women and in psychosocial adversity [1] are:
- being responsible for the care of three or more young children
- lack of a confiding relationship
- lack of a job outside the home
- separation from own mother before the age of 11.

Table 27 Common exogenous causes of depression.

Psychosocial factors (mainly loss)	Medical conditions (any devastating illness)	Drugs
Bereavement	Cerebrovascular accident	Reserpine
Unemployment	Carcinoma of pancreas	Beta-blockers
Divorce/separation	and bronchus	Calcium antagonists
Mutilating surgery	Hypothyroidism	Oral contraceptives
Disability	Cushing's disease	Corticosteroids
	Systemic lupus	Alcohol
	erythematosus	Cocaine withdrawal
	Parkinson's disease	Amphetamine
	Multiple sclerosis	withdrawal

These vulnerability factors sensitize the individual to major adverse life events which are characterized by loss or threat of loss, e.g.
- redundancy
- physical illness.

Other aetiological factors are:
- Genetic—identical twins reared apart show 60% more concordance than dizygotic twins
- Brain physiology—decrease in REM latency
- Endocrine—cortisol suppression, i.e. overactivity of hypothalamic–pituary–adrenocortical system, but is this primary or secondary?
- Psychological—learned helplessness, based on model of harnessed dogs subjected to recurrent aversive stimuli who become apathetic and fail to escape when restraints are removed [1].

See also Section 2.10.2, p. 197.

Epidemiology

Five per cent of the general population will experience an episode of moderate to severe depression. Prevalence is 2–3% of men and up to 9% of women. It is commoner in lower socio-economic groups because of chronic adversity.

Clinical presentation

Mood disorders can be bipolar or unipolar. Unipolar disorder is much commoner than bipolar.
- Bipolar disorder—there are episodes of persistent lowering of mood interspersed with bouts of sustained elation and overactivity
- Unipolar disorder—there are only downward mood swings.

Common

A common mixture of psychological and biological symptoms present most days for at least 2 weeks (Table 28). Patients may be agitated or retarded (Table 29).

Table 28 Clinical presentation of major depression.

Psychological symptoms
Persistent lowering of mood, often worse in the mornings
Slowing of thought and speech
Pessimism, self criticism, guilt and worthlessness
Helplessness and hopelessness
Poor concentration and memory
Loss of a sense of enjoyment (anhedonia)
Loss of interest
Thoughts of death and/or suicide
Suicide attempts

Biological symptoms
Insomnia with early morning
Diminished appetite with weight loss (occasionally increased appetite)
Loss of sex drive
Lack of drive, energy and motivation

Table 29 Signs of psychomotor agitation and retardation.

Psychomotor agitation
Pacing hand wringing
Repetitive and futile activity
Quest for reassurance

Psychomotor retardation
Avoidance of company
Self neglect
Mutism

Uncommon

Psychotic depression

Depression can be of psychotic intensity with delusional convictions of disease, putrefaction, poverty, contaminating others or causing evil. There may also be hallucinations, especially accusing or derogatory voices.

Seasonal affective disorder

There is a female to male ratio of 6 : 1. Onset is in the mid-twenties. Depression tends to occur in the winter months and is often accompanied by oversleeping and overeating. It can be treated with antidepressants and photo-therapy, which artificially lengthens the day and maintains biological rhythms.

Recurrent brief depressions

Bouts of brief (2–5 days) but intense depression occurring every month or so but not related to menstruation.

Atypical depression

Hypersomnia and increased appetite *or* psychological symptoms but no biological features.

Anxiety and depression often coexist.

Treatment

Treatment should be both psychological and pharmacological.
• Psychological—cognitive therapy
• Pharmacological—antidepressant ± ECT. Add antipsychotic drug for delusions and/or hallucinations.

⚡ Caution in treatment of depression in bipolar affective disorder—there is a risk of inducing mania.

Antidepressants

These tend to be more effective in severe depression and where biological symptoms are prominent.
• Tricyclics, e.g. amitriptyline, lofepramine (less cardiotoxic)
• SSRIs, e.g. fluoxetine
• MAOIs—inhibit reuptake of NA and 5HT increasing amount of available neurotransmitter at the synapse.

🔑 **Management of depression**

• Assess for suicide risk (see Section 1.4, p. 168); if the risk is high admission to psychiatric unit is indicated, if necessary under Mental Health Act (see Section 2.14, p. 203).
• Social isolation, severe self neglect and failure to eat or drink also require hospital admission.
• Mobilization of support from carers and mental health professionals, especially community psychiatric nurses (CPN).

⚡ **Monoamine oxidase inhibitors**

Risk of tyramine response ('cheese reaction') causing dangerous rise in blood pressure. Also incompatability with opioids, especially pethidine.

Tricyclics

Side effects of tricyclics are:
• anticholinergic, e.g. dry mouth, blurred vision, constipation, ileus, precipitation of glaucoma, urinary retention, delirium in the elderly
• noradrenergic, e.g. postural hypotension
• cardiac dysrhythmias
• lowering the seizure threshold
• cardiotoxicity in overdose
• weight gain
• sexual dysfunction.

Selective serotonin reuptake inhibitors

These have fewer cardiovascular effects than tricyclics and are less sedative. They also have no anticholinergic side effects, but they can cause gastrointestinal problems, agitation, insomnia and headache.

Tricyclics and SSRIs are probably of equal efficacy. In depression of psychotic intensity, a neuroleptic should be added to the antidepressant.

Electroconvulsive therapy

This is the treatment of choice in:
• severe depression
• refusal to eat or drink
• grave suicide risk
• failure of other treatment methods.

⚡ **ECT**

Contraindications: raised intracranial pressure, a recent myocardial infarction or cerebrovascular accident, or recent ventricular dysrhythmia.

ECT is applied under general anaesthetic with muscle relaxants [2]. The usual course is six to eight applications, with two applications per week. Major risk factors are those of general anaesthetic. Side effects include:
• headache
• short-term amnesia
• seizures between treatments
• delirium in the elderly
• cardiovascular complications.

Prognosis

Most episodes of depression remit within 6 months. Fifteen per cent experience chronic symptoms. There is a high risk of recurrence if recovery from a particular episode is incomplete. Risk of recurrence increases with age. Mortality due to suicide is 15%.

Prevention

• Cognitive therapy reduces the risk of further episodes.
• Also consider continuation treatment with antidepressants and mood stabilizers (see Section 2.12, p. 201).

Williams JMG. Depression. In: Clark DM, Fairburn CG. *Science and Practice of Cognitive Behaviour Therapy.* Oxford: Oxford University Press, 1997: 259–285.

Wolpert L. *Malignant Sadness: the anatomy of depression.* London: Faber, 1999.

1 Brown GW, Harris TO. *Social Origins of Depression.* London: Tavistock, 1978.

2 Wijeratne C, Halliday GS, Lyndon RW. The present status of electroconvulsive therapy: a systematic review. *Med J Aust* 1999; 171: 250–254.

2.12 Bipolar affective disorder

This consists of recurrent episodes of mania and depression. Episodes of elevated mood are called manic if they are severe and have psychotic features (delusions and hallucinations). Less severe cases are labelled hypomanic. Minimum duration of symptoms is 4 days.

Aetiology/psychopathology

There is a concordance rate of about 75% in monozygotic twins and about 54% in dizygotic twins. A cyclothymic personality is a predisposing factor.

Mania might be secondary to the following:
- antidepressant treatment
- head injury
- stroke
- amphetamine.

Epidemiology

The lifetime risk of mania is 0.6–1%. Mean age of onset is 30. The incidence is the same in men and women. The age of onset is earlier than in the unipolar disorder.

Clinical presentation

Mania is characterized by the following:
- sustained elevation of mood or irritability
- abundant energy
- disinhibition
- reckless behaviour with extravagant spending, fast driving and promiscuity
- pressure of speech
- increased self esteem
- grandiose and self-important ideas
- sometimes a sense of special mission
- acceleration of thinking and flight of ideas
- reduced need for sleep
- poor concentration
- distractibility
- lack of insight
- sometimes delusions of grandeur
- auditory hallucinations in the second person (i.e. talking to the patient).

 Mixed affective states (i.e. co-occurrence of depression and manic symptoms) can occur in at least 16% of manic–depressive patients, usually while the mood is shifting between poles.

Schizoaffective disorder

This diagnostic category is used for manic or depressive symptoms and schizophrenic symptoms occurring concurrently or within a few days of each other.

Rapid-cycling bipolar affective disorder

This is uncommon. There are more than four episodes of severe affective disorder in a year. It is commoner in women and commoner when taking antidepressants.

Differential diagnosis

Differential diagnosis of hypomania and mania is:
- drug-induced overactivity and euphoria—amphetamines, cocaine, ecstasy
- organic states—hypothyroidism (surprisingly), HIV, general paralysis of the insane (GPI), multiple sclerosis.

Treatment

- Haloperidol 15–25 mg three times a day.
- Rarely (and paradoxically) ECT three times a week.

🔑 For mania, admission to hospital, compulsory if necessary, is usually indicated to prevent personal and social damage due to frenetic and reckless behaviour [1]. Hypomania might be contained at home provided the patient can be supervised and is prepared to take regular medication.

⚡ Watch for severe depressive downswing with risk of suicide.

Prophylaxis

Lithium is indicated after two severe episodes within 2 years. Check renal and thyroid function, and ECG because of risk of cardiac dysrhythmias in older patients. Monitor serum lithium levels, aiming for a level of 0.6–0.8 mmol/L. Watch for hypothyroidism (treat with L-thyroxine) and nephrogenic diabetes insipidus.

 Lithium

Lithium is effective prophylactically in 70% of cases of bipolar affective disorder. Alternatives are carbamazepine and sodium valproate. Lithium is teratogenic (see Section 2.10, p. 197).

Complications

- Risk of death from suicide in depressive phase
- Risk of death from exhaustion after weeks of untreated mania
- Manic stupor.

Prognosis

Untreated episodes might last between 3 and 6 months. Untreated there is significant mortality from exhaustion. Over 50% will have further episodes if the disorder begins before the age of 30.

el-Mallakh RS. Bipolar illness. *South Med J* 1997; 90: 775–779.

Goodwin FK, Jamison KR. *Manic–Depressive Illness*. Oxford: Oxford University Press, 1990.

McElroy SL, Keck PE, Strakowski SM. Mania, psychosis, and antipsychotics. *J Clin Psychiatry* 1999; 57: 14–26.

1 Tohen M, Grundy S. Management of acute mania. *J Clin Psychiatry* 1999; 60: 31–34.

2.13 Delusional disorder

Epidemiology

Delusional disorder is less common than schizophrenia. It can occur at any age, but onset is most frequent between 34 and 45 years. Prevalence is 0.03% in the general population [1].

Clinical presentation

Patients usually do not perceive themselves as having a mental illness and are accepted as eccentric, hence they often do not present for treatment. Their delusions frequently have internal logic and are systematized. They may have olfactory and tactile hallucinations that provide confirmatory evidence to their beliefs, but hallucinations are generally not prominent. Apart from the delusions and their ramifications, the patient's functioning is not markedly impaired. However, the condition should be taken seriously as patients may be at risk of impulsivity, suicide and homicide [2]. The different subtypes of delusional disorder are shown in Table 30.

Risk factors

- Social isolation
- Stress of immigration/exile
- Family history
- Personality disorder.

Table 30 Different subtypes of delusional disorder [1].

Subtype	Typical preoccupation
Somatic type	Undiagnosed disease
Persecutory type	Conspiracy
Grandiose type	Missionary zeal
Jealous type	Morbid jealously (Othello syndrome)
Erotomanic type	Impossible love relationship (de Clerambault's syndrome)

Differential diagnosis

The following conditions present with either delusional thinking or preoccupations that can be confused with delusional thinking [2].

- Schizophrenia and other psychotic disorders (see Section 2.3, p. 182)
- Mood disorders
- Dementia (see Section 2.2, p. 180)
- Somatoform disorders (see Section 1.6, p. 172)
- Obsessive–compulsive disorder (see Section 2.8, p. 193)
- Neurological disorders, e.g. after head injury
- Substance abuse (see Section 1.8, p. 175).

Treatment

Reassurance, compassion and support. Cognitive therapy may ameliorate delusional thinking. Antipsychotic medication and SSRIs have been shown to be of some value. Hospitalize if there are concerns about aggression, suicide, homicide or extreme impulsivity.

Morbid jealously carries significant risk of violence, and concurrent alcohol abuse increases this risk.

Prognosis

Often a chronic lifelong problem. Thirty-three to fifty per cent of cases go into remission [2].

1 American Psychiatric Association. *Diagnostic and Statistical Manual of Mental Disorders* (4th edn). Washington: American Psychiatric Association, 1994.

2 Manschreck TC. Delusional disorder: the recognition and management of paranoia. *J Clin Psychiatry* 1996; 57 (Suppl. 3): 32–38.

2.14 The Mental Health Act (1983)

The Mental Health Act deals with the compulsory detention and treatment of people suffering from mental disorders who are considered to be:
- a danger to themselves and/or
- a danger to others and/or
- at risk of severe self neglect.

The term 'mental disorder' includes all the psychiatric disorders described in this module, with two important exceptions:
- Substance abuse or acute intoxication with drugs and/or alcohol *per se*. Note that psychiatric disorders arising out of substance misuse, such as alcoholic hallucinosis or drug-induced psychosis, are covered by the Act.
- Individuals whose personality disorder is regarded as untreatable. Note that although a particular patient's personality disorder might be deemed untreatable, patients with comorbidity, such as a sociopathic patient with a major depressive illness, would be covered by the Act. Thus, a person with a sociopathic personality who is suicidally depressed can be compulsorily detained and treated.

Physicians only need to be familiar with a limited number of Sections ('Sections' referring to main paragraph numbers of the Act). Clinicians may encounter psychiatric emergency situations in a wide range of settings:
- A&E departments (see Sections 1.4, p. 168, 1.5, p. 170, 1.9, p. 177)
- medical and surgical intensive care and high-dependency units (see Section 1.1, p. 163)
- general medical and surgical wards
- obstetric wards (see Section 2.10, p. 197).

Accident and emergency departments

This is probably the commonest setting for psychiatric emergencies and the most frequent situation is the gravely suicidal patient who declines to be admitted for observation and treatment.

Action:
- Ensure that a member of staff stays with the patient at all times.
- Call the duty psychiatrist.
- If the suicidal patient attempts to abscond from A&E before or during psychiatric assessment, the staff of A&E have a duty under Common Law to restrain the patient.

If the duty psychiatrist (who has to be formally approved by the Department of Health as having special experience in the diagnosis and treatment of mental disorder) concludes that the patient requires compulsory admission for observation and/or treatment, he or she will arrange for a second medical assessment to be carried out.

Ideally this second medical assessment would be carried out by the patient's own general practitioner. However, since many patients attending the A&E department in these circumstances are not actually registered with a general practitioner or might have one who is unavailable, the psychiatrist will summon a second psychiatrist (who must work at a different hospital to prevent 'collusion').

If they all agree that compulsory admission is indeed necessary they will complete Section 2 or Section 3 documentation.
- Section 2 authorizes admission for observation (and any necessary treatment) for up to 28 days.
- Section 3 authorizes admission for treatment for up to 6 months.

Patients have the right to appeal against both Sections.

Other medical and surgical wards

If the patient is already being nursed on a medical, surgical or obstetric ward, or in an intensive care or high-dependency unit, and they develop a mental illness *de novo*, or have an exacerbation or relapse of a pre-existing disorder, their physician or surgeon can authorize their compulsory detention for up to 72 h under Section 5(2) of the Mental Health Act. The Section form can be obtained from the nearest inpatient psychiatric unit.

During those 72 h the medical or surgical team must request a formal assessment by:
- a consultant psychiatrist
- the patient's own general practitioner, and
- an approved social worker.

Again, if the general practitioner is not available, the patient's own surgeon or physician is authorized to complete the Section.

 It is important to note that the patient may be detained under the Mental Health Act on the grounds of health and safety alone, i.e. the patient does not necessarily have to constitute a danger to themselves and/or others.

3 Self-assessment

Answers on pp. 216–218

Question 1
1 What are the essential differences between anorexia nervosa and bulimia nervosa?
2 Name four endocrine conditions that may present with a physical picture similar to anorexia nervosa.

Question 2
1 In chronic fatigue syndrome, what symptoms, other than fatigue, need to be identified to make a diagnosis?
2 In the treatment of chronic fatigue syndrome, consider the following statements (T/F):
A patients should rest as much as is possible
B graded exercise is the mainstay of treatment
C immunotherapy has been shown to be beneficial
D antidepressants are very effective and should be used
E dietary supplements should be prescribed.

Question 3
1 Would three glasses of wine every day of the week be within recommended limits of safe alcohol use advised by the Department of Health?
2 What is the CAGE mnemonic?

Question 4
In substance misuse consider the following (T/F):
A heroin can be smoked
B babies born to addicted mothers may take months to recover fully from opioid withdrawal
C in methadone replacement therapy, the dose is calculated according to the amount of heroin the patient has been using
D naltrexone is used long-term after opioid withdrawal to reduce the relapse rate
E hepatitis C is an increasingly common problem.

Question 5
1 What are the core features of schizophrenia?
2 What are the core features of neuroleptic malignant syndrome?
3 What adverse effect of clozapine is most worrying?

Question 6
In schizophrenia, consider the following statements (T/F):
A it is more common in men
B it is characterized by violence

C there are neuroradiological changes
D there is a significant risk of suicide
E psychological therapies can be used to treat psychotic symptoms.

Question 7
1 Briefly describe what a personality disorder is.
2 Consider the following statements with regard to personality disorder (T/F):
A personality disorders are untreatable
B borderline personality is more common in women
C the psychopathology of schizophrenia includes a split in personality
D people with personality disorders often suffer from depression as well
E psychotherapy is not effective in personality disorder.

Question 8
An acute organic reaction (T/F):
A is unlikely to be caused by a subdural haematoma in the absence of a severe head injury
B is unlikely to be associated with Wernicke's encephalopathy if examination of external ocular movements shows no abnormality
C can occur in SLE
D can be caused by *all* of the following drugs: procyclidine, tricyclic antidepressants, L-dopa, bromocriptine, digoxin, cimetidine and theophylline, efavirenz (Sustiva)
E can be caused by *all* of the following: hyperthyroid crisis, myxoedema, Addisonian crisis, hypopituitarism, hypoparathyroidism, hyperparathyroidism.

Question 9
Panic attacks commonly occur in (T/F):
A simple partial seizures
B carcinoid syndrome
C mastocytosis
D withdrawal from paroxetine
E LSD use.

Question 10
In HIV-associated dementia (T/F):
A AZT might have a preventative effect
B CNS abnormalities might include ataxia, dysarthria and a snout reflex
C before the introduction of combination therapy the median life expectancy after the development of HIV dementia was 6 months

D has a prevalence rate of over 25%
E risk factors for developing HIV-associated dementia include a CD4 count below 200.

Question 11
In the assessment of suicide risk (T/F):
A risk factors are highly specific
B risk factors are highly sensitive
C young men are increasingly at risk
D those who talk about committing suicide rarely carry it out
E people who commit suicide rarely seek medical help before taking their own lives.

Question 12
In anorexia nervosa (T/F):
A patients cannot receive nasogastric tube feeding under the Mental Health Act
B patients have always suffered sexual abuse
C patients may present with delusions
D only women are affected
E neuropathy is a possible complication.

Question 13
Chronic fatigue syndrome (T/F):
A is more common in women
B cognitive behaviour therapy can be helpful
C should be treated with antidepressants
D membership of a self-help group is associated with a good prognosis
E may present with memory impairment.

Question 14
Consider the following statements regarding alcohol withdrawal symptoms (T/F):
A it always indicates dependence
B formication may occur
C confusion is inevitable and not very worrying
D it occurs in men who drink more than 21 units per week
E ophthalmoplegia may occur.

Question 15
The following are symptoms of opioid withdrawal (T/F):
A constricted pupils
B pyrexia
C hypothermia
D abdominal cramps
E hallucinations.

Question 16
Consider the following statements in relation to the management of violent patients (T/F):

A intramuscular chlorpromazine is a good choice for sedation
B let the patient know who is in charge and their behaviour will not be tolerated
C patients with schizophrenia are dangerous
D it is lawful to restrain and sedate violent patients
E police have a duty to assist with violence in A&E.

Question 17
Consider the following statements (T/F):
A dementia is characterized by a state of altered consciousness
B dementia is a disease of old age
C frontal lobe dementia is associated with personality changes
D depression may be confused with dementia
E donepezil is a cholinesterase inhibitor used in Alzheimer's disease.

Question 18
In patients with general medical conditions who also have psychiatric symptoms, consider the following statements (T/F):
A serious mental health problems are unusual on general medical wards
B these psychiatric symptoms should be vigorously treated
C demyelinating disorders may present with psychiatric symptoms
D reassurance and providing information may be the only treatment that is required
E malingering is common.

Question 19
1 What are the risk factors that increase the likelihood of someone developing delusional disorder?
2 In delusional disorder, consider the following statements (T/F):
A it has a prevalence of about 0.03% in the general population
B it is a type of schizophrenia
C psychological strategies may lessen delusional thinking
D hallucinations do not occur
E antipsychotics are used to treat it.

Question 20
Lithium carbonate (T/F):
A the prophylactic serum level is 0.6–0.8 mmol/L
B acute toxicity develops with a serum of level of 1.5 mmol/L or above
C long-term administration can cause thyrotoxicosis
D long-term administration can cause diabetes mellitus
E can be used to augment tricyclic antidepressants in the treatment of refractory depression.

Answers to Self-assessment

Neurology

Answer to Question 1

E

S1 radiculopathy may present with an absent ankle jerk and weakness of plantar flexion. Both a high common peroneal nerve lesion and an L5 radiculopathy may present with a similar pattern of sensory disturbance.

Inversion is performed by tibialis posterior (L4, 5 via the tibial nerve) and eversion by peroneus longus and brevis (L5, S1 via the superficial peroneal nerve, a branch of the common peroneal nerve).

Associated weakness of eversion only would therefore be suggestive of a common peroneal nerve lesion.

Answer to Question 2

The most likely diagnosis is of a paraneoplastic subacute sensory neuroneopathy secondary to an underlying small-cell lung carcinoma.

Investigations may show a raised CSF protein with a mild pleocytosis, anti-Hu antibodies in blood and confirmation of the neuroneopathy on nerve conduction studies. Paraneoplastic conditions present when the driving tumour is small, therefore a CT chest rather than chest X-ray alone may be required to detect a malignancy.

Although not always successful, the best chance of disease stabilization or cure is complete resection of the underlying cancer if possible.

Answer to Question 3

This is not the clinical picture of DMD in which patients present in the first decade and are wheelchair bound in the second. Although CK is raised in DMD, this is not specific. Dystrophin is absent in almost all DMD patients. There need not be a positive family history; the dystrophin gene is large so new mutations account for approximately one-third of cases of both DMD and the allelic Becker's muscular dystrophy (BMD). Alternatively, as the dystrophin gene is carried on the X chromosome, the patient's mother and any of his sisters may be asymptomatic carriers.

The most likely diagnosis is of BMD, although other rarer autosomal recessive limb girdle muscular dystrophies cannot be excluded given the above information.

Diagnosis may be made by genetic analysis. Mutations in the dystrophin gene are found in both DMD and BMD. DMD is characterized by an out-of-frame delection/mutation or duplication resulting in no protein, whereas in BMD, there is an in-frame abnormality leading to a truncated or abnormal dystrophin protein.

Answer to Question 4

1 A, B, E

2 H

3 D, F, I

4 C, F, G

Answer to Question 5

1 D, H

2 A

3 A, F

4 B

Answer to Question 6

F, T, T, T, F

Idiopathic Parkinson's disease usually has a unilateral onset.

A parkinsonian syndrome and tardive dyskinesia are associated with neuroleptic use.

Bradykinesia and rigidity in the absence of tremor and failure to respond to L-dopa are major clinical pointers to a parkinsonian syndrome rather than idiopathic disease.

The majority of patients taking L-DOPA for a prolonged period will develop dyskinesias. (90% of young PD patients on L-DOPA report dyskinesias and motor fluctuations after 5 years; see Schrag *et al. Mov Disord* 1998; 6: 885–894.).

Answer to Question 7

1 Bell's palsy

2 Hyperacusis, impaired lacrimation and decreased salivation

3 Ramsay Hunt syndrome.

Bell's palsy is an idiopathic cause of acute lower motor neurone facial paralysis. The facial nerve supplies the muscles of facial expression, anterior two-thirds of the tongue, stapedius muscle in the inner ear, lacrimal gland and sublingual and submandibular salivary glands. Ramsay Hunt syndrome is a presumed infection of the geniculate ganglion with the herpes zoster virus, resulting in facial nerve palsy in association with a vesicular eruption involving the ear, palate, pharynx or neck.

Answer to Question 8

1 F

2 A, B

3 C, E

4 C, D, E, F

Amyloid and diabetes can both cause a painful neuropathy. However, this tends to be chronic rather than subacute.

Approximately two-thirds of HMSN 1 have a duplication or point mutation of PMP22.

Mutation in the connexin 32 gene is responsible for X-linked dominant HMSN X.

The vasculitides usually have a subacute presentation but can occasionally present more chronically.

Answer to Question 9

1 Bilateral internuclear ophthalmoplegia
2 Medial longitudinal fasciculus
3 Relapsing–remitting multiple sclerosis
4 MRI of the brain
  Cerebrospinal fluid examination for oligoclonal bands.
  Bilateral internuclear ophthalmoplegia, especially in a young adult, strongly suggests MS. The lack of disease progression between attacks points towards relapsing–remitting MS in this patient. It is worth remembering that investigations only aid in making the diagnosis. The diagnosis of MS is based fundamentally on clinical evidence requiring the demonstration of CNS lesions disseminated in time and place.

Answer to Question 10

1 A
2 D
3 A, C
Certain antiepileptics increase the metabolism of the OCP.
  Blood plasma levels of antiepileptics fall in the later stages of pregnancy due to expanded blood volume and altered protein binding and metabolism.
  Lack of sleep can provoke seizures despite good compliance and stable plasma concentrations.

Answer to Question 11

Patients with a CPS will usually be aware that an attack has occurred and may experience postictal confusion unlike a typical absence attack. CPSs usually last longer (minutes rather than seconds) and are preceded by an aura. An electroencephalogram (EEG) is likely to show 3 Hz spike-and-wave activity consistent with an idiopathic aetiology, in the patient with typical absence.

Answer to Question 12

No significant weakness (motor fibres are large myelinated axons).
  Preserved reflexes (the fibres subserving the afferent limb of the muscle stretch reflex arc are large myelinated axons, as are the efferent motor fibres).
  Preserved balance (proprioceptive information is conducted in large myelinated axons).
  Reduced pinprick and temperature sensation.
  Sometimes autonomic disturbance.

Answer to Question 13

L4 is affected by the L3/L4 disc, and L5 by the L4/L5 disc. See Fig. 3.

Answer to Question 14

If the following features apply, then it is likely that the cause is vascular.
1 Focal neurological symptoms and signs.
2 Predominantly negative features (e.g. loss of power and sensation).
3 Sudden-onset symptoms.
4 Symptoms maximal within minutes to hours.

Answer to Question 15

F, F, T, T, F
Motor involvement, e.g. ataxia and weakness indicates a poorer prognosis.
  Dominant visual symptoms are a good prognostic indicator.
  Women fare better than men.
  The relapsing–remitting form of the disease at the onset is a better prognostic factor.
  Early age of onset implies a more favourable prognosis.

Answer to Question 16

T, F, T, F, F
It typically affects young women.
  It is rarely bilateral.
  However, in chronic cases the pupils may become constricted.
  It is associated with depressed deep tendon reflexes.
  Neurosyphilis is the usual cause of Argyll–Robertson pupils.

Answer to Question 17

1 F
2 D
3 E
4 B

Answer to Question 18

1 B
2 C
3 D
4 A

Answer to Question 19

D
The lateral cutaneous nerve is a pure sensory nerve. Involvement of the femoral nerve will cause weakness of the quadriceps muscle (weak hip flexion and knee extension), impaired knee jerk and sensory disturbances over the anterior and medial aspects of the thigh and medial aspect of the lower leg.

Answer to Question 20

1 Spinal epidural abscess.
2 MRI of the spine; blood cultures.

3 Surgical decompression; intravenous antibiotics (empirically will need to include a penicillin to cover *S. aureus*).

Answer to Question 21

F, F, F, T, T

Inhibition of DDC increases CNS bioavailability.

Dopamine agonists may be poorly tolerated due to cognitive problems as well as nausea and vomiting.

Levodopa preparations contain a DDC inhibitor to reduce peripheral metabolism.

COMT inhibition further increases available levodopa and may help to stabilize clinical fluctuations between doses.

Answer to Question 22

T, F, F, F, T

Patients with Alzheimer's disease typically have fluent speech with semantic or anomic errors.

Repetition is usually preserved in Alzheimer's disease but impaired in lesions of Brocca's area.

The classical amnesia of Alzheimer's disease is one of antegrade, episodic memory, i.e., memory of events subsequent to the onset of the disease.

Concrete thinking is found in fronto-temporal dementias.

Impaired category fluency ('how many animals can you name in a minute?') reflects the anomia.

Answer to Question 23

T, F, T, T, F

A and C highlight the important complications of autonomic involvement.

Pulmonary emboli are a complication of any disease causing immobilization.

GBS is usually monophasic, although relapses have been reported.

Answer to Question 24

1 C8 and T1.

2 Dissociated sensory loss.

3 Syringomyelia.

4 MRI of the cervical spine.

5 Horner's syndrome.

Syringomyelia is cavitation of the spinal cord. Characteristically, there is dissociated sensory loss (loss of pain and temperature sensation but preserved light touch) and lower motor neurone signs at the level of the lesion. There may be a pyramidal deficit below the level of the lesion, sphincter abnormalities and sympathetic dysfunction (Horner's syndrome). MRI confirms the diagnosis.

Answer to Question 25

F, T, F, T, T

Metabolic muscle disease characteristically gives pain on exercise.

Sustained exercise may induce muscle necrosis; myoglobinuria is secondary to rhabdomyolysis.

Gower's manoeuvre is a feature of early-onset dystrophies with severe proximal weakness.

Mitochondria contain their own DNA and as we inherit our mitochondria through the maternal line, disorders of such show maternal inheritance.

Patients with disorders of glycogen metabolism may learn to 'pace themselves' and exercise gradually through the pain while energy sources switch to lipid metabolism.

Answer to Question 26

1 S2, S3 and S4.

2 Cauda equina.

The cauda equina (horse's tail) includes the terminal spinal cord, nerve roots from T12 to S5 and the filum terminale. Features suggesting a cauda equina lesion include asymmetrical lower motor neurone signs in the legs, loss of sensation in the saddle distribution (which may be asymmetrical), sphincter disturbances and impairment of male sexual function.

Answer to Question 27

F, T, T, F, T, T, T

The following factors increase the chances of recurrence of seizures if medication is withdrawn:

- Age over 16
- Taking more than one antiepileptic drug
- A history of seizures after starting antiepileptic drugs
- A history of tonic–clonic seizures
- A history of myoclonic seizures
- An abnormal EEG in the previous year.

The most important aspects considered by the patient will be side effects of the drugs, and how dependent they are on driving. If driving is important for their work, for example, they are unlikely to want to withdraw the medication (if they are seizure free and have a driving license), however small the risk.

Answer to Question 28

1 Chest X-ray; high-frequency repetitive nerve stimulation during electromyography.

2 Lambert–Eaton syndrome.

3 Small-cell lung carcinoma.

4 Antibodies against primary antigen in small-cell carcimoma cross-react with voltage-gated Ca^{2+} channels at the presynaptic nerve terminal, causing an insufficient presynaptic release of acetylcholine.

The Lambert–Eaton syndrome is a myasthenic syndrome with a well-recognized association with malignancy (50–60% of cases), most commonly small-cell lung carcinoma. It is characterized by proximal muscle weakness which improves for a short while after exercise (postexercise facilitation) and depressed or absent deep tendon reflexes which may enhance with repeated muscle contraction. Autonomic disturbances (e.g. dry mouth and impotence in the above case) may occur. Extraocular and bulbar muscles are usually spared. High-frequency repetitive nerve stimulation results in incremental response of the compound muscle action potential because accumulation of presynaptic calcium facilitates acetylcholine release.

Answer to Question 29
T, F, T, T, T, T

Myoclonus is a cardinal feature of CJD but is found only late, if at all, in new variant CJD (nvCJD).

Answer to Question 30
1 Familial amyotrophic lateral sclerosis.
2 Electromyography.

The combination of mixed upper and lower motor neurone features together with the absence of eye, sphincter and sensory disturbances point towards amyotrophic lateral sclerosis. The condition is familial in this case because of the family history. Electromyography shows evidence of widespread of denervation and reinnervation.

Answer to Question 31:
T, F, T, T, T

Thyrotoxicosis is associated with insomnia.
Insomnia is a common side effect of phenytoin.

Answer to Question 32
1 Myasthenic crisis; cholinergic crisis.
2 Administration of edrophonium chloride.
3 For myasthenic crisis, intravenous immunoglobulin or plasmapheresis.

For cholinergic crisis, discontinue pyridostigmine bromide.

It is important to be aware that respiratory failure in a patient with myasthenia gravis may be due to the disease itself/inadequate doses of anticholinesterases (myasthenic crisis) or to overdose of anticholinesterases (cholinergic crisis). The former improves with intravenous edrophonium but the latter worsens. However, in practice it can be difficult to distinguish between these two conditions and discontinuation of all anticholinesterases and ventilatory support may be needed.

Answer to Question 33
F, T, T, F, F

Faced with a subacute, painful neuropathy, one must always think of vasculitic and paraneoplastic conditions. Guillain–Barré syndrome is not typically painful, but lower back and proximal leg pain certainly may occur.

Answer to Question 34
1 Bilateral idiopathic brachial plexopathy.
2 C5 and C6.

Idiopathic brachial plexopathy is usually unilateral, but can be bilateral. It often involves the C5 and C6 segments of the brachial plexus. It begins abruptly with a severe stabbing pain which may last from hours to weeks. There is often associated weakness and profound wasting of the muscles involved. Occasionally, there is a precipitating event, e.g. an upper respiratory tract infection, immunization or minor injury. Recovery may take months to years and may be incomplete.

Answer to Question 35
T, F, F, T, F
The dorsal column tracts responsible for proprioception and vibration sense ascend without crossing in the spinal cord.

The lateral spinothalamic tract which conveys pain and temperature sensation cross in the spinal tract.

There is ipsilateral upper motor neurone paralysis below T1 as the pyramidal tract decussates in the medulla.

Ipsilateral lower motor neurone paralysis at the level of the lesion is part of the Brown–Séquard syndrome.

The ipsilateral abdominal reflex is diminished as it is part of the upper motor neurone paralysis below T1.

Answer to Question 36
1 Frontotemporal dementia.
2 Frontal lobe pathology.

Frontotemporal dementia is associated with early personality change with impairment of memory and frontal executive tasks. Speech gradually deteriorates and some patients may present with aphasia. Pathologically there is frontotemporal lobar atrophy. Other frontal release signs include glabellar, palmomental, pout and suck reflexes.

Answer to Question 37
T, T, T, F, T

Mean of onset is 29 years in new variant Creutzfeldt–Jakob disease and 60 years in sporadic Creutzfeldt–Jakob disease.

Psychiatric and sensory symptoms are prominent early features in new variant CJD.

Upgaze paresis is uncommon in sporadic CJD.

Dementia is a prominent early feature in sporadic CJD.

Mean disease duration is 14 months in new variant CJD and 5 months in sporadic CJD.

Answer to Question 38
F, T, T, T, T

The waking pattern consists mainly of α and β activity.
The α rhythm is also attenuated by mental activity.
In sleep there is increasing δ activity with increasing depth of sleep.

α activity is 8–12 Hz, δ activity is 1–3 Hz and θ activity is 4–7 Hz.

In drowsiness there is also increased θ and β activities.

Answer to Question 39

1D, 2E, 3A, 4A, 5B

The oculomotor, trochlear and abducens nerves, ophthalmic division of trigeminal nerve and superior ophthalmic vein pass through the superior orbital fissure. The mandibular division of trigeminal nerve passes through the foramen ovale. The facial and vestibulocochlear nerves, and internal auditory artery pass through the internal acoustic meatus. The glossopharyngeal, vagus and spinal accessory nerves, and sigmoid sinus pass through the jugular foramen. The medulla, meninges, spinal accessory nerve, vertebral arteries, anterior and posterior spinal arteries pass through the foramen magnum.

Answer to Question 40

1D, 2B, 3E, 4G, 5A

In conduction aphasia, verbal fluency and auditory comprehension are intact, but repetition and naming are impaired. In transcortical aphasias, repetition is intact but auditory comprehension is impaired. Fluency is intact in sensory transcortical aphasia, but not in motor transcortical aphasia. Global aphasia is caused by a lesion in the central speech area (Broca's area, Wernicke's area and interconnecting arcuate fasciculus). Sensory transcortical aphasia is caused by a lesion surrounding the superior temporal gyrus. Mixed transcortical aphasia is caused by a lesion surrounding both Broca's and Wernicke's areas.

Answer to Question 41

T, T, F, F, T

C: The visual hallucinations of peduncular hallucinosis are purely visual, appear in natural form and colour, move as in an animation and are considered by the patient to be unreal. They are most often associated with lesions of the thalamus or midbrain.

D: Epileptic visual hallucinations are more likely to be simple.

Answer to Question 42

1A, 2E, 3D

The spread of positive sensory phenomena would be against TIA in the first case, and is more in keeping with a migrainous aura with or without the headache. The second case represents the dysarthria–clumsy hand syndrome, a common lacunar syndrome for which diabetes and hypertension are a common risk factor. The three features of case 3 are those classically described in spontaneous internal carotid artery dissection, one of the commoner causes of stroke in young people. Look specifically for a left-sided Hor-ner's syndrome in this patient to confirm your clinical suspicion.

Answer to Question 43

F, F, T, F, T

A: Most forms of vertigo are worsened by movement, and so this feature is non-specific.

B: A positive Hallpike's manoeuvre is indicated by the onset, after a latency of some seconds, of torsional nystagmus associated with vertigo. The result will fatigue on repeat testing. For the result to suggest a diagnosis of BPV, both latency and fatigability must be present.

D: Although this is often the case, antiepileptic drugs may cause nystagmus in any direction.

E: Consider Arnold–Chiari malformation, meningioma and Paget's disease.

Answer to Question 44

B

This history is absolutely typical for transient global amnesia. The bewilderment and amnesia, with relative preservation of the sense of self and of intellectual functioning, without clouding of consciousness is characteristic. The aetiology is not entirely clear, but patients do not seem at higher risk of stroke or epilepsy, and the recurrence risk is low (approximately 5% per annum). Reassurance is the mainstay of treatment.

Answer to Question 45

1 Right incomplete third nerve palsy with pupillary involvement.

2 Pupillary involvement suggests that the underlying cause is a compressive lesion since the parasympathetic fibres travel along the outside of the third nerve.

3 Posterior communicating artery aneurysm.

4 Cerebral angiography.

The key to this question is recognizing that this patient has incomplete third nerve palsy. The incomplete third nerve palsy is affecting the right superior rectus muscle which is responsible for elevation of the abducted eye. Pupillary sparing usually occurs when the pathology is infarction of the third nerve trunk. A posterior communicating artery aneurysm is the most likely cause of a compressive lesion in this case, in view of the age of the patient. It is useful to note that although aneurysms usually cause periocular pain, pain is not decisive in differentiating aneurysmal from ischaemic causes of third nerve palsy, as up to 50% of patients suffering ischaemic third nerve palsies have pain. Conventional cerebral angiography remains the most reliable method of detecting aneurysms.

Answer to Question 46

F, T, T, F, T

Metoclopramide is an anti-emetic that acts by blockade

of dopamine receptors in the chemoreceptor trigger zone and in the upper GI tract, where it has a prokinetic action. However, the drug crosses the blood-brain barrier and would be expected to exacerbate the symptoms of Parkinson's disease by blockade of dopamine receptors in the nigrostriatal pathway. L-DOPA is always administered with an inhibitor of DOPA-decarboxylase that inhibits the peripheral metabolism of L-DOPA and allows a much lower dose of L-DOPA to be used. This is an example of a favourable drug interaction and one of the select instances when the use of a combination tablet (in this case co-beneldopa or co-careldopa) is regarded as beneficial. Dyskinesias are a recognised adverse effect of therapy with L-DOPA that are more prominent with long-term therapy. Many neurologists delay treatment with L-DOPA for this reason. Ropinirole is a newer generation dopamine receptor agonist which, in a recent randomized controlled trial, was shown to be as effective as L-DOPA in the first-line treatment of Parkinson's disease but was associated with a delay in the development of dyskinesias (*N Engl J Med* 2000; 342: 1484–1491). Anticholinergic drugs successfully treat the tremor of Parkinson's disease but are associated with the development of anti-cholinergic side-effects such as visual disturbance, dry mouth, constipation, urinary retention and confusion).

Answer to Question 47

1F, 2A, 3C, 4E

Edrophonium is a short-acting acetylcholinesterase inhibitor used for the diagnosis of myasthenia gravis. Pyridostigmine is a longer acting acetylcholinesterase inhibitor used in the treatment of this disorder. Organophosphates act by producing 'irreversible' cholinesterase inhibition. Pralidoxime mesylate is cholinesterase reactivator used as an antidote in organophosphate poisoning. Atropine may also be a useful adjunctive measure to reduce the miosis, ocular pain, ciliary spasm, bronchoconstriction, bronchial hypersecretion, involuntary defaecation, sweating, and excess salivation that are the consequence of profound cholinesterase inhibition. Pilocapine is a muscarinic receptor agonist used with acetazolamide in the treatment of acute angle closure glaucoma. Pilocarpine induces miosis and in so doing aids aqueous drainage.

Answer to Question 48

1B, 3D, 3B, 4E.

Ophthalmology

Answer to Question 1

1B, 1K, 2C, 3A, 4E, 4I, 4K, 5D

- Amiodarone and hydroxychloroquine may be deposited in the cornea (cornea verticillata), but this is rarely symptomatic. Ethambutol may cause an optic neuropathy in doses of >15 mg/kg or if drug metabolism is impaired, such as in renal failure. Corticosteroids are cataractogenic given systemically.
- Tamoxifen and canthaxanthin may be deposited in the retina at the macula, appearing as small white (tamoxifen) or golden (canthaxanthin) crystals. Hydroxychloroquine is very rarely associated with a toxic maculopathy, which was much more common with chloroquine, which it has replaced as a drug for arthritis. Routine screening for ocular toxicity of hydroxychloroquine is not now recommended. Rifabutin may cause severe uveitis, especially when prescribed concomitantly with clarithromycin.
- Thalidomide is associated with coloboma of the iris and Duane's syndrome, an unusual ocular motility problem. Sildenafil use may be associated with transient visual disturbance, thought to result from its effect on cGMP (cyclic guanosine monophosphate), an important component in phototransduction. Cyclosporin is not associated with ocular side effects, and can be a valuable drug in the management of severe sight-threatening ocular inflammation.

Answer to Question 2

T, F, F, F, F

- Diabetes is the most common cause of blindness and visual impairment in the developed world in people of working age; it is also the most common preventable cause of blindness.
- Diabetic maculopathy is the most common cause of irreversible visual impairment, outnumbering proliferative disease by 6 : 1, which reflects the higher incidence of type 2 diabetes.
- Maculopathy is treated by laser photocoagulation, and lipid-lowering drugs have no impact on the incidence of maculopathy.
- Background retinopathy by definition does not require treatment because this is required only if maculopathy or proliferative disease develops. Screening for diabetic retinopathy can identify eyes at risk of sight loss before visual symptoms develop.
- Screening for diabetic retinopathy is highly cost-effective, and admirably fulfils the WHO criteria: it can be reliably diagnosed, effective treatment is available and it is of major economic importance because approximately 3% of the world's population has diabetes.

Answer to Question 3

F, F, T, T, F

- Palsy of nerve III causes an efferent pupil defect, where the pupil is dilated and unresponsive to light or accommodation.
- There is no ptosis or ocular motility abnormality in an eye with an RAPD.
- The pupil abnormality is caused by either major retinal

disease (retinal artery occlusion, ischaemic vein occlusion or major retinal detachment) or optic nerve lesion (arteritic or non-arteritic ischaemic optic neuropathy, advanced glaucoma, optic neuritis or optic nerve compression).
• The pupil sizes are normal and equal, even if one eye is blind, unless there is a separate cause of anisocoria, such as an efferent pupillary defect.

Answer to Question 4
D
• The haemorrhages found in accelerated hypertension are often flame shaped and associated with cotton-wool spots. The retinal changes in proliferative diabetic retinopathy consist of new vessels, not seen here.
• Subarachnoid haemorrhage can cause bilateral dense retinal haemorrhages, but Roth's spots are not a feature.
• The slide shows multiple dense retinal haemorrhages, the two larger each demonstrating a pale centre. These are Roth's spots which are a classic feature of infective endocarditis. *Streptococcus viridans* endocarditis was subsequently confirmed, as a result of infection of a previously unidentified bifid aortic valve after dental surgery.
• Similar haemorrhages may occasionally be seen in severe anaemia, thrombocytopenia and myeloproliferative disorders, but not in carotid disease, which usually presents as a retinal arterial occlusion, sometimes with intraluminal emboli visible.

Answer to Question 5
F, F, T, F
• Tamoxifen may appear as fine crystalline deposits at the macula, which are not seen here. There are no features of diabetic retinopathy, and laser treatment is not indicated.
• The figures show three well-defined, rounded, raised, choroidal lesions typical of metastases from carcinoma of the breast. Choroidal secondaries are more common than is clinically recognized because they do not necessarily affect vision.
• Radiotherapy is an effective palliation, improving vision. The risks of cataract and radiation retinopathy are irrelevant in this probably terminal situation.

Answer to Question 6
T, F, T, T, T
• There are two well-defined haemorrhages deep to the retinal vessels, but the vitreous is clear. Such haemorrhage is a feature of blunt injury to the eye.
• Radiating from the disc and below the retina are multiple, fine and slightly irregular red lines of angioid streaks, one of which runs between the haemorrhages.
• This young man with previously undiagnosed pseudoxanthoma elasticum had sustained blunt trauma to his right eye in a playground fight at school, after which he was aware of blurred vision.

Answer to Question 7
D
• There is a dense white opacity involving the disc margin from 2 to 8 o'clock, which also obscures the inferonasal retinal vessels. This is pathognomonic of myelinated nerve fibres.
• The upper visible edge of the disc is well defined, excluding papilloedema and disc ischaemia.
• Toxoplasma chorioretinitis may involve the disc, but the chorioretinal scar shows areas of pigment clumping and atrophy, and not the feathery ivory white appearance seen here.
• The retina shows no changes suggestive of hypertension such as haemorrhages or microinfarcts.

Answer to Question 8
T, T, T, T, F
• The picture shows a horizontally subluxed lens, which is consistent with Marfan's syndrome, homocystinuria and blunt injury. Classically, the lens in Marfan's syndrome subluxes upwards, in contrast to the homocystinuric lens which subluxes downwards.
• Eyes with subluxed lenses may maintain good vision, although this may require spectacle or contact lens correction when the lens has moved beyond the visual axis.
• There is an increased risk of retinal detachment with any cause of lens dislocation or subluxation because the eye interior is unstable.
• Firefighters have the highest professional standard of vision, requiring 6/6 uncorrected vision in each eye.
• The cause of this appearance was Marfan's syndrome. The patient's father had died aged 35 with an aortic dissection.

Answer to Question 9
B
• There is a well-circumscribed intraretinal haemorrhage adjacent to, but just sparing, the fovea. The cherry red spot of retinal artery occlusion (and Tay–Sachs disease) arises at the fovea itself.
• There are no other retinal microvascular changes such as microaneurysms or haemorrhages to suggest diabetic retinopathy, and an intraretinal haemorrhage of this size would be very unusual in diabetes.
• The optic disc is normal.
• Valsalva haemorrhages resolve spontaneously, although secondary bleeding can occur which may break through into the vitreous. Aspirin should be avoided to reduce the risk of secondary haemorrhage, as should heavy lifting, but normal daily activities can be undertaken.

Answer to Question 10
F, T, T, F, T
• The pigmentary disturbance is typical of the focal scars from panretinal photocoagulation performed for

proliferative diabetic retinopathy, with obvious disc new vessels persisting despite treatment.
• A preretinal haemorrhage is present on the nasal side of the disc as a result of bleeding from disc new vessels, which collects between the vitreous and retina.
• The haemorrhage is of low risk and not itself sight threatening, but further laser treatment is needed to control neovascularization and reduce the risk of recurrent bleeding. This may be rendered impossible if bleeding later breaks into the vitreous itself and obscures the retinal view.
• The macula appears healthy, without haemorrhages or hard exudate and, if the vitreous is also clear, the vision will remain normal.

Answer to Question 11
T, F, F, F, T
• There is a mild degree of upper lid retraction and bilateral lower lid retraction is present, although a similar appearance may also arise from exophthalmos.
• Lid lag is a dynamic sign and can be elicited only during examination.
• There is no evidence of ptosis because the upper lids are well above the pupils.
• Optic nerve compression could be present, but cannot be determined simply by inspecting the external eye. Critical information includes visual acuity, colour vision and pupillary reactions.
• This appearance is consistent with thyroid eye disease, despite the currently normal thyroid function.

Psychiatry

Answer to Question 1
1 Anorexia nervosa is characterized by self-induced weight loss to a weight below 15% of expected weight, resulting in endocrine changes associated with starvation. Patients have a body image distortion that is so intense it is almost delusional. In bulimia nervosa, the main features are the recurrent episodes of binge eating and compensatory behaviours to prevent weight gain.
2 Thyrotoxicosis, hypopituitarism, diabetes and Addison's disease.

Answer to Question 2
1 The following symptoms are important to identify as they are included in the diagnostic criteria: subjective memory impairment, tender lymph nodes, muscle pain, joint pain, headache, unrefreshing sleep, postexertional malaise.
2 F, T, F, F, F
There is no dramatically effective treatment for chronic

fatigue syndrome, and new strategies are being explored. Excessive rest is detrimental and reinforces the fatigue, but graded exercise programmes have been shown to be effective. Immunotherapy has not convincingly been shown to be effective and antidepressants should only be used if the patient has concurrent major depressive disorder. Dietary supplements or restricting diets are frequently advised in the lay press, but there is no reliable information to support their use.

Answer to Question 3
1 This would be within the limit for men, but in women it is at the upper end of the limit and above the limit recommended by the Royal College of Psychiatrists.
2 It is a set of four clinical pointers to assist clinicians screen for alcohol abuse that have been shown to have good validity. These are as follows:
C—cutting down: has been trying
A—annoyed by someone commenting on their drinking
G—guilty feelings about drinking
E—eye openers: drinking first thing in the morning.

Answer to Question 4
T, T, F, T, T
Heroin is inhaled either by heating it on foil or adding it to tobacco or cannabis. Babies can continue to be irritable as a result of opioid dependence for 6 months or longer after birth. Never calculate the methadone dose according to what the patient tells you, always titrate it slowly and carefully. Naltrexone significantly reduces the relapse rate. Hepatitis C may be transmitted through sharing injecting equipment and its prevalence among intravenous drug users is increasing.

Answer to Question 5
1 Delusions, hallucinations, disorganized speech, disorganized behaviour and/or negative symptoms occurring over at least a 6-month period.
2 Muscle rigidity, hyperthermia, fluctuating level of consciousness and autonomic dysfunction, leucocytosis, elevated CPK.
3 Agranulocytosis, which occurs in about 2% of people using clozapine.

Answer to Question 6
F, F, T, T, T
It is equally common in men and women. Most people with schizophrenia are not violent and the vast majority of violent crime is not committed by individuals with this diagnosis despite myths propagated by the mass media. Structural changes are seen in MRI, single-photon emission computed tomography (SPECT) and positron emission tomography (PET) scanning. Up to 50% of people with schizophrenia attempt suicide and 10% succeed in killing themselves. Cognitive and family therapy have both been

shown to be significantly effective in, respectively, treating delusions and preventing relapse.

Answer to Question 7

1 A personality disorder is an enduring pattern of inner experience and behaviour, that deviates markedly from the expectations of the individual's culture, is pervasive and inflexible, has an onset in adolescence or early adulthood, is stable over time, and leads to distress or impairment.

2 F, T, F, T, F

In personality disorders cure may be elusive, but the severity of these disorders can be ameliorated with treatment. Borderline personality disorder is twice as common in women. Schizophrenia is a psychotic disorder and has nothing to do with a split personality. People with personality disorders are more likely to suffer from depression than the general population. Psychotherapy is the mainstay of treatment of personality disorders.

Answer to Question 8

F, F, T, T, T

Even a trivial injury can cause a subdural haematoma in a patient with arteriosclerosis. Furthermore, the alcoholic patient may have forgotten that they sustained such an injury. In Wernicke's encephalopathy sixth nerve palsies might be transient. The commonest neuropsychiatric syndromes encountered in SLE are acute organic reactions. Dementia can also occur while schizophrenic and affective psychoses are not uncommon. Anxiety, depression and personality change are also encountered.

Answer to Question 9

T, F, F, T, T

In simple partial seizures the patient may experience 'forced fear' accompanied by autonomic symptoms with no impairment of consciousness. In carcinoid syndrome there is flushing, diarrhoea and attacks of wheezing but panic is not a prominent feature. In mastocytosis there are episodes of intense flushing together with light-headedness, palpitations, headache, shortness of breath, chest pain and nausea but intense fear is not a dominant symptom. Abrupt withdrawal of the SSRI antidepressant, paroxetine (Seroxat), can cause anxiety, agitation, insomnia, paraesthesia, dizziness, tremor and sweating. LSD can cause intense anxiety and depersonalization. It has sympathomimetic effects producing tachycardia, dilated pupils and raised blood pressure.

Answer to Question 10

T, T, T, F, T

Early studies of HIV-associated dementia suggested prevalence rates of up to 38%. However, these reports used broad criteria for the diagnosis of this condition and included selected populations from neurology clinics.

Current estimates show a prevalence of under 10%. Kaposi's sarcoma may actually have a neuroprotective effect.

McArthur JC, Hoover DR, Bacellar H, Miller EN, Cohen BA & Becker JT. Dementia in AIDS patients: incidence and risk factors. *Neurology* 1993; 43: 2245–2252.

Baldeweg T, Catalan J & Gazzard BG. Reduced risk of HIV dementia and opportunistic brain disease in AIDS associated with zidovudine use for up to 18 months. *J Neurol* 1998; 65: 34–41.

Answer to Question 11

F, F, T, F, F

The statistical correlates of suicide have low specificity and sensitivity. In one study the risk factors for suicide when combined had a sensitivity of only 60% and a specificity of 61%.

Answer to Question 12

F, F, F, F, T

The Mental Health Act and nasogastric tube feeding should only be used if the patient's situation is life threatening and there is no other way of gaining her co-operation. A history of sexual abuse may be common but it is not universal. Distorted beliefs about her body may be almost delusional in intensity, but these are not considered delusional and do not respond to neuroleptic drugs. Females are predominantly affected with a sex ratio of 10 : 1. Mild neuropathy is a complication of starvation.

Answer to Question 13

T, T, F, F, T

The relative risk of a woman having chronic fatigue syndrome is 1.3–1.7. Antidepressants should only be used to treat depression and may have a role in treating insomnia and myalgia. With current available information it is most useful to classify it as a somatoform disorder. Patients may present with memory impairment which is subjective.

Sharpe M. Cognitive behaviour therapy for chronic fatigue syndrome: efficacy and implications. *Am J Med* 1998; 105(3A): 104S–109S.

Answer to Question 14

T, T, F, F, T

Withdrawal symptoms do indicate physical dependence, but dependence is a much more complex concept than just physical dependence. Formication is a type of tactile hallucination that feels like insects crawling on the skin and it is frequently experienced by people in alcohol with-drawal. Confusion is a worrying symptom and patients with confusion may have severe medical complications, e.g. Wernicke's, seizures. Dependence is related to genetic predisposition, time and amount of drinking and psychological factors. These factors vary between individuals. Ocular palsies and nystagmus are signs of Wernicke's encephalopathy.

Answer to Question 15

F, T, T, T, F

Pupils are constricted with opioid intoxication. Temperature dysregulation is a feature of withdrawal as are abdominal cramps usually accompanying diarrhoea, nausea and vomiting. Hallucinations are not typical of opioid withdrawal.

Answer to Question 16

F, F, F, T, T

Chlorpromazine should not be used, especially not intra-muscularly, as it has been associated with sudden cardiac deaths. A firm approach is appropriate but you should also be understanding and reassuring as they may not be in full control of their actions. Threatening the patient is unhelp-ful. Only a small percentage of patients with schizophrenia are dangerous, but threats of violence by people with schizophrenia should be taken very seriously indeed. Violent patients may be restrained and sedated under Common Law only as an emergency. An assessment by a psychiatrist should then be arranged for further treat-ment under the Mental Health Act. The police do assist with violence in A&E.

Answer to Question 17

F, F, T, T, T

People with dementia typically do not have any impair-ment of consciousness, although in dementia with Lewy bodies transient episodes of loss of consciousness may occur. Dementia can occur at any age depending on the aetiology. Personality changes are often the first present-ing symptom of frontal lobe dementia. Depression may present with cognitive difficulties that may mimic dementia. Donepezil is the first cholinesterase inhibitor licensed in the UK for use in Alzheimer's disease.

Answer to Question 18

F, F, T, T, F

On general medical wards conditions like delirium, depression and anxiety are common. Psychiatric symptoms in the presence of a general medical condition should be carefully evaluated as clinical judgement will dictate management. Conditions like multiple sclerosis may present with inappropriate mood, depression or personality changes. Patients who are low in mood and anxious as a result of being in hospital may respond to explanation and reassur-ance. Malingering is unusual and should be carefully evaluated if suspected.

Answer to Question 19

1 Risk factors for developing delusional disorder are social isolation, the stress of immigration or exile, a family history of delusional disorder and having a personality disorder (especially of the paranoid or litigious types).
2 T, F, T, F, T

This is a rare condition. Delusional disorder is a type of psychotic disorder, but it is a separate condition to schiz-ophrenia. Cognitive–behavioural therapy has been shown to ameliorate delusional thinking. Hallucinations may occur and usually support the content of the delusions, but they are not predominant. Response to antipsychotics is variable, but sometimes they are effective.

Answer to Question 20

T, T, F, F, T

The symptoms of acute lithium toxicity are as follows: ataxia, poor co-ordination, muscle twitching, dysarthria, confusion, coma and convulsions. Vomiting and diarrhoea also occur. Hypothyroidism with raised thyroid-stimulating hormone can occur in up to 20% of patients on long-term lithium. It is commoner in women. Nephrogenic diabetes insipidus can occur in less than 10%.

The Medical Masterclass series

Infectious Diseases and Dermatology

Infectious Diseases

Cardiology and Respiratory Medicine

Cardiology

Neurology, Ophthalmology and Psychiatry

Neurology

Nephrology

Rheumatology and Clinical Immunology

Index

229

beta-interferons 79
internal capsule 90, *91*
International Classification of Diseases
 (ICD) 10 165
 anorexia nervosa 170
interpersonal therapy 185
intervertebral disc
 minor bulges 8
 protrusion *6*
intracerebral haemorrhage 96–100
 clinical presentation 97
 complications 98
 epidemiology 97
 hydrocephalus 98
 hypertensive 96
 investigations 97–8
 pathology 96
 physical signs 97
 prognosis 98
 stroke differential diagnosis 92
 treatment 98
intracranial aneurysm 140
intracranial haemorrhage 47
 neck stiffness 48
intracranial hypertension, idiopathic 42, 43
 tension-type headache differential
  diagnosis 84
intracranial lesions 84
intracranial pressure, raised 41
 double vision 140
 idiopathic intracranial hypertension 42
 papilloedema 48
intraocular inflammation 129, 130
intraocular pressure measurement 130
intraretinal microvascular abnormalities
 (IRMAs) 149
intravenous immunoglobulin (IvIg)
 Guillain–Barré syndrome 63
 myasthenia gravis 71
iris neovascularization 143, 146, 150
iritis 36, 37, 129, 130, 141–2
 causes **141**
 scleritis differential diagnosis 142
 treatment 130, 141

jealousy, morbid 202

Kaposi's sarcoma 166, 167
Kayser–Fleischer rings 10
Kennedy's disease 64

Lambert–Eaton myasthenic syndrome
 71, 104, 105
language
 assessment 111
 therapy 51
laser photocoagulation 145
Lazarus syndrome 167
Leber's optic neuropathy 146
leg pain 5, *6*, 7–8
 imaging 7
 nerve conduction studies 7–8
legs
 cutaneous nerve supply *8*
 peripheral neuropathies 58, **59**
 sensory abnormalities 7
 tremor 9
 weakness 7, 23–5
letter fluency 111
levator disinsertion 34, 36
levodopa 73, 107
Lewy bodies
 Parkinson's disease 72
 see also dementia, with Lewy bodies
Lewy body disease, diffuse 51
limb girdle muscular dystrophy 68, 69
lipid metabolism disorders 66–7

lithium
 bipolar affective disorder 201
 breast feeding 198
 cluster headache 83
 pregnancy 198
liver disease, chronic 5
lofepramine 200
lofexidine 177
lower limbs *see* legs
LSD 107, 108
lumbar canal stenosis 7
 muscle pain **14**, 15
lumbar puncture 112–13
 complications 113
 indications 112
 normal findings 112
 subarachnoid haemorrhage 116
 technique 112–13
lumbosacral plexus lesion 7
lung carcinoma, small-cell
 Lambert–Eaton myasthenic syndrome 105
 paraneoplastic encephalitis 104
 paraneoplastic vasculitic neuropathy 105
 subacute sensory neuropathy 105
Lyme disease 63
lymphoma 142
lymphoproliferative disorders 64
lysuride 107

macular oedema 137, 138, 139
magnetic resonance angiography 116–17
 carotid artery stenosis 119
magnetic resonance imaging (MRI) 115,
 116–17
malignancy
 hemiparesis 47
 Lambert–Eaton myasthenic syndrome 71
 lumbar puncture 112
 neck and shoulder pain 26, 28
 peripheral neuropathy 59
 ptosis 35, 36
malingering 53–4
 mental disorder signs/symptoms 186
mania 167, 168
 bipolar affective disorder differential
  diagnosis 201
 risk of death 202
 treatment 201
marche à petit pas 11
 dysarthria 50
maternity blues 197
McArdle's disease **14**, 15, 66
MDMA (ecstasy) 107
medical wards, Mental Health Act 203
medulla oblongata lesions 22
memory
 assessment 111
 difficulties 19–20
Ménière's disease 44
meninges, malignant infiltration 4, 7
meningitis
 communicating hydrocephalus 42
 mental disorder signs/symptoms 185
 MRI 116
meningoradiculitis 63
mental disorders
 compulsory detention 203
 medication/medical conditions 185–6
Mental Health Act (1983) 172, 178, 200,
 203
metabolic disturbance 63
metachromatic leukodystrophy 78
metastases
 gait disorders 12
 paraneoplastic conditions 106
 vertebrae 7
methadone 176–7

methotrexate
 multiple sclerosis 79
 scleritis 142
alpha-methyldopa 109
methysergide 81
metoclopramide
 migraine 80
 nausea/vomiting 107
micrographia 10
micturition pathways 29, *30*
migraine 79–81
 aura 79, 80
 differential diagnosis 80
 equivalents 80, 132–3
 hemiplegic 80
 hormone replacement therapy 81
 Horner's syndrome 36
 investigations 80
 ophthalmoplegic 33, 40, 80
 pregnancy 81
 presentation 41–2, 79–80
 prognosis 81
 prophylaxis 81
 retinal 80
 site of pain *43*
 TIA differential diagnosis 96
 treatment 80–1
 variants 80
 vertebrobasilar 80
 vision loss 132–3
 visual hallucinations 51
Miller–Fisher variant of Guillain–Barré
 syndrome 62
mind, body, behaviour interactions 186
Mini-Mental State Exam 111
mitochondrial disorders **14**, 15, 67
 maternal inheritance 15
mitoxantrone 79
moclobemide 108, 110
Modafinil 18
monoamine oxidase inhibitors (MAOIs) 200
 action 198
 breast feeding 198
 depression 108
 dietary tyramine 110
 tyramine reaction 110, 200
mononeuritis multiplex 3
mood
 delirium 164
 HIV-associated disturbance 167–8
mood disorder
 alcoholism 174
 delusional disorder differential diagnosis 202
 underlying medical condition/
  medication 185
 violence 178
morphine 109
motor neurone disease 57, 63–5
 aetiology 63
 cranial nerves 64
 differential diagnosis 64
 dysphagia 21, 22–3
 epidemiology 63–4
 investigations 64
 prognosis 65
 treatment 65
motor neurone signs 22
motor neuropathy 105
 multifocal 64
movements
 involuntary 12–14
 see also eye, movements
multiple sclerosis 54–6, 77–9
 acute cord syndromes 24
 bipolar affective disorder differential
  diagnosis 201
 chorea 13